Clinical Asthma

Clinical Asthma

Editor: Brendol Keith

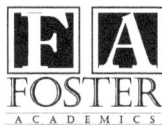

FOSTER
ACADEMICS

www.fosteracademics.com

www.fosteracademics.com

FA FOSTER
ACADEMICS

Cataloging-in-Publication Data

Clinical asthma / edited by Brendol Keith.
      p. cm.
Includes bibliographical references and index.
ISBN 978-1-63242-799-1
1. Asthma. 2. Asthma--Treatment. 3. Bronchi--Diseases. 4. Lungs--Diseases, Obstructive.
5. Respiratory allergy. I. Keith, Brendol.
RC591 .C55 2019
616.238--dc23

Foster Academics,
118-35 Queens Blvd., Suite 400,
Forest Hills, NY 11375, USA

ISBN 978-1-63242-799-1 (Hardback)

Contents

Permissions

List of Contributors

Index

Preface

This book has been a concerted effort by a group of academicians, researchers and scientists, who have contributed their research works for the realization of the book. This book has materialized in the wake of emerging advancements and innovations in this field. Therefore, the need of the hour was to compile all the required researches and disseminate the knowledge to a broad spectrum of people comprising of students, researchers and specialists of the field.

Asthma is a chronic inflammatory disease of the lungs. It is associated with the blockage of the airways and bronchospasm. Its symptoms include chest tightness, shortness of breath, coughing and wheezing. People suffering from asthma are more likely to develop obstructive sleep apnea, anxiety disorders, rhinosinusitis and gastro-esophageal reflux disease. Asthma can be caused by a combination of genetic and environmental factors. Some of the most common microbes causing asthma include Chlamydophila pneumoniae, Mycoplasma pneumoniae and human rhinoviruses. People having eczema, hay fever, atopic disease, urticaria and eosinophilic granulomatosis with polyangiitis have a greater risk of developing asthma. This book aims to shed light on some of the unexplored aspects of clinical asthma and the recent researches related to it. It includes some of the vital pieces of work being conducted across the world, on various topics related to clinical asthma. This book will serve as a reference to a broad spectrum of readers.

At the end of the preface, I would like to thank the authors for their brilliant chapters and the publisher for guiding us all-through the making of the book till its final stage. Also, I would like to thank my family for providing the support and encouragement throughout my academic career and research projects.

Editor

Role of T cells in a gp91^{phox} knockout murine model of acute allergic asthma

Ena Ray Banerjee[1,2]* and William R Henderson Jr[1]

Abstract

Objective: Molecular regulation of inflammation, especially, the role of effector cells in NADPH oxidase-mediated redox reactions for producing O$_2$ (superoxide anion) is a critical step. This study explores the roles of macrophages and neutrophils and their cross-talk with extra-cellular matrix components in the light of the role essayed by T cells. Materials and Methods and Treatment: To clarify the role of NADPH oxidase in the pathophysiology of T cell-initiatedmacrophage-associated allergic asthma, we induced allergen dependent inflammation in a gp91^{phox}−/− SKO (single knockout) and a gp91^{phox}−/− MMP-12−/− DKO (double knockout) mouse and analysed trafficking and functionality of various cell types, the T cell function and T cell-macrophage interaction being given special emphasis.

Results: Composite asthma symptoms expressed in a more aggravated manner in both the KO (SKO and DKO) mice compared to WT indicating that some redundancy may exist in the response pathways of gp91phox and MMP-12. On the one hand, upregulation in macrophage functions such as proliferation, mixed lymphocyte reaction, and MCP-1 directed chemotaxis, may indicate that a regulatory cross-talk is switched on between T cell and macrophage and on the other, downregulation of respiratory burst response hints at a dichotomy in their signaling pathways. Increased B7.1 but reduced B7.2 and MHC class II expression on KO alveolar macrophages may suggest that a switching on-off mechanism is operative where alteration of co-stimulatory molecule expression selectively activating T cell is a critical step.

Inference: T cell mediated functions such as Th2 cytokine secretion, and T cell proliferation in response to OVA were upregulated synchronous with the overall robustness of the asthma phenotype.

Conclusions: As far as cell-cell interaction is concerned, the data is indicative of the existence of a plethora of networks where molecular switches may exist that selectively induce activation and deactivation of regulatory pathways that ultimately manifest in the overall response. gp91^{phox} and MMP-12 either redundantly or synergistically but not additively, provide a regulatory checkpoint for restricting T cell cross-talk with macrophages and keep excessive tissue damage and ECM degradation during acute allergic inflammation under control.

Introduction

The production of superoxide anions (O$_2^-$) by neutrophils and other phagocytes is an important step in our body's innate immune response. [1,2]. These act as microbicidal agents and kill invading micro-organisms either directly or through the activation of proteases [3,4]. O$_2^-$ is produced by the NADPH oxidase, a multi-protein enzyme complex, which is inactive in resting phagocytes, but becomes activated after interaction of the phagocyte with pathogens and their subsequent engulfment in the phagosome [5]. Defects in the function of the NADPH oxidase result in a severe immunodeficiency, and individuals suffering from CGD (chronic granulomatous disease), a rare genetic disorder that is caused by mutations in NADPH oxidase genes, are highly susceptible to frequent and often life-threatening infections by bacteria and fungi [6,7].

NADPH oxidase, the primary source of reactive oxygen species is a strong candidate for the development of therapeutic agents to ameliorate inflammation and

* Correspondence: enarb1@gmail.com
[1]Department of Medicine, Division of Allergy and Infectious Diseases, Center for Allergy and Inflammation, University of Washington, Room 254, 850 Republican Street, Seattle, WA 98109, USA
[2]Department of Zoology, University of Calcutta, 35 Ballygunge Circular Road, Kolkata 700019, West Bengal, India

end-organ damage [8,9]. Additionally, the study of cytochrome isolated from patients with X-linked CGD has contributed to our current understanding of its function [10,11].

Involvement of the gp91phox subunit in oxidative burst response by PMNs as well as Macrophages is not clear. Macrophages use a membrane-associated NADPH oxidase to generate an array of oxidizing intermediates. In some studies, it has been demonstrated that oxidants potently and efficiently inactivate matrilysin (MMP-7) by cross-linking adjacent tryptophan-glycine residues within the catalytic domain of the enzyme. These *in vitro* observations suggest that MMP inactivation can occur on or near phagocytes that produce both MMPs and reactive intermediates. In the absence of reactive intermediates, unrestrained proteolytic activity might lead to detrimental tissue damage. Indeed, inherited deficiency of $gp91^{phox}$, a phagocyte-specific component of the NADPH oxidase required for oxidant production, and targeted deletion of its mouse homologue result in granuloma formation and excessive tissue destruction [12].

This study addresses for the first time the relationship between gp91phox and MMP-12 in the development of T cell mediated acute allergic asthma in a mouse model using genetic knockout mice, gp91phox–/– which will be referred to as NOX–/– or SKO and MMP-12-NOX DKO. The study focuses on the cross-talk between T cells and macrophages and shows that gp91phox most likely has a regulatory role in the onset and maintenance of the composite asthma phenotype in mouse and deletion of gp91phox may alter expression of co-stimulatory /co-inhibitory molecules B7.1 (increased) and B7.2 (decreased) and MHCII expression (increased) which may explain the mechanism by which macrophages despite increased migration to the inflammatory foci *in vivo* and increased migration in a chemotaxis chamber to MCP-1, and enhanced proliferation to syngeneic or allogeneic stimulus *in vitro*, fail to execute oxidative burst response. MMP-12 seems to be either redundant, not contributing to the overall asthma phenotype or has a synergistic (not additive) role in the process.

Materials and Methods
Mice
Both $gp91^{phox-/-}$ mice [13,14] were on a C57Bl/6J background and had been outcrossed and then intercrossed for three generations to generate animals deficient in both genes. C57BL6 mice (Taconic) were used as the control group and are called wildtype. In total the following number of animals were used in each group: WT (14), NOX –/– (14), MMP-12NOX–/–(16) in the control group and WT (16), NOX–/– (15), MMP-12NOX–/–(14).

Allergen sensitization and challenge
Mice were sensitized and later challenged with OVA (Thermo Scientific Pierce Protein Research Products, Rockford, IL) as described previously [15].

Tissue analyses
The mouse underwent exsanguination by intra-orbital arterial bleeding and cells, obtained by bronchoalveolar lavage and those from lung parenchyma (obtained by lung mincing and digestion was performed after lavage as described previously [15] with 100u/ml collagenase for 1 hr at 37°C, and filtered through a 60# sieve (-Aldrich Corporation, St. Louis, Sigma) were evaluated after air drying, by staining with Wright-Giemsa (Biochemical Sciences Inc, Swedesboro, NJ) and their differential count was taken under a light microscope at 40X magnification. Cell number refers to that obtained from lavage of both lungs/ mouse. In addition, cells from hemolysed peripheral blood (PB), bone marrow(BM), bronchoalveolar lavage (BAL), lung parenchyma (LP), spleen, mesenteric lymph nodes (MLN), cervical lymph nodes (CLN), axillary lymph nodes (LNX) and inguinal lymph nodes (LNI) were analyzed on a FACSCalibur (BD Immunocytometry Systems, San Jose, CA) by using the CELLQuest program. Staining was performed by using antibodies conjugated to fluorescin isothiocyanate (FITC), phycoerythrin (PE), allophucocyanin (APC), Peridinin Chlorophyll Protein (Per CP-Cy5.5) and Cy-chrome (PE-Cy5 and PE-Cy7). The following BD pharmingen (San Diego, CA) antibodies were used for cell surface staining : APC-conjugated CD45 (30F-11), FITC-conjugated CD3(145-2C11), PE-Cy5 conjugated CD4 (RM4-5),PE-conjugated CD45RC (DNL-1.9), APC-conjugated CD8(53–6.7), PE-Cy5 conjugated B220 (RA3-6B2), FITC-conjugated IgM, PE-conjugated CD19 (ID3), PE-conjugated CD21(7G6), FITC-conjugated CD23 (B3B4), APC-conjugated GR-1(RB6-8C5), and PE-conjugated Mac1 (M1/70). PE-Cy5 conjugated F4/80 (Cl:A3-1(F4/80)) was obtained from Serotec Ltd., Oxford, UK. PE-conjugated anti-α4 integrin (PS2) and anti-VCAM-1(M/K-2) was from Southern Biotechnology, Birmingham, Ala. Irrelevant isotype-matched antibodies were used as controls.

Chemotaxis assay
Chemotaxis assay was performed with 10 million macrophages pooled from 4 mice/experimental group. Macrophages were prepared by adhering BALf cells in high glucose medium for 2 hours followed by detachment by mechanical scraping and resuspension in Phenol red-free high glucose DMEM (Gibco) with 5% FBS with 0.5μg/ml Calcein-AM (1:2000 dilution) and incubation for 20 min at 37°C. MCP-1 at dilutions ranging from 0.1-25mM were used and 15 mM was taken to be the optimum dose. 96 well Neuroprobe CTX plates (Chemicon, Temecula,CA) were used. 29μl MCP-1

Table 1 List of mouse primers for real time PCR

Cell marker	Gene	Forward primer	Reverse primer
House- keeping genes	GAPDH	CGTCCCGTAGACAAAATGGT	TCAATGAAGGGGTCGTTGAT
	β-actin	GTGGGCCGCTCTAGGCACCAA	CTCTTTGATGTCACGCACGATTTC
Cytokine genes	IFN-γ	GCGTCATTGAATCACACCTG	TGAGCTCATTGAATGCTTGG
	IL-1α	TCAAGATGGCCAAAGTTCCT	TGCAAGTCTCATGAAGTGAGC
	IL-1β	TGAAGCAGCTATGGCAACTG	GGGTCCGTCAACTTCAAAGA
	IL-2	AACCTGAAACTCCCCAGGAT	CGCAGAGGTCCAAGTTCATC
	IL-3	CCGTTTAACCAGAACGTTGAA	CCACGAATTTGGACAGGTTT
	IL-4	GGCATTTTGAACGAGGTCAC	AAATATGCGAAGCACCTTGG
	IL-5	ATGGAGATTCCCATGAGCAC	AGCCCCTGAAAGATTTCTCC
	IL-6	AACGATGATGCACTTGCAGA	GGTACTCCAGAAGACCAGAGGA
	IL-10	TGAATTCCCTGGGTGAGAAG	TGGCCTTGTAGACACCTTGG
	IL-12β	ATCGTTTTGCTGGTGTCTCC	CATCTTCTTCAGGCGTGTCA
	IL-13	CCTCTGACCCTTAAGGAGCTT	ATGTTGGTCAGGGAATCCAG
	MCP-3	TCTGTGCCTGCTGCTCATAG	CTTTGGAGTTGGGGTTTTCA
Growth factor genes	TGFβ2	GGAGGTTTATAAAATCGACATGC	GGCATATGTAGAGGTGCCATC
	VEGFa	TACCTCCACCATGCCAAG	TGGTAGACATCCATGAACTTGA
	VEGFb	GGCTTAGAGCTCAACCCAGA	TGGAAAGCAGCTTGTCACTTT
	VEGFc	GGGAAGAAGTTCCACCATCA	TCGCACACGGTCTTCTGTAA

(15mM) was added as a single convex drop and the polycarbonate filter placed gently over it and incubated at 37°C for 30 min. Cell suspension was added in designated slots over the filter membrane also in 29μl volume. The chamber was incubated at 37°C in humidified CO_2 incubator for 2h. Excess cells were wiped off with kimwipes at the end of the incubation period. Migrated cells were quantified by fluorescence (excitation at 488 nm, emission at 520 nm) using a Victor 3V (Perkin Elmer laboratories) using a Wallac1420 software.

Oxidative burst reposnse
Alveolar leukocytes (0.5×10^6 cells) were stained with F4/80-Cy-Chrome and Gr1-APC for 30 min on ice, washed in PBS, warmed up at 37°C for 5 min and loaded with 5mM dihydrorhodamine 123 (Molecular Probes, Eugene, OR). After 10 min at 370C, cells were split in two equal aliquots, and PMA (Sigma, St. Louis, MO) was added to one aliquot at final concentration of 1mM. After 10 min incubation cells were washed in ice-cold PBS and immediately subjected to FACS analysis. Cells were gated on neutrophils (Gr1hi), or monocyte/macrophages (F4/80+) and percentage of cells positive for dihydrorhodamine 123 fluorescence with or without PMA treatment was determined for each gate.

Real time-PCR analysis
For real time PCR analysis of mRNA expression of particular genes in differentiating human ESC as well as in the

lungs of recipient animals in transplantation experiments, total RNA was extracted from cells (<500/sample) by PicoPure RNA isolation kit from Arcturus, Mountainview, CA) and those from lungs (kept in RNA later (Ambion) at -80°C), by RNA extraction kit (RNeasy) from Qiagen and cDNA made from it using superscript III system from Invitrogen (Life Technologies, Grand Island, NY). The PCR

Table 2 Recruitment index

		T cells	B cells	Macs	PMNs	Eos	Basophils
Lungs	WO	0.6	0.015	0.22	0.18	3	0.04
	NOXO	0.6	0.19*	1.3*	0.49*	3.8	0.16*
	DKOO	0.58	0.05*	1.1*	0.44*	3.4	0.13*
BALf	WO	0.22	0.25	0.77	0.107	5.75	0.03
	NOXO	0.32*	0.17	0.85	0.27	6.3	0.09
	DKOO	0.51*	0.16	0.78	0.26	5.8	0.08

Upregulation of inflammatory recruitment index in lung and airways of KO post-OVA. Cell number was counted using a Z1 particle counter from Beckman Coulter. Blood (PB) was obtained by infra-orbital bleeding and extrapolated to a 2 ml volume as the total volume of blood in a 20gm mouse, from the volume of blood actually obtained, perfused lung was minced and digested with collagenase IV and single cell suspension made of both lungs, and brochoalveolar lavage fluid (BALf) was obtained from both lungs, and the cell numbers counted. Recruitment index was calculated as a ratio of number of cells in lung parenchyma tissue versus number of the same cell subtypes in peripheral circulating blood and similarly in lung interstitium versus circulating cells. This denotes the fraction of inflammatory cells recruited from blood and migrated to lung. The data shown have been derived from 3 independent experiments and expressed as mean values ± SEM. *denotes p value<0.01 compared to post-OVA wildtype values. Abbreviations used are: WT=wildtype, NOX=gp91phox–/–, DKO=gp91phox-MMP-12 double knockout, WA=WT+alum, WO=WT+OVA, NOXA=gp91phox–/–+alum, NOXO=gp91phox–/–+OVA, DKOA= gp91phox-MMP-12 double knockout+alum, DKOO= gp91phox-MMP-12 double knockout+OVA.

Table 3 Enhanced cytokine gene expression in KO lung

	IFN-γ	IL-1α	IL-1β	IL-2	IL-4	IL-5	IL-6	IL-10	IL-12β	IL-13
CWT	4.67±1.70	71.27±6.47	3.79±0.32	2.57±0.02	44.26±12.70	27.15±1.70	3.59±1.65	4.21±2.60	7.27±5.25	4.72±1.38
WTO	4.96±1.85	411.67±2.46	21.17±8.11	65.56±13.28	65.42±13.58	103.45±30.68	20.04±9.80	23.61±3.66	21421.95±15756.71	45.15±9.45
CKO	1.18±0.271	62.81±0.68	6.20±1.58	2.65±1.61	33.72±19.35	43.12±0.90	3.74±0.96	1.76±0.65	29.23±21.91	4.68±1.32
KOO	2.06±0.60	6037.51+5.50	33.65±1.74	8.63+1.72	92.78+1.02	147.74±1.42	20.58±8.28	134.96+3.43	306948.33+107868.44	90.59+14.51

Real time PCR analysis shows expression of mRNA for the particular genes as calculated by relative index of Ct values normalized to GAPDH by real time PCR. PCR was carried out using the comparative Ct method (Applied Biosystems software) with SYBR Green PCRcore reagents (Applied Biosystems) and anlysed using Applied Biosystems 7900HT Real-Time PCR System software SDS 2.2.1. All primers used were specific to mouse. The graphs in * denotes p value <0.01 compared to bleo-treated untransplanted group. Mean denotes the avergae of 2 independent experiments (n=4/group). Underlined numbers denote mRNA expression in relative units normalized to mouse GAPDH that have p value<0.05 compared to wildtype post-OVA. Abbreviations used are: cWT= saline treated wildtype, WTO=wildtype post-OVA treatment, CKO=saline treated gp91phox knockout, KOO= OVA treated gp91phox knockout, CKO=OVA treated control.

reaction solution contained 0.5 μg of total RNA, 6-mM magnesium chloride, and 0.5-μM of each primer (primer oligo sequences are in Table 1). Other components in the reverse transcriptase–PCR master mix included buffer, enzyme, SYBR Green I, and deoxyribonucleotide triphosphate. For reverse transcription, the 20 μL of reaction capillaries were incubated at 50°C for 2 min followed by a denaturation at 95°C for 10 min. Polymerase chain reaction by an initial denaturation at 95°C for 15 s and then annealing at 60°C 1 min, repeat 45 cycles. Finally, a melting curve analysis was perfomed by following the final cycle with incubation at 95°C for 15 s, at 60°C for 15 s, then 95°C for 15 s. Negative control samples for the reverse transcriptase–PCR analysis, which contained all reaction components except RNA, were performed simultaneously to determine when the nonspecific exponential amplification cycle number was reached. Forward and reverse primers are as in Table 1 and were synthesized by the University of Washington Biochemistry services using the Primer Express software. PCR was carried out using the comparative Ct method (Applied Biosystems software) with SYBR Green PCRcore reagents (Applied Biosystems Life Technologies) and anlysed using Applied Biosystems 7900HT Real-Time PCR System software SDS 2.2.1.

Statistical analysis

Statistical differences among samples were tested by Student t test. P value less than 0.05 was considered statistically significant.

Results

Inflammatory recruitment index in KO mice post-OVA compared to WT

The various nuances of allergic asthma developed fully and more exaggeratedly in both gp91^{phox}–/– and MMP-

12-gp91^{phox} double knockout mice post OVA treatment compared to WT as described in detail in [16]. Absolute inflammatory migration profile measured by increase in cell number in tissues versus their sites of poiesis and circulation, i.e.bone marrow and peripheral blood respectively was increased (Table 2). In bone marrow, NOX–/– post OVA has 1.4-fold more cells (data not shown), in peripheral blood, 1.3-fold more cells, spleen had 1.3-fold more cells (data not shown), lung parenchyma had 1.8-fold more cells, and BALf: 2-fold more cells compared to post-OVA WT. Of note, 2.4-fold more PMNs, 1.96-fold more B lymphocytes, 5-fold more eosinophils in post-OVA NOX–/– and DKO compared to post-OVA WT BALf was found [17].

Over-expression of Th2 cytokine gene expression in the lung

Cytokine concentrations present in BALf was measured by ELISA and protein concentrations were presented in [16]. Table 3 shows that actual mRNA upregulation was 1.4-fold for IL-4 gene and 1.9-fold for IL-13 genes in the lung parenchyma tissue which are Th2 specific. There was also upregulation in IL-1α, IL-10 and IL-12α, the dignificance of which is not clear at this point. Figure 1 shows 2.75-fold increase in IL-13 gene expression in gp91phox–/– mice post-OVA compared to WT post-OVA. IL-4 was increased All other Th2 cytokines showed values similar to post-OVA WT BALf. Overall, IL-4: NOX–/– post OVA has 1.2-fold more protein and 2-fold more mRNA; IL-5: NOX–/– post OVA has 2-fold more protein and 2.8-fold more mRNA; IL-13: NOX–/– post OVA has 3-fold more protein and 5.6-fold more mRNA. Therefore, both by protein concentration and mRNA expression, Th2 cytokines show manifold increase in gp91phox–/– post-OVA compared to WT.

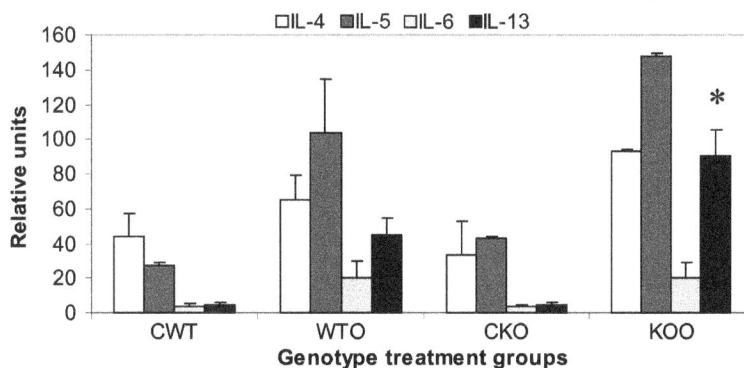

Figure 1 Alteration of TH cytokine gene expression in lung. Real time PCR analysis was used to quantitate expression of mRNA for the particular genes as calculated by relative index of Ct values normalized to GAPDH by real time PCR. PCR was carried out using the comparative Ct method (Applied Biosystems software) with SYBR Green PCRcore reagents (Applied Biosystems) and anlysed using Applied Biosystems 7900HT Real-Time PCR System software SDS 2.2.1. All primers used were specific to mouse. Data expressed here are mean ± SEM. n = 5/group. While all other Th2 cytokine levels were comparable to WT+OVA, IL-13 concentration was increased 2.7-fold over post-OVA WT values. Abbreviations used are: CWT = saline treated control wildtype, WTO = WT+OVA, CKO = gp91phox–/–+alum, KOO = gp91phox–/–+OVA. MMP-12.

Table 4 Alteration in growth factor genes in KO lung post-OVA

	MCP-3	TGFβ2	VEGFa	VEGFb	VEGFc
CWT	4.63±1.63	18.03±15.34	1973.06±1549.62	176.39±2.24z	2283.58±1671.63
WTO	7.14±1.94	44.67±22.84	4260.86±1982.14	334.59±3.56	4500.67±1827.83
CKO	20901.40±6361.97	32.88±9.71	34.40±13.79	106.73±80.67	15.11±0.97
KOO	166575.87±119300.10	28.30±23.65	297.97±234.29	744.17±61.60	35.15±11.41

Real time PCR data shows expression of mRNA for the particular genes as calculated by relative index of Ct values normalized to GAPDH by real time PCR. PCR was carried out using the comparative Ct method (Applied Biosystems software) with SYBR Green PCRcore reagents (Applied Biosystems) and anlysed using Applied Biosystems 7900HT Real-Time PCR System software SDS 2.2.1. All primers used were specific to mouse. The underlined numbers p value <0.01 compared to OVA -treated wildtype group. Abbreviations used are: cWT= saline treated wildtype, WTO=wildtype post-OVA treatment, CKO=saline treated gp91phox knockout, KOO= CKO=OVA treated gp91phox knockout.

Chemokine and growth factor gene expression

MCP-3 is a known macrophage chemotactic protein. Its gene expression was found to be upregulated manifolds both in the saline treated control lung as well as post-OVA. The reson for this may be that in the absence of gp91phox, there is spontaneous upregulation of the chemokine gene. VEGFb was upregulated by 2.2-fold. Surprisingly, there was downregulation of TGFβ. MMP-12 (Table 4).

Expression of Rho kinase and MMPs associated with inflammation

Since this is an inflammatory response to the allergen, we hypothesized that other pro-inflammatory kinases and proteases may also be intimately involved in the pathway. Figure 2 and 3 shows RT-PCR analysis of gene expression of Rho kinase, known to have anti-

inflammatory functions. Genes for MMP7, 10 and 28 were similarly downregulated as well.

Functionality of T cells

Proliferation of MACS-purified (>86-92%) CD4+ and CD8+ splenocytes by MTT incorporation assay and OD measurement at 545nm of anti CD3/CD28 (0.01-1ug/ml)induced proliferation of CD4+ shows a 8.4-folds increase in post-OVA WT compared to a 7.4-fold increase in both KO mice. In CD8+ while post-OVA WT increased by 6.4-fold, the KO mice showed 7.9-fold increase compared to the corresponding saline treated mice. With PMA/ionomycin (10ng/ml), CD4+ (post-OVA WT was 2.3-fold more than that in NOX–/–) while CD8+ was 1.5-fold more in post-OVA WT than in either KO mice. Overall, whereas proliferation of both T cell subsets to anti CD3/CD28 is comparable, response to PMA/ionomycin

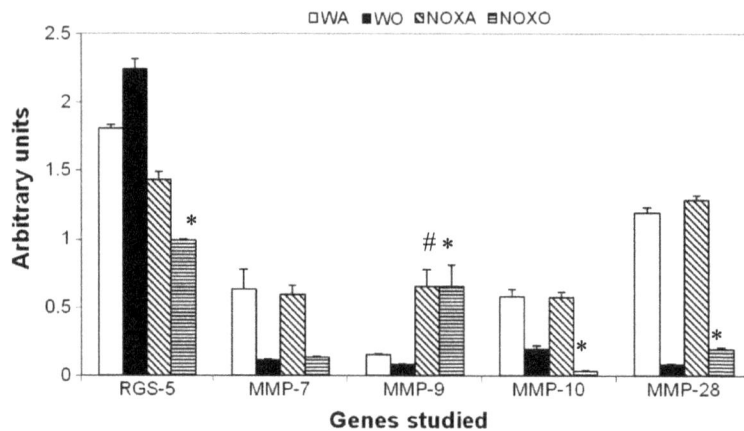

Figure 2 Downregulation Rho kinase RGS-5 and MMP10 but upregulation of MMP9 and MMP28 genes in KO lung. Real time PCR analysis was used to quantitate expression of mRNA for the particular genes as calculated by relative index of Ct values normalized to GAPDH by real time PCR. PCR was carried out using the comparative Ct method (Applied Biosystems software) with SYBR Green PCRcore reagents (Applied Biosystems) and anlysed using Applied Biosystems 7900HT Real-Time PCR System software SDS 2.2.1. All primers used were specific to mouse. * denotes p value<0.01 compared to WT+OVA values. # denotes p value<0.01 compared to WT+alum (control baseline values). n=5/group pooled from 2 experiments. Expression of the gene of interest was expressed in relative values normalized to the values obtained for mouse GAPDH. Compared to post-OVA WT values, Rho kinase RGS-5 mRNA was decreased 2.3-folds and MMp-10 3-fold, while MMP-9 was increased 8-fold and MMP-28 increased 2.3-fold (*denotes p value<0.05 compared to post-OVA WT).

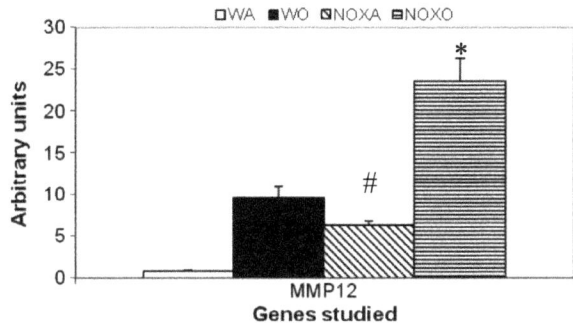

Figure 3 Upregulation of MMP-12 gene in post-OVA in KO lung. Real time PCR analysis was used to quantitate expression of mRNA for the particular genes as calculated by relative index of Ct values normalized to GAPDH by real time PCR. PCR was carried out using the comparative Ct method (Applied Biosystems software) with SYBR Green PCRcore reagents (Applied Biosystems) and anlysed using Applied Biosystems 7900HT Real-Time PCR System software SDS 2.2.1. All primers used were specific to mouse. * denotes p value<0.01 compared to WT+OVA values. # denotes p value<0.01 compared to WT+alum (control baseline values). n=5/group pooled from 2 experiments. Expression of the gene of interest was expressed in relative values normalized to the values obtained for mouse GAPDH. There was 10-fold increase in the gene expression of MMP-12 in OVA-treated WT vs. control WT whereas saline-treated NOX KO lungs showed 6.5-fold increase over untreated control mouse lung. However, post-OVA treatment, NOX KO mouse lung showed MMP-12 shooting up 4.7-fold over untreated KO. # denotes p value <0.01 compared to control untreated, * denotes p value <0.01 compares untreated KO versus OVA-treated KO lung.

is somewhat compromised in KO post-OVA. (Figure 4 Panels A,B).

Functionality of macrophages (oxidative burst response and chemotaxis to specific stimuli)

Macrophages and neutrophils are the key downstream cells contributing to the inflammation in asthma. Their functions were measured by oxidative burst response to PMA and chemotaxis to MCP-1. Figure 5 shows drastic downregulation of DHR+ cells by FACS gated on both Gr-1+ or F4/80+ populations showing either myeloid population to be incapable of showing respiratory burst response by generating reactive oxygen species by responding to PMA. Figure 6 however, surprisingly shows upregulation calcein fluorophore (proportional to cells showing directed migration or specific chemotaxis) in both gp91phox–/– and DKO alveolar macrophages post-OVA to MCP-1.

T cell-macrophage cross talk by mixed lymphocyte reaction (MLR)

Based on the aforementioned responses of T cells and macrophages it seems apparent that both cells are able to function well in response to OVA on their own at least as far as the asthma phenotype is concerned. They migrate in increased numbers from blood and resident

as well as recruited cells are found in impressive inflammatory exudates around the airways. So the next question was whether there is efficient cross-talk between the T cells upstream and the macrophages downstream. To this end we did a mixed lymphocyte reaction using first the CD4+ T cells as the responders and the γ-irradiated alveolar macrophages as the stimulators from the experimental mice themselves and then used CD4+ T cells from splenocytes of BALB/c mice. Increase in proliferation measured by MTT assay (OD 570nm) (Figure 7) shows increased T cell: APC interaction both when autologous APCs (macrophages from adherent cell population in BALf of the same animal) were used and then APCs from experimental animals were used as stimulators to CD4+ T cells from spleen of BALB/c mice which were the responders.

iNOS expression

iNOS is a surface enzyme expressed by macrophages that are of the M1 or killer phenotype. Figure 8 shows decrease in percent iNOS+ cells in PB, spleen, lung and BALf but not BM of KO mice in comparison to corresponding tissues from WT micemay indicate that there is a skewing of macrophage phenotype from killer to healer phenotype. This corroborates well with data in Figures 5 and 6 that these macrophages although migrating to the inflammatory focus in increased numbers are incapable of typical phagocytic functions which indicates a clear dichotomy in their signaling pathways.

Expression of co-stimulatory molecules

We hypothesized that expression of MHC molecule, which controls T cell activation by APC may be somehow affected in this mechanism. Figure 9 indicates a 1.65-fold increase in post-OVA gp91phox–/– lung parenchyma cells and a 1.38-fold increase in DKO cells in B7.1 positive cells from undetected positive cells in saline treated in any group. B7.2 and MHCII expressions were however decreased in both KO mice with 3.28-fold and 3.18-fold decrease respectively in gp91phox–/– and DKO. MHCII expression was downregulated by 1.18 and 1.13-fold in the two KO mice respectively.

Discussion and conclusions

Deletion of gp91^{phox} results in enhancement of composite asthma phenotype in mouse [17-20]. Double deletion of gp91phoix and MMP-12, a critical enzyme for phagocyte associated inflammation results in no alteration of the phenotype generated in the single deletion of gp91phox. Recruitment index (Table 1) shows statistically significant increase in recruitment of T cells in BALf of KO mice compared to WT but not in lung, while in lung parenchyma of KO mice, macrophage, PMN and basophils are preferentially upregulated compared to

A

B

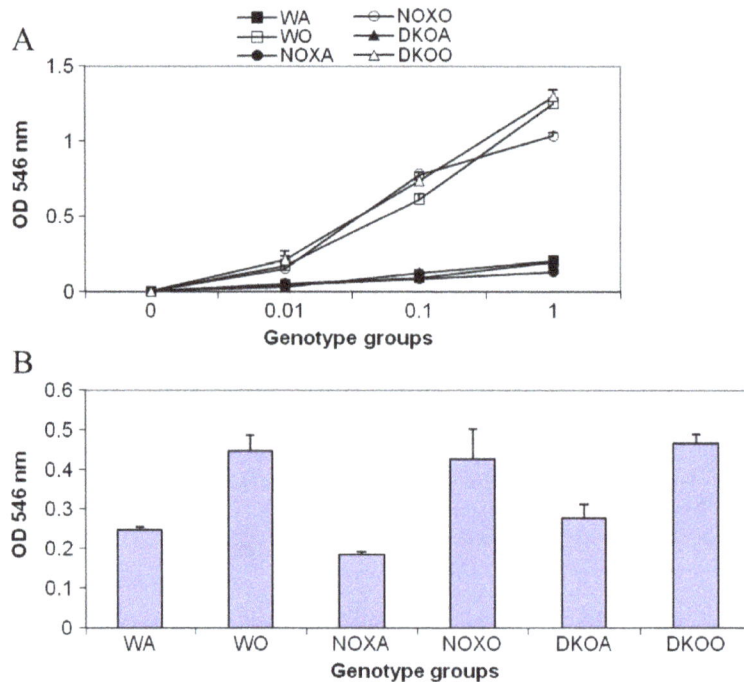

Figure 4 T cells response in WT vs. KO mice. A. Splenocytes from control (saline treated) and OVA treated mice were made into single cell suspensions in DMEM+10% heat-inactivated FCS. 0.1 million cells were plated per well without and with increasing concentrations of anti-CD3 antibody and a constant concentration of anti-CD28 antibody (1µg/ml) and cultured for 3 days. **B.** 1µM PMA and 10ng/ml ionomycin was used to stimulate splenocytes from the above experimental mice and proliferation measured after 3 days. To measure proliferation, MTT assay called CellTiter96 (Promega) was used. OD 546 nm is directly proportional to the number of cells in culture. Abbreviations used are: WT=wildtype, NOX=gp91phox−/−, DKO=gp91phox-MMP-12 double knockout, WA=WT+alum, WO=WT+OVA, NOXA=gp91phox−/−+alum, NOXO=gp91phox−/−+ OVA, DKOA= gp91phox-MMP-12 double knockout+alum, DKOO= gp91phox-MMP-12 double knockout+OVA. Data presented are average of 3 independent experiments ± SEM. (n=5/group).

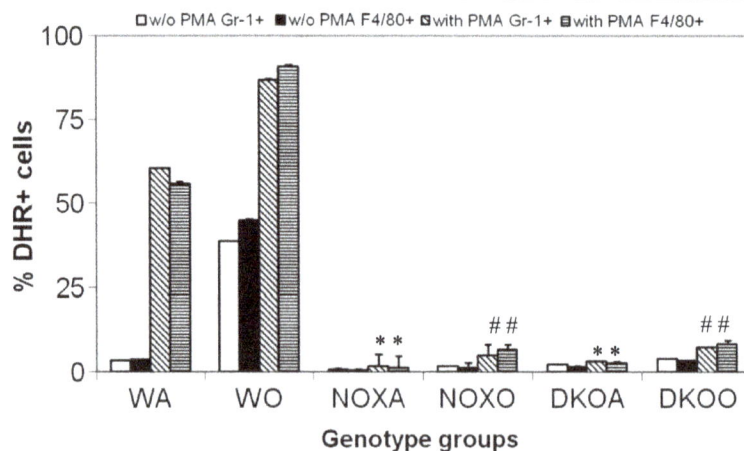

Figure 5 Inhibition of oxidative burst response by KO alveolar leukocytes. Alveolar leukocytes (0.5 × 106 cells) were stained with F4/80-Cy-Chrome and Gr1-APC for 30 min on ice, washed in PBS, warmed up at 370C for 5 min and loaded with 5mM dihydrorhodamine 123 (Molecular Probes, Eugene, OR). After 10 min at 370C, cells were split in two equal aliquots, and PMA (Sigma, St. Louis, MO) was added to one aliquot at final concentration of 1mM. After 10 min incubation cells were washed in ice-cold PBS and immediately subjected to FACS analysis. Cells were gated on neutrophils (Gr1hi), or monocyte/macrophages (F4/80+) and percentage of cells positive for dihydrorhodamine 123 fluorescence with or without PMA treatment was determined for each gate. Results shown are mean of 3 independent experiments ± SEM. (n=5/group). * denotes p value<0.05 compared to WT without PMA treatment and # denotes p value<0.05 compared to WT post-PMA treatment. While WT cells respond to PMA before as well as after OVA challenge, cells from both KO mice before as well as after OVA, failed to respond appreciably. DHR was measured at Fluorescent channel 1 in using a BD Facscaliber and DHR+ cells (CD45+gated and Gr-1+ gated or F4/80+ gated) were analyzed using CellQuestpro software.

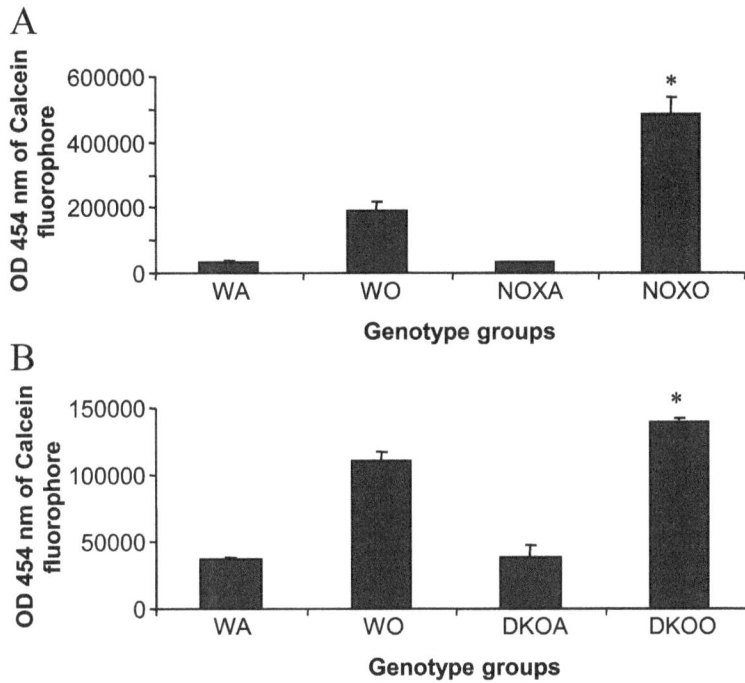

Figure 6 Inhibition of MCP-1-driven chemotaxis of alveolar macrophages in post-OVA KO mice. 15mM MCP-1 was put in 29µl volume in the lower well and 10 × 106 alveolar macrophages (from 4 mice/experimental group), also in 29µl volume in the upper wells of a 96 well Neuroprobe CTX plates (Chemicon) in high glucose medium for 2 h followed by detachment by mechanical scraping and resuspension in Phenol red-free high glucose DMEM (Gibco) with 5% FBS with 0.5µg/ml Calcein-AM (1:2000 dilution) and incubation for 20 min at 370C. Migrated cells were quantified by fluorescence (excitation at 488 nm, emission at 520 nm) using a Victor 3V (Perkin Elmer laboratories) using a Wallac1420 software. 2.5-fold and 1.26-fold increase in OD (proportinate to number of fluorescing cells in the upper well equivalent to the number of cells migrated) was found in post-OVA gp91phox−/− and DKO mice respectively. * denotes p value<0.05 compared to values in OVA-treated wildtype group.

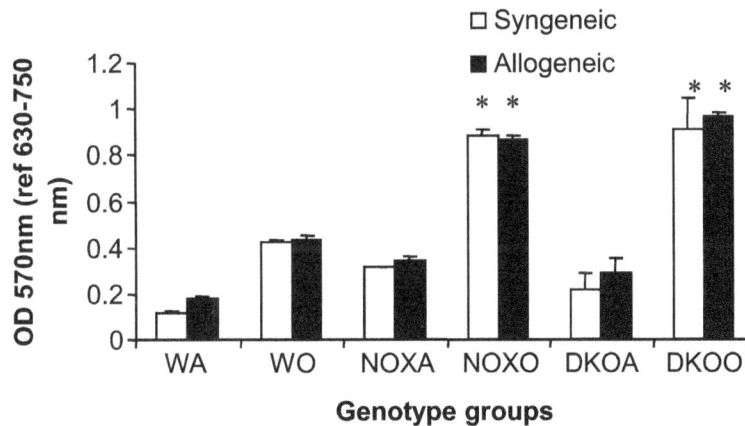

Figure 7 Altered Mixed Lymphocyte Reaction in post-OVA KO mice. 0.1 × 105 CD4+ T cells isolated by magnetic activated cell separation (MACS) by positive selection from spleen of the mice were co-cultured with γ-irradiated 0.1x103 adhering alveolar macrophages from BALf of the same experimental animal. Both cell types were from the experimental animals themselves viz. C57Bl/6 WT and KO mice. This is Syngeneic MLR where the APCs (alveolar macrophages) were γ-irradiated (3300rads). Allogeneic MLR reaction involves co-culturing 0.1x105 CD4+ T cells from the spleen of BALB/c mice with 0.1x103 γ-irradiated APCs from BALf of the experimental mice. Both control (saline-treated) and OVA-treated of each group were tested. Each culture was incubated with 1µg/ml OVA.The responders here are the T cells and the stimulators are the APCs, viz. alveolar macrophages which are γ-irradiated to inhibit their own proliferation. Since acute allergic asthma is a Th2 mediated phenomenon, interaction between T cells and macrophages will elucidate functional cross-talk between the two cell types when responders are autologous as well as when they are from a different species. 2-fold increase in post-OVA NOX vs. post-OVA WT and 2.16-fold increase in post OVA-DKO vs. post-OVA shows that T cell:APC interaction is actually more efficient in the absence of the gp91phox and MMP-12 as well as gp91phox.

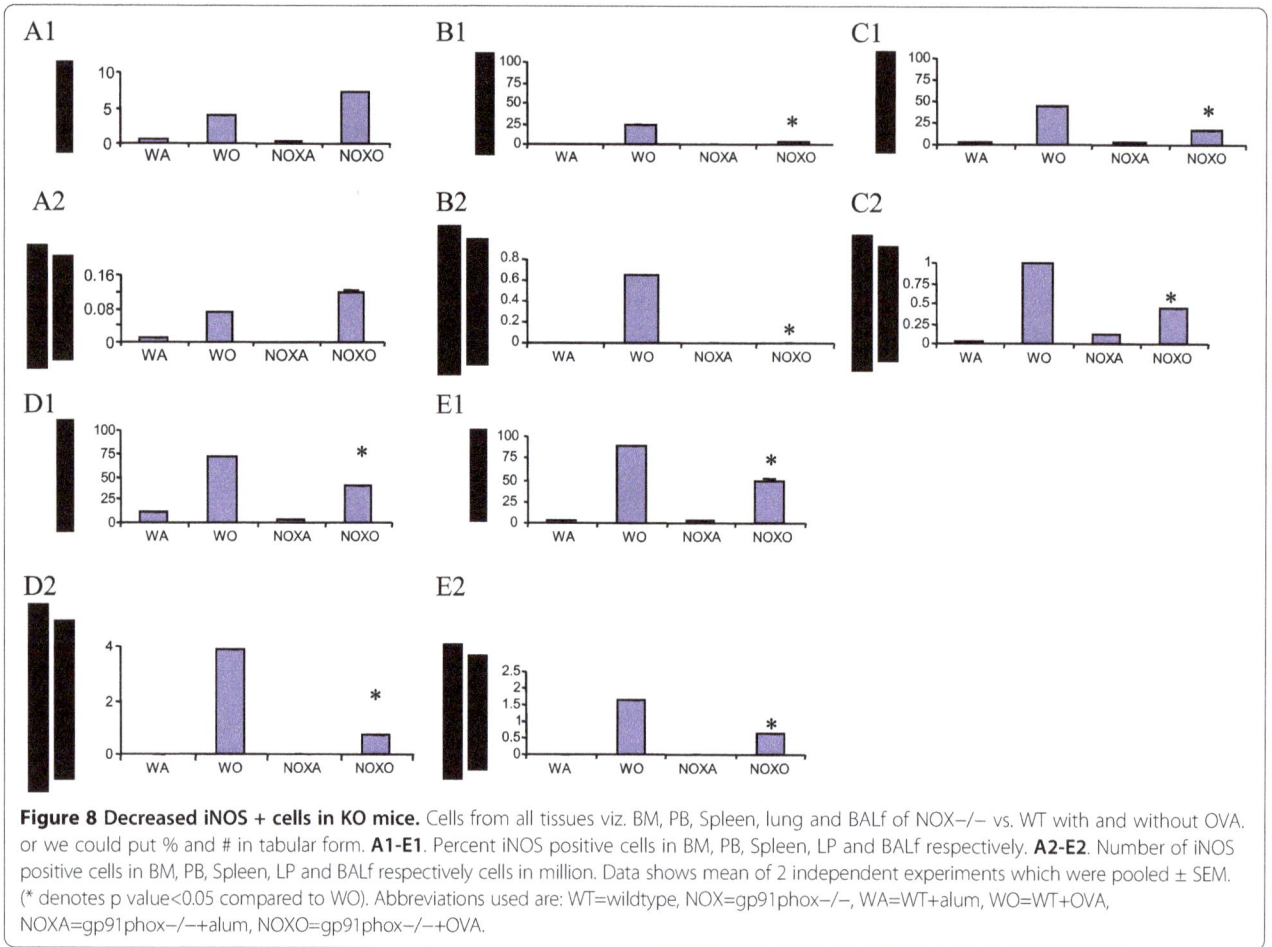

Figure 8 Decreased iNOS + cells in KO mice. Cells from all tissues viz. BM, PB, Spleen, lung and BALf of NOX–/– vs. WT with and without OVA. or we could put % and # in tabular form. **A1-E1**. Percent iNOS positive cells in BM, PB, Spleen, LP and BALf respectively. **A2-E2**. Number of iNOS positive cells in BM, PB, Spleen, LP and BALf respectively cells in million. Data shows mean of 2 independent experiments which were pooled ± SEM. (* denotes p value<0.05 compared to WO). Abbreviations used are: WT=wildtype, NOX=gp91phox–/–, WA=WT+alum, WO=WT+OVA, NOXA=gp91phox–/–+alum, NOXO=gp91phox–/–+OVA.

WT. Overall systemic response, inflammatory recruitment from blood to inflammation in lung is more in KO mice compared to WT (Table 2). Selective upregulation of both cytokine protein and cytokine mRNA of IL-13 indicates a preferential T cell mediated pathway which is unregulated in the gp91phox knockout as well as the DKO mouse. (Table 3, Figure 1) Surprisingly, there was downregulation

of TGFβ which may indicate that in keeping with decreased iNOS expression and the consequent shift in macrophage phenotype to M1 (killer) from M2 (healer), TGFβ expression was also downregulated indicating a possible regulatory role for gp91phox in the development of Th2 phenotype and that deletion of the same disrupts the control or moderating effect involving cross-talk

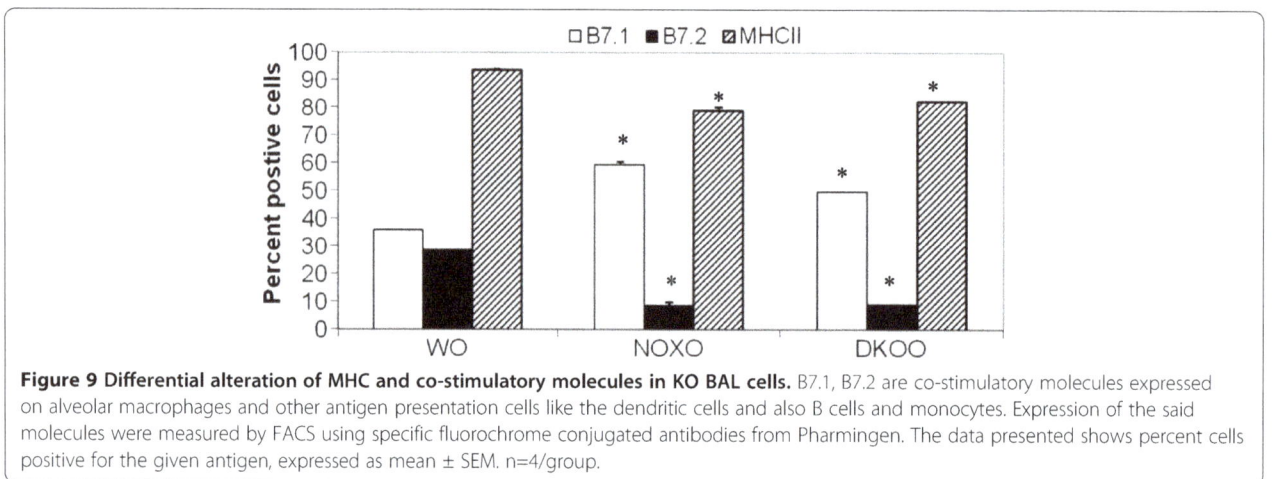

Figure 9 Differential alteration of MHC and co-stimulatory molecules in KO BAL cells. B7.1, B7.2 are co-stimulatory molecules expressed on alveolar macrophages and other antigen presentation cells like the dendritic cells and also B cells and monocytes. Expression of the said molecules were measured by FACS using specific fluorochrome conjugated antibodies from Pharmingen. The data presented shows percent cells positive for the given antigen, expressed as mean ± SEM. n=4/group.

between T cells. Consequently, the phagocytes down-stream that need NADPH enzyme for the respiratory burst response and proliferation are affected. Increased chemotaxis to MCP-1 may be explained by the increased expression of MCP-3. Upregulation of MMP-12 in gp91phox−/− both before and after OVA, may indicate a compensatory mechanism in the regulation of Th2 response (Table 4). Downmodulation of genes for MMP-7, 9, 10, and 28 in post-OVA SKO and DKO lungs may indicate that these metalloproteases which are also known regulators of inflammation, when downregulated in a situation of gp91phox deletion, may have disrupted a critical control mechanism on the development of Th2 mediated inflammation in lung.(Figure 2 and 3) T cells in SKO and DKO mice were functionally competent as revealed by functional tests. (Figure 4) Contradictory up- and down-modulation data of different functional responses, viz. oxidative burst response by a heterogeneous population of phagocytes in the lung and directed migration to MCP-1 gradient in a chemotaxis assay done with alveolar macrophages, indicate a dichotomy in the signaling of the same cells when different stimuli are present. (Figure 5 and 6) There was unregulated oxidative burst response (Figure 5), enhanced chemotaxis to MCP-1(Figure 6) and increased MLR (both syngeneic and allogeneic) (Figure 7), probably indicating relation to the role of these molecules in the cross-talk between T cells and alveolar macrophages, a phenomenon which can account for the "unregulated" recruitment of KO T cells to the lung interstitium which is what finally dictates development of lung inflammation in Th2 mediated allergy [16,21-25]. The overall Th2 response was enhanced possibly due to a lack of control over T cell: APC cross-talk in the KO mice as shown by the results of the MLR assay. Increased B7.1 but decreased B7.2 and MHCII expression may provide possible mechanistic insights into the regulatory function of gp91^{phox} and MMP-12 [26,27]. iNOS upregulation has always been construed as indicator of heightened inflammation by the participating cells [28-30]. Recruitment of B cells, monocytes, neutrophils and basophils are increased in lungs of both knockout mice compared to post-OVA wildtype while that of T cells, neutrophils and basophils in BALf are increased in the knockout vs. the OVA-treated wildtype (Table 2). MMP-12 controls migration of monocytes and macrophages to inflammatory sites and airway remodeling by degrading ECM proteins [31]. It is supposed to have a protective effect in emphysema [32]. B7.1, a co-stimulatory signal necessary for the activation of T cells, are expressed on cell surface by B cells, dendritic cells and macrophages, the so-called antigen presenting cells. It is associated with activation of cell mediated response, especially Th2 response. At baseline, they are not expressed but upon activation are upregulated. In our model, upregulation of B7.1 but downregulation of B7.2

and MHCII shows a possible mechanism by which gp91^{phox} and MMP-12, may synergistically regulate Th2 responsiveness and deletion of the same possibly disrupts this pathway. Mature T lymphocytes become activated to perform their effector functions when stimulated by appropriate APC bearing MHC class I or class II molecules. So antagonistic alterations in B7 family of receptors in the acute asthma pathway may indicate a definite role for either gp91phox or both gp91^{phox} and MMP-12 in controlling the co-stimulatory activating pathway in T cell activation in Th2 response.

The data presented above in this study indicate the following regulatory role for gp91^{phox} and MMP-12 in the etiology of T cell mediated acute allergic asthma pathophysiology:

(i) gp91^{phox} specifically may be regulating IL-13 gene activation in the lung tissue as well as translation into protein secreted into the airways. This may be associative.

(ii) The direction of stimulus to → response seems to be T cells to →macrophages and not vice versa. In other words, gp91^{phox} alone or gp91^{phox} and MMP-12 together regulate/translate T cell directive to macrophages for clinical manifestation of the Th2-initiated, macrophage-mediated allergic phenomenon.

(iii) Downmodulation of respiratory burst response in neutrophils and macrophages isolated from lung but upregulation of MCP-1 directed chemotaxis by alveolar macrophages collected from lung interstitium and airways, indicate a dichotomy in the role of gp91^{phox} in controlling macrophages responses to divergent stimuli in a cell specific or tissue specific manner. Upmodulated B7.1expression but downmodulateded B7.2 and MHC class II expression in KO alveolar macrophages may indicate that alteration of co-stimulatory molecule expression may give critical signals for T cell activation.

(iv) There seems to be some redundancy in their regulatory capacity for Th2 activation but gp91^{phox} and MMP-12 do seem to provide a regulatory checkpoint (possibly sequentially but not additively) to restrict T cell cross-talk with macrophages and keeps excessive tissue damage and ECM degradation during acute allergic inflammation under control.

Abbreviations
WT: Wildtype; NOX: gp91^{phox} KO; OVA: Ovalbumin; AM: Alveolar macrophage; BM: Bone marrow; PB: Peripheral blood; BALf: Bronchoalveolar lavage fluid; LP: Lung parenchyma; AHR: Airway hyper-reactivity/responsiveness; i.t.: Intra-tracheal; i.v.: Intravenous; i.p.: Intraperitoneal; H&E: Hematoxylin and Eosin; Penh: Enhanced pause; WBP: Whole body plethysmography; KO: Knockout;

ROS: Reactive oxygen species; NOX: NADPH oxidase; SKO: Single knockout; DKO: Double knockout; TCR: T cell receptor.

Competing interest
The authors have declared that no conflict of interest exists.

Authors' contributions
WRH initiated and funded the project and gave key suggestions in its execution and read this manuscript. ERB conceptualized, designed and executed all experiments and analyzed all data and wrote this manuscript. All authors read and approved the final manuscript.

Acknowledgements
This work was supported by National Institute of Health grants 62–9208 and 62–9538 (WRH). We thank J. W. Heinecke for the Cybb–/– mice that were bred in his laboratory by Z. Sagawa and R. Norris for initial editing of this manuscript. The author also acknowledges contribution of Tim Burkland, Ph. D. and Eman Sadoun, Ph.D. respectively for carrying out the real time PCR analysis of the MMP and RGS genes. Some confirmatory assays were performed in the ERB lab at the University of Calcutta, India and editing of the final manuscript done by fellows of ERB lab- Kaustab Mukherjee, Debalina Mukhopadhyay, Shankha Subhra Chatterjee, Gaytri Datta, Anjan Ghosh and Anisha Polley. Finally I wish to thank Dr. Umesh Singh and my children Urbi, Adit and baby Arit for their support all the way.

References
1. Dikalov SI, Li W, Doughan AK, Blanco RR, Zafari AM: Mitochondrial reactive oxygen species and calcium uptake regulate activation of phagocytic NADPH oxidase. *Am J Physiol Regul Integr Comp Physiol* 2012, Epub ahead of print.
2. Groemping Y, Rittiner K: Activation and assembly of the NADPH oxidase: a structural perspective. *Biochem J* 2005, 386:401–416.
3. Henriet SS, Hermans PW, Verweij PE, Simonetti E, Holland SM, Sugui JA, Kwon-Chung KJ, Warris A: Human leucocytes kill Aspergillus nidulans by ROS-independent mechanisms. *Infect Immun* 2010.
4. Bylund J, Brown KL, Movitz C, Dahlgren C, Karlsson A: Intracellular generation of superoxide by the phagocyte NADPH oxidase: How, where, and what for? *Free Radic Biol Med* 2010, 49(12):1834–1845.
5. Kumar S, Patel S, Jyoti A, Keshari RS, Verma A, Barthwal MK, Dikshit M: Nitric oxide-mediated augmentation of neutrophil reactive oxygen and nitrogen species formation: Critical use of probes. *Cytometry A.* 2010, 77(11):1038–1048.
6. De Ravin SS, Zarember KA, Long-Priel D, Chan KC, Fox SD, Gallin JI, Kuhns DB, Malech HL: Tryptophan/kynurenine metabolism in human leukocytes is independent of superoxide and is fully maintained in chronic granulomatous disease. *Blood* 2010, 116(10):1755–1760.
7. Chan EC, Dusting GJ, Guo N, Peshavariya HM, Taylor CJ, Dilley R, Narumiya S, Jiang F: Prostacyclin receptor suppresses cardiac fibrosis: role of CREB phosphorylation. *J Mol Cell Cardiol* 2010, 49(2):176–185.
8. Schröder K, Zhang M, Benkhoff S, Mieth A, Pliquett R, Kosowski J, Kruse C, Lüdike P, Michaelis UR, Weissmann N, Dimmeler S, Shah AM, Brandes RP: Nox4 Is a protective reactive oxygen species generating vascular NADPH oxidase. *Circ Res* 2012, Epub ahead of print.
9. Leverence JT, Medhora M, Konduri GG, Sampath V: Lipopolysaccharide-induced cytokine expression in alveolar epithelial cells: Role of PKCζ-mediated p47phox phosphorylation. *Chem Biol Interact* 2010, 189(1-2):72–81.
10. Kim Y, Zhou M, Moy S, Morales J, Cunningham MA, Joachimiak A: High-resolution structure of the nitrile reductase QueF combined with molecular simulations provide insight into enzyme mechanism. *J Mol Biol* 2010, 404(1):127–137.
11. Kang EM, Malech HL: Gene therapy for chronic granulomatous disease. *Methods Enzymol* 2012, 507:125–154.
12. Santilli G, Almarza E, Brendel C, Choi U, Beilin C, Blundell MP, Haria S, Parsley KL, Kinnon C, Malech HL, Bueren JA, Grez M, Thrasher AJ: Biochemical correction of X-CGD by a novel Chimeric promoter regulating high levels of transgene expression in myeloid cells. *Mol Ther* 2010, 19(1):122–132.
13. Pollock JD: Mouse model of X-linked chronic granulomatous disease,an inherited defect in phagocyte superoxide production. *Nat Genet* 1995, 9:202.
14. Shipley JM: Metalloelastase is required for macrophage-mediated proteolysis and matrix invasion in mice. *Proc Natl Acad Sci U S A* 1996, 93:3942–3946.
15. Ray Banerjee E: Triple selectin knockout (ELP–/–) mice fail to develop OVA-induced acute asthma phenotype. *J Inflamm* 2011, 8:19.
16. Ray Banerjee E, LaFlamme MA, Papayannopoulou T, Kahn M, Murry CE, Henderson WR Jr: Human embryonic stem cells differentiated to lung lineage-specific cells ameliorate pulmonary fibrosis in a xenograft transplant mouse model (2012). *PLoS One* 2012, e33165(3):1–15.
17. Banerjee ER, Henderson WR Jr: NADPH oxidase has a regulatory role in acute allergic asthma. *J Adv Lab Res Biol* 2011, 2(3):103–120. ISSN 0976-7614.
18. Ena Ray B, Banerjee ER, Henderson WR Jr: Defining the molecular role of gp91phox in the manifestation of acute allergic asthma using a preclinical murine model. *Clin Mol Allergy* 2012, 10(1):2–16.
19. Kassim SY, Fu X, Liles WC, Shapiro SD, Parks WC, Heinecke JW: NADPH oxidase restrains the matrix metalloproteinase activity of macrophages. *J Biol Chem* 2005, 280(34):30201–30205.
20. Lanone S, Zheng T, Zhu Z, Liu W, Lee CG, Ma B, Chen Q, Homer RJ, Wang J, Rabach LA, Rabach ME, Shipley JM, Shapiro SD, Senior RM, Elias JA: Overlapping and enzyme-specific contributions of matrix metalloproteinases-9 and –12 in IL-13–induced inflammation and remodelling. *J Clin Invest* 2002, 110(4):463–474.
21. Banerjee ER, Jiang Y, Henderson WR Jr, Scott LM, Papayannopoulou T: Alpha4 and beta2 integrins have non-overlapping roles in asthma development, but for optimal allergen sensitization only alpha4 is critical. *Exp Hematol* 2007, 35(4):605–617.
22. Banerjee ER, Jiang Y, Henderson WR Jr, Latchman YL, Papayannopoulou T: Absence of α4 but not β2 integrins restrains the development of chronic allergic asthma using mouse genetic models. *Exp Hematol* 2009, 37:715–727.
23. Ray Banerjee E, Latchman YL, Jiang Y, Priestley GV, Papayannopoulou T: Distinct changes in adult lymphopoiesis in Rag2–/– mice fully reconstituted by α4-deficinet adult bone marrow cells. *Exp Hematol* 2008, 36(8):1004–1013.
24. Ulyanova T, Ray Banerjee E, Priestley GV, Scott LM, Papayannopoulou T: Unique and redundant roles of alpha4 and beta2 integrins in kinetics of recruitment of lymphoid vs myeloid cell subsets to the inflamed peritoneum revealed by studies of genetically deficient mice. *Exp Hematol* 2007, 35(8):1256–1265.
25. Henderson WR, Banerjee ER, Chi EY: Differential effects of (S)- and (R)-enantiomers of Albuterol in mouse asthma model. *J Allergy Clin Immunol* 2005, 116:332–340.
26. Nurieva RI, Mai XM, Forbush K, Bevan MJ, Dong C: B7h is required for T cell activation, differentiation,and effector function. *PNAS* 2003, 100:14163.
27. Wang S, Zhu G, Chapoval AI, Dong H, Tamada K, Ni J, Che L: Costimulation of T cells by B7-H2, a B7-like molecule that binds ICOS. *Blood* 2000, 96(8):2808–2810.
28. Suh WK, Tafuri A, Berg-Brown NN, Shahinian A, Plyte S, Duncan GS, Okada H, Wakeham A, Odermatt B, Ohashi P, Mak TW: The inducible costimulator plays the major costimulatory role in humoral immune responses in the absence of CD28. *J Immunol* 2004, 172(10):5917–5923.
29. Hutloff A, Dittrich AM, Beier KC, Eljaschewitsch B, Kraft R, Anagnostopoulos I, Kroczek RA: ICOS is an inducible T-cell co-stimulator structurally and functionally related to CD28. *Nature* 1999, 397(6716):263–266.
30. Yoshinaga SK: T-cell co-stimulation through B7RP-1 and ICOS. *Nature* 1999, 402(6763):827–832.
31. Qian X, Agematsu K, Freeman GJ, Tagawa Y, Sugane K, Hayashi T: The ICOS-ligand B7-H2, expressed on human type II alveolar epithelial cells, plays a role in the pulmonary host defense system. *Eur J Immunol* 2006 Apr, 36(4):906–918.
32. Schuyler M, Gott K, Edwards B: Th1 Cells that adoptively transfer experimental hypersensitivity pneumonitis are activated memory cells. *Cell Immunol* 1999, 177(6):377–389.

2

Asthma: Gln27Glu and Arg16Gly polymorphisms of the beta2-adrenergic receptor gene as risk factors

Ana Carolina Zimiani de Paiva[1†], Fernando Augusto de Lima Marson[1,2*†], José Dirceu Ribeiro[2] and Carmen Sílvia Bertuzzo[1]

Abstract

Background: Asthma is caused by both environmental and genetic factors. The *ADRB2* gene, which encodes the beta 2-adrenergic receptor, is one of the most extensively studied genes with respect to asthma prevalence and severity. The Arg16Gly (+46A > G) and Gln27Glu (+79C > G) polymorphisms in the *ADRB2* gene cause changes in the amino acids flanking the receptor ligand site, altering the response to bronchodilators and the risk of asthma through complex pathways. The *ADRB2* polymorphisms affect beta-adrenergic bronchodilator action and are a tool to identify at-risk populations.

Objective: To determine the frequency of these two polymorphisms in allergic asthma patients and healthy subjects and to correlate these data with the occurrence and severity of asthma.

Methods: Eighty-eight allergic asthma patients and 141 healthy subjects were included in this study. The *ADRB2* polymorphisms were analyzed using the amplification-refractory mutation system – polymerase chain reaction (ARMS-PCR) technique. The statistical analysis was performed with the SPSS 21.0 software using the Fisher's Exact and χ^2 tests.

Results: The *ADRB2* polymorphisms were associated with asthma occurrence. The Arg16Arg, Gln27Gln and Gln27Glu genotypes were risk factors; the odds ratios were 6.782 (CI = 3.07 to 16.03), 2.120 (CI = 1.22 to 3.71) and 8.096 (CI = 3.90 to 17.77), respectively. For the Gly16Gly and Glu27Glu genotypes, the odds ratios were 0.312 (CI = 0.17 to 0.56) and 0.084 (CI = 0.04 to 0.17), respectively. The haplotype analysis showed that there were associations between the following groups: Arg16Arg-Gln27Gln (OR = 5.108, CI = 1.82 to 16.37), Gly16Gly-Glu27Glu (OR = 2.816, CI = 1.25 to 6.54), Arg16Gly-Gln27Glu (OR = 0.048, CI = 0.01 to 0.14) and Gly16Gly-Gln27Glu (OR = 0.1036, CI = 0.02 to 0.39). The polymorphism Gln27Glu was associated with asthma severity, as the Gln27Gln genotype was a risk factor for severe asthma (OR = 2.798, CI = 1.099 to 6.674) and the Gln27Glu genotype was a protective factor for mild (OR = 3.063, CI = 1.037 to 9.041) and severe (OR = 0.182, CI = 0.048 to 0.691) asthma.

Conclusions: The Arg16Gly and Gln27Glu polymorphisms in the *ADRB2* gene are associated with asthma presence and severity.

Keywords: Asthma, *ADRB2* gene, Lung disease, Arg16Gly, Gln27Glu

* Correspondence: fernandolimamarson@hotmail.com
†Equal contributors
[1]Department of Medical Genetics, Faculty of Medical Sciences, State University of Campinas (Unicamp), Campinas, São Paulo zip code: 13081-970, Brazil
[2]Department of Pediatrics, Faculty of Medical Sciences, State University of Campinas (Unicamp), Tessália Vieira de Camargo, 126, Campinas, SP zip code: 13081-970, Brazil

Background

Asthma is a chronic inflammatory disease of the airways defined by clinical, physiological and pathological characteristics. The main traits of allergic asthma in children are shortness of breath, wheezing, obstruction and inflammation of airways, and atopy [1]. Genetically, asthma is a complex disease in which multiple genes interact among themselves and with the environment [1].

Asthma affects approximately 300 million people worldwide (1 to 18% of the population in different countries) [2,3] and is associated with 250,000 deaths per year. In Brazil, 20% of the population is affected, with approximately 350,000 hospitalizations per year or 2.3% of the hospital admissions in the Public Health System [4]. Asthma-related mortality has been growing over the last 10 years but does not correlate with disease prevalence. Asthma causes 5 to 10% of the respiratory-related deaths, with a high number of deaths occurring at home [4].

There are several factors that influence the development of asthma, including genes that predispose an individual to atopy and airway hyperresponsiveness; obesity; sex; and environmental causes, such as allergens (house dust mites, animal fur, and fungi), viral infections, occupational sensitizers, tobacco smoke, air pollution and eating habits. Additionally, some immunological characteristics, such as immune system maturation and the number of exposures to infectious agents during the first years of life, are factors that affect the risk of developing asthma. Another characteristic linked to an increased risk of asthma is ethnicity, which reflects vast genetic differences as well as significant social and economic variations that affect exposure to allergens and access to health services [1,5-10].

Asthma severity is assessed by analyzing the frequency and intensity of symptoms and examining pulmonary function. Based on these criteria, asthma is classified as either intermittent or persistent asthma, the latter of which can be mild, moderate or severe [1].

The pathophysiological characteristic present in asthmatic patients is bronchial inflammation, which is the result of complex interactions between the inflammatory cells, cell-derived mediators, and airway cells [11].

An important factor studied in asthma-related research is the beta-2-adrenergic receptor, which is encoded by the ADRB2 gene [12]. The ADRB2 gene is a small gene on chromosome 5q31-q32 [13], a region genetically linked to asthma [14]. Nine coding polymorphisms were originally described in the ADRB2 gene, including four that cause non-synonymous changes in the amino acid sequence (Gly16Arg, Gln27Glu, Val34Met and Thr164Ile).

The β2 receptors (β2-AR) are widely expressed in the respiratory tract, particularly in the airway smooth muscles [12,15-17]. They are members of a family of seven-transmembrane receptors [18] and are 413 amino acids long [19]. Once activated, the most clinically relevant effect of the β2-ARs in the pulmonary smooth muscle is relaxation, which may be caused by β2-AR agonists. Chronic exposure to these agonists leads to a significant reduction in the number of β2-ARs on the cell surface [16,17]. This down-regulation is reflected in vivo as a tolerance to the effects of the β2-AR agonists [20-24].

In airway smooth muscle cells, the β2-AR agonists activate adenylyl cyclase through membrane-coupled G-proteins; this activation increases the intracellular cAMP (cyclic adenosine monophosphate) concentration and relaxes the airway tonus [25]. The β2-AR agonists may also affect Ca^{2+} and K^+ channels in smooth muscles and lead to relaxation independently of cAMP [26].

The two most frequent deleterious polymorphisms in the ADRB2 gene are Arg16Gly (+46A > G; rs1042713) and Gln27Glu (+79C > G; rs1042714). The Arg16Gly and Gln27Glu polymorphisms are near the receptor's ligand-binding site [27]. The frequency of Gly16 is greater than that of Arg16, which is considered the normal allele. The allelic frequency described for the Arg16 variant ranges from 67% to 72% in different populations [28,29].

In the Brazilian population, to the best of our knowledge, there are no studies on asthma and the frequency of the Arg16Gly and Gln27Glu polymorphisms that take into account asthma risk and clinical severity. Therefore, our study included asthma patients and healthy subjects, and the associations between both groups and each polymorphism were assessed during the same analysis. The clinical evaluation of asthma severity was associated with the Arg16Gly and Gln27Glu polymorphisms.

Methods
Patients and healthy controls

A cross-sectional prospective study including 88 asthmatic patients was conducted at the Pediatric Pulmonology Clinic at the University Hospital.

The mean age was 10.38 (±2.93) years with a range of 7 to 16 years. All patients enrolled had allergic asthma according to the GINA criteria [1]. The allergy classification was defined by co-occurrence with asthma, atopic dermatitis, a positive skin test in response to allergens (dust mites, fungi, or house dust components), increased IgE serum levels, greater than 4% eosinophils in the peripheral blood in the absence of parasites and clinical history. All patients were subjected to three parasitological stool examinations three months prior to the onset of the study and were treated with albendazole as necessary.

The control group was composed of 141 healthy subjects ranging in age from 18 to 25 years who donated blood at the Unicamp University Hospital. In our data, all controls were examined for allergic asthma and a family history of asthma. In the case of a family history of asthma, the subject was excluded from our control group.

Table 1 Association of *ADRB2* polymorphisms [Arg16Gly (c.46A > G) and Gln27Glu (c.79C > G)] with asthma risk

Polymorphism	Genotype	Patient	Control	OR	95% CI
Arg16Gly (c.46A > G) [1,2]	Homozygous Arg16	28	9	**6.782**	**3.07-16.03**
	Heterozygous	38	59	1.056	0.61-1.81
	Homozygous Gly16	22	73	**0.312**	**0.17-0.56**
	Total	**88**	**141**		
Gln27Glu(c.79C > G) [3,4]	Homozygous Gln27	41	41	**2.120**	**1.22-3.71**
	Heterozygous	36	11	**8.096**	**3.90-17.77**
	Homozygous Glu27	11	89	**0.084**	**0.04-0.17**
	Total	**88**	**141**		

ADR2 = alpha2-adrenergic receptor; Arg = arginine; Gly = Glycine; Gln = Glutamine; Glu = Glutamic acid; A = Adenine; G = Guanine; T = Thymine; OR = Odds Ratio; CI = Confidence Interval.
Hardy-Weinberg equilibrium was calculated using the OEGE tool (http://www.oege.org/software/hardy-weinberg.html), being: (1 - patient) χ^2 = 1.54, p-value > 0.05; (2 - control) χ^2 = 0.48, p-value > 0.05; (3 - patient) χ^2 = 0.41, p-value > 0.05; (4 - control) χ^2 = 95.62, p-value < 0.001.
The OR was calculated using the Open-Epi tool (http://www.openepi.com). The OR and 95% CI values were obtained using the Mild-P test. For all data analyzed, α = 0.05 was used. The significant p-values are in bold.

The project was approved by the University Ethics Committee (#267/2005), and all patients and/or their guardians signed an informed consent.

Arg16Gly and Gln27Glu polymorphism analyses

Genomic DNA was extracted from the venous blood samples using phenol-chloroform. The DNA concentration was determined using a GE NanoVue™ Spectrophotometer (GE Healthcare Biosciences, Pittsburgh, USA), and 50 ng/mL of each sample was used for the analysis.

Polymorphism analysis of the *ADRB2* gene was performed by the polymerase (PCR) allele specific (ARMS) reaction [30,31]. Four reactions were performed (ARMS1a,

Table 2 Association of *ADRB2* polymorphism [Arg16Gly (c.46A > G) and Gln27Glu (c.79C > G)] combinations with asthma risk

Polymorphisms	Genotypes groups*	Patient	Control	OR	95% CI
Gly16 – Gln27	1	19	23	1.411	0.71-2.79
Arg16 – Glu27	1	10	0	-	-
Arg16 – Gln27	0	14	5	**5.108**	**1.82-16.37**
Gly16 – Glu27	2	17	11	**2.816**	**1.25-6.54**
Het16 – Gln27	0	10	12	1.376	0.55-3.38
Het16 – Glu27	1	9	0	-	-
Het16 – Het27	0	3	60	**0.048**	**0.01-0.14**
Arg16 – Het27	0	4	4	1.627	0.36-7.39
Gly16 – Het27	1	2	26	**0.1036**	**0.02-0.39**

ADRB2 = alpha2-adrenergic receptor; Arg = arginine; Gly = Glycine; Gln = Glutamine; Glu = Glutamic acid; A = Adenine; G = Guanine; T = Thymine; Het = heterozygotes; OR = Odds Ratio; CI = Confidence Interval.
*The groups were created by counting each homozygous guanine allele at the Arg16Gly (c.46A > G) and Gln27Glu (c.79C > G) polymorphisms: (0) Arg16Arg + Gln27Gln genotype combination; (1) Gly16Gly or Glu27Glu genotype presence; (2) Gly16Gly + Glu27Glu genotype combination.
The OR was calculated using the Open-Epi tool (http://www.openepi.com). The OR and 95% CI values were obtained using the Mild-P test. For all data analyzed, α = 0.05 was used. The significant p-values are in bold.

ARMS2a, ARMS1b and ARMS2b), each containing a common primer (5′-AGG CCC ATG ACC AGA TCA GCA CAG GCC AG-3′) and one allele-specific primer [ARMS1a (5′- ACG GCA GCG CCT TCT TGC TGG CAC CCA AAA-3′), ARMS2a (5′-ACG GCA GCG CCT TCT TGC TGG CAC CCA AAG-3′), ARMS1b (5′-GCC ATG CGC CGG ACC ACG ACG TCA CGC ATC-3′) and ARMS2b (5′-GCC ATG CGC CGG ACC ACG ACG TCA CGC AAG-3′)]. All four reactions were performed under the same conditions. Each 10 μL reaction contained 1 × 4 PCR buffer, 200 μM of dNTPs, 5.0 nM of MgCl$_2$, 0.4 U of Taq polymerase, 0.2 pmol of each primer and 1.0 μL (approximately 50 ng) of genomic DNA.

The PCR amplification conditions consisted of 5 minutes at 94°C followed by 35 cycles of 94°C for 1 minute, 60°C (46A or G, 16Arg or Gly) or 67°C (70C or G, 27 Gln or Glu), and 72°C for 1 minute followed by 72°C for 10 minutes.

The amplicons were subjected to electrophoresis on a 12% acrylamide gel and stained with ethidium bromide.

Statistical analysis

Statistical analysis was performed using the software SPSS (Statistical Package for the Social Sciences) version 21.0 (Armonk, NY: IBM Corp), Open Epi [32] and R version 2.12 (Comprehensive R Archive Network, 2011). The statistical power calculation for the sample was performed using the GPOWER 3.1 software [33] and demonstrated statistical power above 80% for the analysis conducted. An alpha level of 0.05 was used in all of the data analyses.

The Fisher's Exact and chi-squared (χ^2) tests were performed to determine the association between the polymorphisms analyzed and the presence and severity of asthma.

The Hardy-Weinberg equilibrium was calculated using the Online Encyclopedia for Genetic Epidemiology (OEGE) software (http://www.oege.org/software/hardy-weinberg.html).

Table 3 Association of *ADRB2* polymorphisms [Arg16Gly (c.46A > G) and Gln27Glu (c.79C > G)] with asthma risk based on the presence of Guanine alleles

Genotypes groups*	Patient	Control	OR	95% CI
0	31	81	**0.405**	**0.23-0.70**
1	40	49	1.562	0.90-2.70
2	17	11	**2.816**	**1.25-6.54**

ADRB2 = alpha2-adrenergic receptor; Arg = arginine; Gly = Glycine; Gln = Glutamine; Glu = Glutamic acid; A = Adenine; G = Guanine; T = Thymine; OR = Odds Ratio; CI = Confidence Interval.
*The groups were created by counting each homozygous guanine allele at the Arg16Gly (c.46A > G) and Gln27Glu (c.79C > G) polymorphisms: (0) Arg16Arg + Gln27Gln genotype combination; (1) Gly16Gly or Glu27Glu genotype presence; (2) Gly16Gly + Glu27Glu genotype combination.
The OR was calculated using the Open-Epi tool (http://www.openepi.com). The OR and 95% CI values were obtained using the Mild-P test. For all data analyzed, α = 0.05 was used. The significant p-values are in bold.

To calculate the sample power, the GPower*3.1.6 program was used [33]. In the calculation, we considered the minor allele frequency (MAF) to establish the sample size. According to the NCBI (National Center for Biotechnology Information - http://www.ncbi.nlm.nih.gov/) database, the frequencies of the A and C alleles at the 46A > G and 79C > G polymorphisms were 0.471 and 0.238, respectively. With the frequency of 0.238, α = 0.05 and β = 0.80, the power calculation estimates the patient sample size should be 193 patients based on using a χ^2 test for the comparisons to be performed. In our study, we included 229 patients and controls and with our population obtained a β-error of 0.846.

To evaluate the genetic interactions among the polymorphisms in our sample, we used the Multifactor Dimensionality Reduction (MDR) model, which is a nonparametric and genetic model-free data mining tool for nonlinear interaction identification among genetic and environmental attributes [34-36]. To adjust the results for multiple comparisons, we performed a MDR permutation test on our data using 100,000 permutations.

Results

The allelic frequencies for the Arg16Gly polymorphism were 94 (53.4%) and 82 (46.6%) for the A and G alleles, respectively, in the asthma group and 77 (27.3%) and 205 (72.7%), respectively, in the healthy subjects. For the Gln27Glu polymorphism, the allelic frequencies for the C and G alleles were 118 (67.0%) and 48 (33.0%), respectively, in the asthma group and 93 (33.0%) and 189 (67%), respectively, in the healthy subjects.

The polymorphisms are in Hardy-Weinberg equilibrium except for the Gln27Glu polymorphism, which is not in equilibrium in the healthy subject population. The complete genotype data and the Hardy-Weinberg equilibriums are shown in Table 1.

In our data, the *ADRB2* polymorphisms were associated with the occurrence of asthma. For the Arg16Arg, Gln27Gln and Gln27Glu genotypes, the risk factor odds ratios were 6.782 (CI = 3.07 to 16.03), 2.120 (CI = 1.22 to 3.71) and 8.096 (CI = 3.90 to 17.77), respectively. For the Gly16Gly and Glu27Glu genotypes, the odds ratios were

Table 4 Association of asthma severity with *ADRB2* polymorphisms [Arg16Gly (c.46A > G) and Gln27Glu (c.79C > G)]

Severity	Arg16Gly (c.46A > G) polymorphism							χ^2	p-value
	Arg16Arg	OR (95% CI)	Arg16Gly	OR (95% CI)	Gly16Gly	OR (95% CI)	Total		
Severe	14 (37.8%)	1.258 (0.508 - 3.114)	3 (8.1%)	**0.25 (0.064 - 0.966)**	20 (54.1%)	1.672 (0.698 - 4.003)	37 (100%)	4.674	0.322
Moderate	7(33.3%)	0.909 (0.319 - 2.587)	5 (23.8%)	1.625 (0.484 - 5.454)	9 (42.9%)	0.703 (0.259 - 1.906)	21 (100%)		
Mild	8 (32%)	0.829 (0.306 - 2.246)	7 (28%)	2.431 (0.771 - 7.665)	10 (40%)	0.667 (0.258 - 1.726)	25 (100%)		
	Gln27Glu (c.79C > G) polymorphism								
	Gln27Gln	OR (95% CI)	Gln27Glu	OR (95% CI)	Glu27Glu	OR (95% CI)	Total		
Severe	25 (67.6%)	**2.708 (1.099 - 6.674)**	3 (8.1%)	**0.182 (0.048 - 0.691)**	9 (24.3%)	1.023 (0.372 - 2.812)	37 (100%)	8.285	0.082
Moderate	10 (47.6%)	0.701 (0.26 - 1.892)	6 (28.6%)	1.667 (0.534 - 5.197)	5 (23.8%)	0.979 (0.307 - 3.124)	21 (100%)		
Mild	10 (40%)	0.438 (0.168 - 1.141)	9 (36%)	**3.063 (1.037 - 9.041)**	6 (24%)	0.9925 (0.331 - 2.973)	25 (100%)		
	Arg16Gly (c.46A > G) and Gln27Glu (c.79C > G) polymorphisms in combination*								
	0	OR (95% CI)	1	OR (95% CI)	2	OR (95% CI)	Total		
Severe	12 (32.4%)	0.571 (0.232 - 1.406)	21 (56.8%)	1.706 (0.712 - 4.086)	4 (10.8%)	0.994 (0.247 - 4)	37 (100%)	1.908	0.753
Moderate	9 (42.9%)	1.188 (0.435 - 3.241)	10 (47.6%)	0.909 (0.338 - 2.448)	2 (9.5%)	0.827 (0.158 - 4.331)	21 (100%)		
Mild	12 (48%)	1.626 (0.629 - 4.205)	10 (40%)	0.581 (0.224 - 1.504)	3 (12%)	1.182 (0.271 - 5.154)	25 (100%)		

ADRB2 = alpha2-adrenergic receptor; Arg = arginine; Gly = Glycine; Gln = Glutamine; Glu = Glutamic acid; A = Adenine; G = Guanine; T = Thymine; OR = Odds Ratio; CI = Confidence Interval.
*The groups were created by counting each homozygous guanine allele at the Arg16Gly (c.46A > G) and Gln27Glu (c.79C > G) polymorphisms: (0) Arg16Arg + Gln27Gln genotype combination; (1) Gly16Gly or Glu27Glu genotype presence; (2) Gly16Gly + Glu27Glu genotype combination.
The OR was calculated using the Open-Epi tool (http://www.openepi.com). The OR and 95% CI values were obtained using the Mild-P test and in the table the χ^2 value is shown. For all data analyzed, α = 0.05 was used. The significant p-values are in bold.

0.312 (CI = 0.17 to 0.56) and 0.084 (CI = 0.04 to 0.17), respectively. For more details, consult Tables 1 and 2.

The haplotype analysis showed associations between the following polymorphisms: Arg16Arg-Gln27Gln (OR = 5.108, CI = 1.82 to 16.37), Gly16Gly-Glu27Glu (OR = 2.816, CI = 1.25 to 6.54), Arg16Gly-Gln27Glu (OR = 0.048, CI = 0.01 to 0.14) and Gly16Gly-Gln27Glu (OR = 0.1036, CI = 0.02 to 0.39). The complete haplotype analysis is shown in Table 3. To confirm our data, the groups with the highest observed frequency were analyzed in comparison with all of the other possible groups. The complete group data can be found in Table 4.

All of the data and the comparisons between the groups can be found in Figure 1.

When asthma severity was taken into account, the polymorphism Gln27Glu was a risk factor for severe asthma when the Gln27Gln genotype was present (OR = 2.798, CI = 1.099 to 6.674) and a protective factor for mild (OR =

3.063, CI = 1.037 to 9.041) and severe asthma (OR = 0.182, CI = 0.048 to 0.691) when the Gln27Glu genotype was present.

The MDR analysis showed evidence of an interaction between Arg16Gly and Gln27Glu as risk factors for asthma [Testing Balance Accuracy = 0.7727; p-value = 0.0000 – 0.0010; Ratio = 0.6377] (Figure 2).

Discussion

Pharmacotherapy that is tailored to an asthmatic patient's genotype should result in a clinically significant increase in efficacy and reduction in adverse events and, therefore, have an important role in disease severity [37]. The β-agonists are the most commonly used agents for asthma treatment [1]. Polymorphisms in the *ADRB2* gene have been screened and found to be associated with altered expression, function and regulation of the β2 receptor. These types of genetically based differences

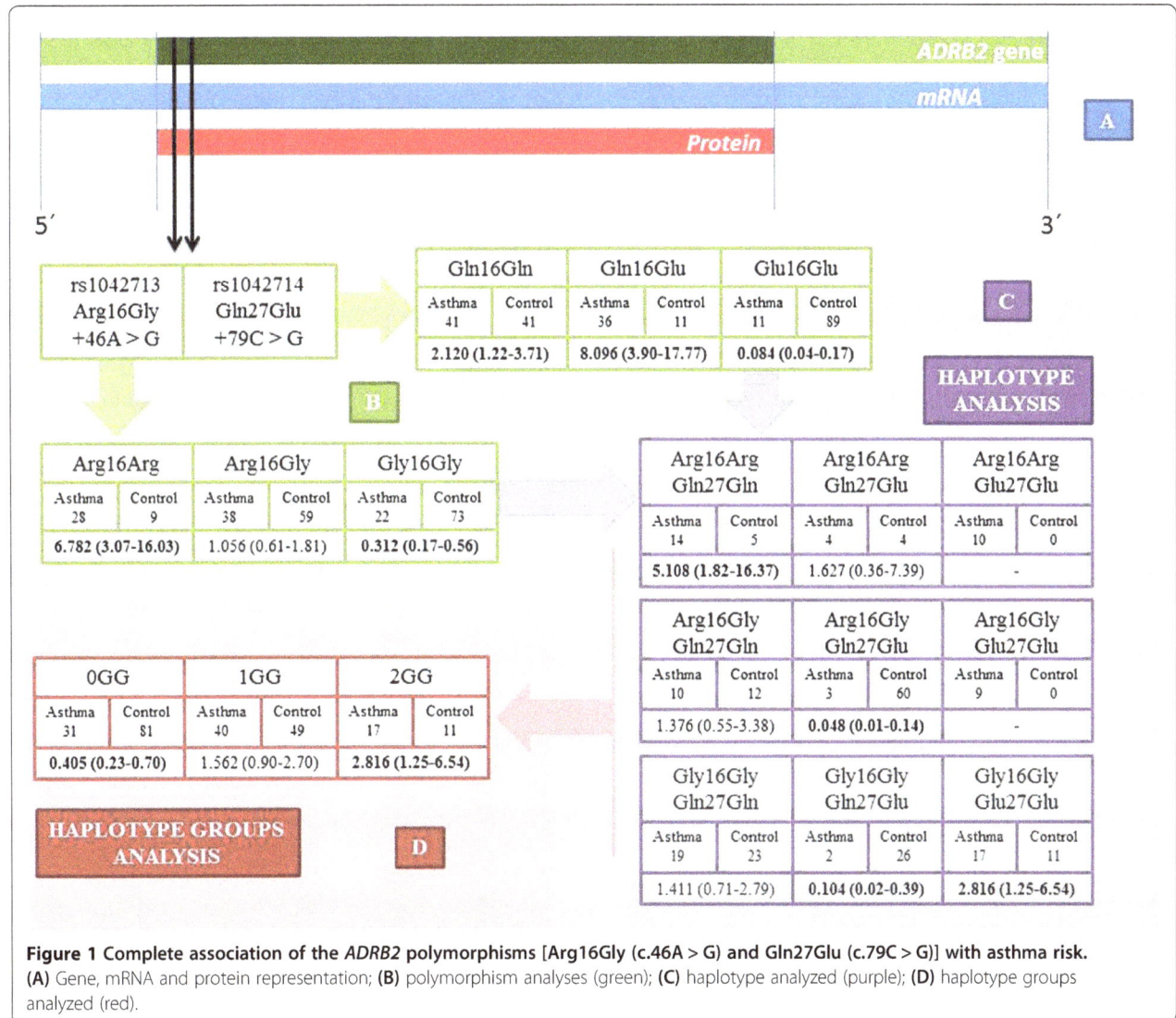

Figure 1 Complete association of the *ADRB2* polymorphisms [Arg16Gly (c.46A > G) and Gln27Glu (c.79C > G)] with asthma risk.
(A) Gene, mRNA and protein representation; (B) polymorphism analyses (green); (C) haplotype analyzed (purple); (D) haplotype groups analyzed (red).

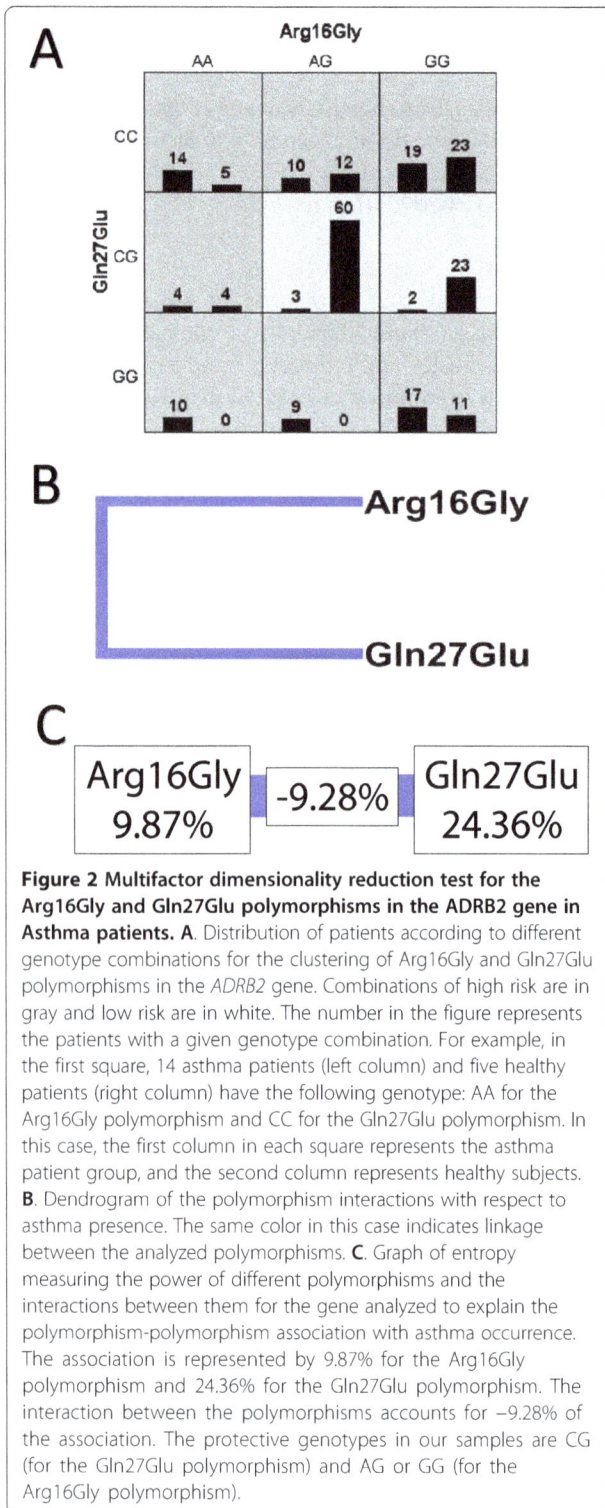

Figure 2 Multifactor dimensionality reduction test for the Arg16Gly and Gln27Glu polymorphisms in the ADRB2 gene in Asthma patients. A. Distribution of patients according to different genotype combinations for the clustering of Arg16Gly and Gln27Glu polymorphisms in the ADRB2 gene. Combinations of high risk are in gray and low risk are in white. The number in the figure represents the patients with a given genotype combination. For example, in the first square, 14 asthma patients (left column) and five healthy patients (right column) have the following genotype: AA for the Arg16Gly polymorphism and CC for the Gln27Glu polymorphism. In this case, the first column in each square represents the asthma patient group, and the second column represents healthy subjects. B. Dendrogram of the polymorphism interactions with respect to asthma presence. The same color in this case indicates linkage between the analyzed polymorphisms. C. Graph of entropy measuring the power of different polymorphisms and the interactions between them for the gene analyzed to explain the polymorphism-polymorphism association with asthma occurrence. The association is represented by 9.87% for the Arg16Gly polymorphism and 24.36% for the Gln27Glu polymorphism. The interaction between the polymorphisms accounts for −9.28% of the association. The protective genotypes in our samples are CG (for the Gln27Glu polymorphism) and AG or GG (for the Arg16Gly polymorphism).

factor associated with bronchodilator response [38-40] but not as a risk factor associated with asthma prevalence within a population.

The allelic frequencies of the Arg16Gly and Gln27Glu SNPs vary with ethnicity [41,42]. The reported allele frequencies for Arg16 in the Caucasian, African American and Asian asthmatic populations were 0.39, 0.50 and 0.40, respectively, while for Gln27, the reported frequencies were 0.57, 0.73 and 0.80, respectively [41]. In the present study, the allelic frequencies of Arg16 were 0.53 in the asthma group and 0.27 in healthy subjects. For the Gln27 allele, the allelic frequencies were 0.67 and 0.33 in the asthma group and the healthy subjects, respectively. We observed that the frequencies found in our study are similar to those found in the African American and Caucasian populations.

The Arg16Gly and Gln27Glu polymorphisms cause differential agonist-stimulated down-regulation of the receptor in transfected cell systems, including human airway smooth muscle cells [43,44]. Many previous studies have investigated possible associations between asthma and polymorphisms in the coding region of the ADRB2 gene, particularly the Arg16Gly and Gln27Glu SNPs; however, these studies have yielded conflicting results [38-40,45-48].

In the present study, associations between the Arg16Arg and Gln27Gln genotypes and susceptibility to asthma were observed.

The Arg16Arg genotype was more frequent in asthma patients than in healthy subjects; the opposite correlation was observed for the homozygous Glu16Glu genotype showing that individuals with the former genotype have an increased susceptibility to the development of asthma. The Gln27Gln and Gln27Glu genotypes were indirectly related to the occurrence of asthma by the fact that the Glu27Glu genotype had a protective effect against asthma. Reinforcing this finding, elevated serum IgE levels have been found in patients carrying the Arg16 and Gln27 homozygous genotypes [49].

Our results contradicted previous data from studies of Japanese [50], African American [51] and North Indian [52] populations but agreed with other studies of Canadian [46], Chinese [53] and British populations [54], as well as a study of African American children [55]. This discrepancy may be the result of racial differences [48].

As expected, the results of the haplotype analysis showed that the haplotype Arg16Arg-Gln27Gln was associated with greater risk and that the Gly16Gly-Glu27Glu haplotype was protective. The haplotype Arg16Arg-Gln27Gln is associated in general with a poor response to the β2-AR agonist and low levels of β2-AR expression. In addition, the good response to exogenous agonists is reflected in a good response to endogenous agonists and a protective effect against asthma [56].

may account for some of the variability in the responses to treatment with ADRB2 agonists and may contribute to the increased mortality in select patient populations, such as cystic fibrosis patients [31]. Several studies have examined the ADRB2 gene as a risk

In a case–control study in the North Indian population, the Gly16Gly genotype conferred a decreased risk of asthma (OR = 0.65; 95% IC = 0.41 − 1.02; p-value = 0.049), while the Gln27Glu polymorphism was not associated with asthma in this population [38]. In our study, we observed a positive association between the Arg16Gly polymorphism and asthma prevalence, but the association is weak. These data do not corroborate another study in a Chinese population in which the Arg16Gly polymorphism was not associated with genetic susceptibility to childhood asthma [39]. A contrasting study showed different evidence: increased risk of nocturnal asthma in Egyptian children was associated with the Gly/Gly genotype of the Arg16Gly polymorphism (OR = 3.2; 95% CI = 1.3–7.7; p-value = 0.03) [40]. In this Egyptian study, as in previous studies, the Gln27Glu polymorphism did not show evidence of association with asthma. In this study, the population analyzed should be considered an important environmental factor that interacts with the polymorphisms in the *ADRB2* gene.

Specific data can be reviewed for the polymorphism-associated responses to short- and long-acting β_2-agonists. For long-acting β_2-agonists, results have shown no positive association between the Arg16Gly polymorphism and bronchodilation, but the Arg16 allele was associated with poor asthma control [57]. Contrasting results were observed in a Chinese population study. In that study, a significantly higher bronchodilator response was observed in patients with the homozygous genotype 46A/A (13.40% ± 3.48%) compared with those patients with the homozygous genotype 46G/G (7.25% ± 3.11%) and the heterozygous genotype 46A/G (7.39% ± 3.14%) (p < 0.0001) [58]. To determine the effects of the polymorphisms on asthma response to bronchodilators, new studies should be performed that include different populations, higher sample numbers and a complete *ADRB2* gene polymorphism analysis. For the direct response to methacholine, no association was found [59].

Based on the data, no consensus has been reached on the relationship between the identified *ADRB2* genetic variations and asthma. The causal alleles that are common in most ethnic groups may have differential effects because of interactions with the environment and/or other genetic variants that are unique to certain ethnic groups. The interpretation of the findings of the genetic association studies of the *ADRB2* polymorphisms is complicated by the inadequate measurement of environmental exposures and differences in the allele and haplotype frequencies of the *ADRB2* gene and asthma severity among different racial groups. The complexity of the observed genotype-response effects limits their clinical applications [60]. In this context, our study has several strengths and limitations: our sample size may be considered small; there is no control for environmental factors;

only two polymorphisms were analyzed; the Brazilian population is admixed; and a region with a specific genotype combination associated with risk may also be associated with a peculiar environmental factor.

The contradictory findings in studies of literature, including the present manuscript, may be associated by: (i) difference in approach to clinical management between centers, (ii) criteria for diagnosis of asthma, (iii) enrolled population of patients (atopic and non-atopic), (iv) population analyzed considering ethnic differences that can alter the genotypic frequency of polymorphisms, (v) clinical variables considered as risk factor (IgE values changed, lung function test, time to diagnosis, evidence of reversibility on spirometry), (vi) presence of non-reported comorbidities, (vii) the characterization of patients taking into account the referral center, whereas non-random sampling for the clinical severity of asthma; (viii) technique for evaluation of polymorphisms in the *ADRB2* gene may have, on rare occasions, erroneous results.

In conclusion, our data show that the Gln27Glu and Arg16Gly polymorphisms of the beta 2-adrenergic receptor gene play an important role in asthma prevalence and severity and are a potential tool for risk analysis in our population. The results reveal the influence of each polymorphism alone and together as a haplotype.

Abbreviations
ADRB2: Beta-2-adrenergic receptor; cAMP: Cyclic adenosine monophosphate; CI: Confidence interval; OEGE: Online Encyclopedia for Genetic Epidemiology; SPSS: Statistical Package for the Social Sciences; Unicamp: State University of Campinas; β2AR: β2 receptors.

Competing interests
The authors declare that they have no competing interests.

Authors' contributions
CZP, FALM: made substantial contributions to conception and design, acquisition of data, and analysis and interpretation of data; involved in drafting the manuscript and revising it for critically important intellectual content. JDR, CSB: made substantial contributions to conception and design, acquisition of data, and analysis and interpretation of data; involved in drafting the manuscript and revising it for critically important intellectual content. In addition, they have given final approval for the publishing of this version. All authors read and approved the final manuscript.

Acknowledgments
Financing agency: CAPES – Coordination for Higher Level Graduate Improvement (PICDT Scholarship) and Fapesp – Fundação de Amparo à Pesquisa do Estado de São Paulo (#2011/18845-1).
Adyléia Dalbo Toro - Center for Investigation in Pediatrics, Pediatrics Department, University of Campinas, São Paulo, Brazil.
Genetic screening: http://www.laboratoriomultiusuario.com.br.

References
1. Global Initiative for Asthma (GINA): *A pocket guide for asthma management and prevention (for adults and children older than 5 years).* 2012. Available from: www.ginasthma.com.
2. Worldwide variation in prevalence of symptoms of asthma, allergic rhinoconjunctivities, and atopic eczema: ISACC: The International Study of

asthma and Allergies in Childhood (ISAAC) - Steering Committee. *Lancet* 1998, 351(111):125–132.

3. Anandan C, Nurmatov U, van Schayck OC, Sheikh A: **Is the prevalence of asthma declining? Systematic review of epidemiological studies.** *Allergy* 2010, 65(2):152–167.

4. Brasil. Ministério da Saúde. Secretaria nacional de Ações Básicas: *Estatísticas de Saúde e Mortalidade.* Brasília: Ministério da Saúde; 2005.

5. Hogg A: **Asthma in children.** *InnovAiT* 2011, 4(3):160–170.

6. Wedes SH, Khatri SB, Zhang R, Wu W, Comhair SA, Wenzel S, Teague WG, Israel E, Erzurum SC, Hazen SL: **Noninvasive markers of airway inflammation in asthma.** *Clin Transl Sci* 2009, 2(2):112–117.

7. Dodig S, Richter D, Zrinski-Topić R: **Inflammatory markers in childhood asthma.** *Clin Chem Lab Med* 2011, 49(4):587–599.

8. Kauffmann F, Castro-Giner F, Smit LAM, Nadif R, Kogevinas M: **Gene-environment interactions in occupational asthma.** In *Occupational Asthma.* Edited by Sigsgaard T, Heederik D. Basel: Birkhäuser; 2010:205–228.

9. Cookson WO, Moffatt MF: **Genetics of complex airway disease.** *Proc Am Thorac Soc* 2011, 8(2):149–153.

10. Barnes KC: **Genetic studies of the etiology of asthma.** *Proc Am Thorac Soc* 2011, 8(2):143–148.

11. Fireman P: **Understanding asthma pathophysiology.** *Allergy Asthma Proc* 2003, 24(2):79–83.

12. Thakkinstian A, McEvoy M, Minelli C, Gibson P, Hancox B, Duffy D, Thompson J, Hall I, Kaufman J, Leung TF, Helms PJ, Hakonarson H, Halpi E, Navon R, Attia J: **Systematic review and meta-analysis of the association between {beta}2-adrenoceptor polymorphisms and asthma: a HuGE review.** *Am J Epidemiol* 2006, 162(3):201–211.

13. NCBI: *National Center for Biotechnology Information.* www.ncbi.nlm.nih.gov/.

14. Hawkins GA, Weiss ST, Bleecker ER: **Clinical consequences of ADRbeta2 polymorphisms.** *Pharmacogenomics* 2008, 9(3):349–358.

15. Johnson M: **The beta-adrenoceptor.** *Am J Respir Crit Care Med* 1998, 158:S146–S153.

16. Hadcock JR, Malbon CC: **Down-regulation of beta-adrenergic receptors: agonist-induced reduction in receptor mRNA levels.** *Proc Natl Acad Sci USA* 1998, 85:5021–5025.

17. Nishikawa M, Mark JC, Barnes PJ: **Effect of short- a long-acting beta-2-adrenoceptor agonists on pulmonary beta-2-adrenoceptor expression in human lung.** *Eur J Pharmacol* 1996, 318:123–129.

18. Kobilka BK, Frielle T, Dohlman HG, Bolanowski MA, Dixon RA, Keller P, Caron MG, Lefkowitz RJ: **Delineation of the intronless nature of the genes for the human and hamster beta-2-adrenergic receptor and their putative promoter regions.** *J Biol Chem* 1987, 262:7321–7327.

19. Henderson R, Baldwin JM, Ceska TA, Zemlin F, Beckmann E, Downing KH: **Model for the structure of bacterorhodopsin based on high-resolution electron cyro-microscopy.** *J Mol Biol* 1990, 213:899–929.

20. Barnes PJ, Liew FY: **Nitric oxide and asthmatic inflammation.** *Immunol Today* 1995, 16(3):128–130.

21. Bhagat R, Kalra S, Swystun VA, Cockcroft DW: **Rapid onset of tolerance to the bronchoprotective effect of salmeterol.** *Chest* 1995, 108:1235–1239.

22. Cheung D, Timmers MC, Zwinderman AH, Bel EH, Dijkman JH, Sterk PJ: **Long terms effect of a long-actin beta-2-adrenoceptor agonist, salmeterol, on airway hiperresponsiveness in patients with mild asthma.** *N Engl J Med* 1992, 327:1198–1203.

23. Van Veen A, Weller FR, Wierenga EA, Jansen HM, Jonkers RE: **A comparison of salmeterol and formoterol in attenuating airway responses to short-acting beta-2-agonists.** *Pulm Pharmacol Ther* 2003, 16:153–161.

24. Yates DH, Kharitonov SA, Barne JP: **An inhaled glucocorticoid does not prevent tolerance to the bronchoprotective effect as a long-acting inhaled beta-2-agonist.** *Am J Respir Crit Care Med* 1996, 154:1603–1607.

25. Liggett SB, Raymond J: **Pharmacology and molecular biology of adrenergic receptors.** *Baillieres Clin Endocrinol Metab* 1993, 7(2):279–306.

26. Kume H, Hall IP, Washabau RJ, Takagi K, Kotlikoff MI: **Beta-adrenergic agonists regulate KCa channels in airway smooth muscle by cAMP dependent and independent mechanisms.** *J Clin Invest* 1994, 93:371–379.

27. Fenech A, Hall IP: **Pharmacogenetics of asthma.** *J Clin Pharmacol* 2002, 53:3–15.

28. Liggett, Stephen B: **Molecular and genetic basis of β -adrenergic receptor function and regulation.** *Asthma* 1997, 1:299–312.

29. Liggett SB: **Polymorphisms of the beta-2-adrenergic receptor and asthma.** *Am J Respir Crit Care Med* 1997, 156(4–2):S156–S162.

30. Tan S, Hall IP, Dewar J, Dow E, Lipworth B: **Association between beta-2-adrenoceptor polymorphism and susceptibility to bronchodilator desensitization in moderately severe stable asthmatics.** *Lancet* 1997, 350(9083):995–999.

31. Marson FA, Bertuzzo CS, Ribeiro AF, Ribeiro JD: **Polymorphisms in *ADRB2* gene can modulate the response to bronchodilators and the severity of cystic fibrosis.** *BMC Pulm Med* 2012, 12:50.

32. Dean AG, Sullivan KM, Soe MM: *OpenEpi. Open Source Epidemiologic Statistics for Public Health, Version 2.3.1.* www.openepi.com, updated 06/2011, accessed 04/2013.

33. Faul F, Erdfelder E, Buchner A, Lang AG: **Statistical power analyses using G*Power 3.1: tests for correlation and regression analyses.** *Behav Res Methods* 2009, 41:1149–1160.

34. Hahn LW, Ritchie MD, Moore JH: **Multifactor dimensionality reduction software for detecting gene-gene and gene-environment interactions.** *Bioinformatics* 2003, 19(3):376–382.

35. Ritchie MD, Hahn LW, Moore JH: **Power of multifactor dimensionality reduction for detecting gene-gene interactions in the presence of genotyping error, mising data, phenocopy, and genetic heterogeneity.** *Genet Epidemiol* 2003, 24(2):150–157.

36. Moore JH, Gilbert JC, Tsai CT, Chiang FT, Holden T, Barney N, White BC: **A flexible computational framework for detecting, characterizing, and interpreting statistical patterns of epistasis in genetic studies of human disease susceptibility.** *J Theor Biol* 2006, 241(2):252–261.

37. Chung LP, Waterer G, Thompson PJ: **Pharmacogenetics of β2 adrenergic receptor gene polymorphisms, long-acting β-agonists and asthma.** *Clin Exp Allergy* 2011, 41(3):312–326.

38. Birbian N, Singh J, Jindal SK, Singla N: **Association of β(2)-adrenergic receptor polymorphisms with asthma in a North Indian population.** *Lung* 2012, 190(5):497–504.

39. Zheng BQ, Wang GL, Yang S, Lu YQ, Liu RJ, Li Y: **Study of genetic susceptibility in 198 children with asthma.** *Zhongguo Dang Dai Er Ke Za Zhi* 2012, 14(11):811–814.

40. Karam RA, Sabbah NA, Zidan HE, Rahman HM: **Association between genetic polymorphisms of beta2 adrenergic receptors and nocturnal asthma in Egyptian children.** *J Investig Allergol Clin Immunol* 2013, 23(4):262–266.

41. Weir TD, Mallek N, Sandford AJ, Bai TR, Awadh N, Fitzgerald JM, Cockcroft D, James A, Liggett SB, Paré PD: **Beta 2-adrenergic receptor haplotypes in mild, moderate and fatal/near fatal asthma.** *Am J Respir Crit Care Med* 1998, 158(3):787–791.

42. Xie HG, Stein CM, Kim RB, Xiao ZS, He N, Zhou HH, Gainer JV, Brown NJ, Haines JL, Wood AJ: **Frequency of functionally important beta-2 adrenoceptor polymorphisms varies markedly among African-American, Caucasian and Chinese individuals.** *Pharmacogenetics* 1999, 9(4):511–516.

43. Moore PE, Laporte JD, Abraham JH, Schwartzman IN, Yandava CN, Silverman ES, Drazen JM, Wand MP, Panettieri RA Jr, Shore SA: **Polymorphism of the beta(2)-adrenergic receptor gene and desensitization in human airway smooth muscle.** *Am J Respir Crit Care Med* 2000, 162(6):2117–2124.

44. Green SA, Turki J, Bejarano P, Hall IP, Liggett SB: **Influence of β2-adrenergic receptor genotypes on signal transduction in human airway smooth muscle cells.** *Am J Respir Cell Mol Biol* 1995, 13(1):25–33.

45. Turki J, Pak J, Green SA, Martin RJ, Liggett SB: **Genetic polymorphisms of the beta-2-adrenergic receptor in nocturnal and nonnocturnal asthma. Evidence that Gly16 correlates with the nocturnal phenotype.** *J Clin Invest* 1995, 95(4):1635–1641.

46. Matheson MC, Ellis JA, Raven J, Johns DP, Walters EH, Abramson MJ: **Beta2-adrenergic receptor polymorphisms are associated with asthma and COPD in adults.** *J Hum Genet* 2006, 51(11):943–951.

47. Asano K, Yamada-Yamasawa W, Kudoh H, Matsuzaki T, Nakajima T, Hakuno H, Hiraoka R, Fukunaga K, Oguma T, Sayama K, Yamaguchi K, Nagabukuro A, Harada Y, Ishizaka A: **Association between beta-adrenoceptor gene polymorphisms and relative response to beta(2)-agonists and anticholinergic dr ugs in Japa-nese asthmatic patients.** *Respirology* 2010, 15(5):849–854.

48. Fu WP, Zhao ZH, Zhong L, Sun C, Fang LZ, Liu L, Zhang JQ, Wang L, Shu JK, Wang XM, Dai LM: **Relationship between polymorphisms in the 5′ leader cistron, positions 16 and 27 of the adrenergic β2 receptor gene and asthma in a Han population from southwest China.** *Respirology* 2011, 16(8):1221–1227.

49. Woszczek G, Borowiec M, Ptasinska A, Kosinski S, Pawliczak R, Kowalski ML: **Beta2-ADR haplotypes/polymorphisms associate with bronchodilator response and total IgE in grass allergy.** *Allergy* 2005, 60(11):1412–1417.

50. Migita O, Noguchi E, Jian Z, Shibasaki M, Migita T, Ichikawa K, Matsui A, Arinami T: *ADRB2* polymorphisms and asthma susceptibility: transmission disequilibrium test and meta-analysis. *Int Arch Allergy Immunol* 2004, **134**(2):150–157.

51. Lima JJ, Holbrook JT, Wang J, Sylvester JE, Blake KV, Blumenthal MN, Castro M, Hanania N, Wise R: The C523A beta2 adrenergic receptor polymorphism associates with markers of asthma severity in African Americans. *J Asthma* 2006, **43**(3):185–191.

52. Bhatnagar P, Gupta S, Guleria R, Kukreti R: Beta2-Adrenergic receptor polymorphisms and asthma in the Nor th Indian population. *Pharmacogenomics* 2005, **6**(7):713–719.

53. Yin KS, Zhang XL, Qiu YY: Association between b2-adrenergic receptor genetic polymorphisms and nocturnal asthmatic patients of Chinese Han nationality. *Respiration* 2006, **73**(4):464–467.

54. Hall IP, Blakey JD, Al Balushi KA, Wheatley A, Sayers I, Pembrey ME, Ring SM, McArdle WL, Strachan DP: Beta2-adrenoceptor polymorphisms and asthma from childhood to middle age in the British 1958 birth cohort: a genetic association study. *Lancet* 2006, **368**(9537):771–779.

55. Elbahlawan L, Binaei S, Christensen ML, Zhang Q, Quasney MW, Dahmer MK: Beta2-adrenergic receptor polymorphisms in African American children with status asthmaticus. *Pediatr Crit Care Med* 2006, **7**(1):15–18.

56. Drysdale CM, McGraw DW, Stack CB, Stephens JC, Judson RS, Nandabalan K, Arnold K, Ruano G, Liggett SB: Complex promoter and coding region beta 2-adrenergic receptor haplotypes alter receptor expression and predict in vivo responsiveness. *Proc Natl Acad Sci U S A* 2000, **97**:10483–10488.

57. Rebordosa C, Kogevinas M, Guerra S, Castro-Giner F, Jarvis D, Cazzoletti L, Pin I, Siroux V, Wjst M, Antò JM, de Marco R, Estivill X, Corsico AG, Nielsen R, Janson C: ADRB2 Gly16Arg polymorphism, asthma control and lung function decline. *Eur Respir J* 2011, **38**(5):1029–1035.

58. Qiu YY, Zhang XL, Qin Y, Yin KS, Zhang DP: Beta(2)-adrenergic receptor haplotype/polymorphisms and asthma susceptibility and clinical phenotype in a Chinese Han population. *Allergy Asthma Proc* 2010, **31**(5):91–97.

59. Manoharan A, Anderson WJ, Lipworth BJ: Influence of β(2)-adrenergic receptor polymorphism on methacholine hyperresponsiveness in asthmatic patients. *Ann Allergy Asthma Immunol* 2013, **110**(3):161–164.

60. Hizawa N: Beta-2 adrenergic receptor genetic polymorphisms and asthma. *J Clin Pharm Ther* 2009, **34**(6):631–643.

3

Electronic health record-based assessment of oral corticosteroid use in a population of primary care patients with asthma

Felicia C Allen-Ramey[1*], Linda M Nelsen[1], Joseph B Leader[2], Dione Mercer[2], Henry Lester Kirchner[3] and James B Jones[2]

Abstract

Background: Oral corticosteroid prescriptions are often used in clinical studies as an indicator of asthma exacerbations. However, there is rarely the ability to link a prescription to its associated diagnosis. The objective of this study was to characterize patterns of oral corticosteroid prescription orders for asthma patients using an electronic health record database, which links each prescription order to the diagnosis assigned at the time the order was placed.

Methods: This was a retrospective cohort study of the electronic health records of asthma patients enrolled in the Geisinger Health System from January 1, 2001 to August 23, 2010. Eligible patients were 12–85 years old, had a primary care physician in the Geisinger Health System, and had asthma. Each oral corticosteroid order was classified as being prescribed for an asthma-related or non-asthma-related condition based on the associated diagnosis. Asthma-related oral corticosteroid use was classified as either chronic or acute. In patient-level analyses, we determined the number of asthma patients with asthma-related and non-asthma-related prescription orders and the number of patients with acute versus chronic use. Prescription-level analyses ascertained the percentages of oral corticosteroid prescription orders that were for asthma-related and non-asthma-related conditions.

Results: Among the 21,199 asthma patients identified in the electronic health record database, 15,017 (70.8%) had an oral corticosteroid prescription order. Many patients (N = 6,827; 45.5%) had prescription orders for both asthma-related and non-asthma-related conditions, but some had prescription orders exclusively for asthma-related (N = 3,450; 23.0%) or non-asthma-related conditions (N = 4,740; 31.6%). Among the patients receiving a prescription order, most (87.5%) could be classified as acute users. A total of 60,355 oral corticosteroid prescription orders were placed for the asthma patients in this study—31,397 (52.0%) for non-asthma-related conditions, 24,487 (40.6%) for asthma-related conditions, and 4,471 (7.4%) for both asthma-related and non-asthma-related conditions.

Conclusions: Oral corticosteroid prescriptions for asthma patients are frequently ordered for conditions unrelated to asthma. A prescription for oral corticosteroids may be an unreliable marker of asthma exacerbations in retrospective studies utilizing administrative claims data. Investigators should consider co-morbid conditions for which oral corticosteroid use may also be indicated and/or different criteria for assessing oral corticosteroid use for asthma.

Keywords: Oral corticosteroids, Asthma, Anti-asthmatic agents, Retrospective studies, Therapeutic use, Managed care programs, Cross-sectional studies

* Correspondence: felicia_ramey@merck.com
[1]Merck & Co. Inc., West Point, PA 19486, USA
Full list of author information is available at the end of the article

Background

The prevention of exacerbations of asthma symptoms is recognized in treatment guidelines as a key component of controlling asthma [1]. An exacerbation is broadly defined as an acute worsening of asthma symptoms requiring a transient change in treatment. There is, however, neither a uniformly accepted definition of an exacerbation nor a consensus on how an exacerbation should be measured [2].

The American Thoracic Society and European Respiratory Society (ATS/ERS) recommended in an official statement that the definition of a severe asthma exacerbation should include the use of systemic corticosteroids [2]. However, this definition applies only in clinical trials [2], and subjects enrolled in major randomized clinical trials of asthma medications are not representative of asthma patients in the general population [3]. Asthma patients in the general population are often studied retrospectively by way of administrative data sets in which surrogate variables are used as a measure of exacerbations.

Observational studies of administrative data sets have used oral corticosteroid prescriptions, either alone or as part of a composite measure with asthma-related emergency department visits and inpatient stays, as a measure of asthma exacerbations [4-10]. The definitions of an exacerbation in these types of studies vary extensively. Finkelstein et al. used the "dispensing of an oral steroid preparation as a proxy for the occurrence of an acute exacerbation" [11]. Friedman defined an asthma exacerbation as an episode requiring "hospitalization, treatment in an emergency room, or an outpatient visit" where the patient "received nebulized medication or a prescription for oral corticosteroids" [12]. More recent studies have been more explicit in terms of days' supply of oral corticosteroid and the timing of a prescription relative to an outpatient visit [7,13,14]. However, the lack of a standardized definition of exacerbations limits the applicability of observational findings to clinical practice.

The NIH and the Agency for Healthcare Research and Quality have drafted recommendations for the standardization of asthma outcome measures for both clinical trials and observational studies [15]. The recommendations define an exacerbation as a "worsening of asthma requiring the use of systemic corticosteroids to prevent a serious outcome" [16]. For exacerbations in patients twelve years of age and older, the core outcome measures for observational studies are the use of systemic corticosteroids (oral, injected, or IV), hospitalization, and emergency department (or urgent care) visits for asthma [16].

One limitation of using oral corticosteroids as a measure of asthma exacerbations is that administrative claims data sets typically do not link a claim for a prescription to the diagnosis prompting the prescription, making it difficult to determine whether a given oral corticosteroid prescription was written for an asthma exacerbation or for a condition unrelated to the patient's asthma. Oral corticosteroids can be prescribed for variety of conditions unrelated to asthma, including systemic inflammatory diseases and pain syndromes. Integrated health care delivery systems that maintain electronic health records of all patient encounters contain the information needed to link a prescription order to the diagnosis assigned at the time the order was placed. Thus, with an electronic health record database, it is possible to determine whether an oral corticosteroid prescription was ordered for an asthma exacerbation or for some other reason.

The objective of this study was to use the electronic health records of an integrated health care delivery system to determine the medical diagnoses associated with oral corticosteroid prescriptions ordered for asthma patients, and thus to characterize the use of oral corticosteroid prescriptions as a measure of asthma exacerbations in a primary care setting.

Methods

Study design and setting

This study was a retrospective cohort analysis of oral corticosteroid use in a population of primary care asthma patients who are members of the Geisinger Health System, an integrated health care delivery system that serves residents in central and northeastern Pennsylvania. The Geisinger Health System includes the Geisinger Clinic, a network of 37 community-based offices staffed by primary care physicians. The Geisinger Clinic network provides primary care to over 400,000 patients. All network offices have used the EpicCare™ electronic health record (EHR) since 2001. The study period was January 1, 2001 to August 23, 2010.

Data sources

Geisinger's longitudinal EHR served as the data source for this study. The EHR includes a patient's "problem list", a dynamic and comprehensive list of all of a patient's medical problems. Each medical problem is entered into the EHR by a provider (e.g., nurse or physician) using a structured vocabulary, the terms of which are automatically linked to the International Classification of Disease (ICD-9) code. Similarly, all patient encounters (e.g., office visits) are assigned at least one diagnostic ICD-9 code by the provider. These provider-entered "encounter diagnosis codes" summarize the specific medical problems addressed during the encounter and are used also for billing purposes. Whereas the problem list is a comprehensive, current list of all of a patient's medical problems and can change over time as problems are resolved and/or new problems are identified, encounter diagnoses are encounter-specific—once assigned to an encounter, they do not change. The EHR includes the date that each problem is added to or removed from the problem list.

At all Geisinger Clinic offices, medication prescriptions must be ordered electronically via the EHR. Each order includes the following items: order date; medication name, dose, and class; prescribed quantity; allowed number of refills; and free-text instructions on dosing and administration (the medication "sig"). In addition, the provider is required to assign one or more diagnostic codes that summarize the conditions the medication is intended to treat. As with the problem list and encounter codes, the reason for the prescription order is entered using a structured vocabulary and mapped to an underlying ICD-9 code.

Patient sample

Potentially eligible patients were identified by searching Geisinger's EHR. The sampling frame included all patients aged 12 to 85 with a primary care provider at one of the Geisinger clinics and an indication of having asthma during the study period. Patients were classified as having asthma if they had any one of the following: ≥2 office visits within a 12-month period with an associated ICD-9 code of 493.xx, an active asthma diagnosis on their problem list during the study period, or a prescription order with an associated asthma diagnosis (493.xx).

Patients were excluded if they had ICD-9 codes for chronic obstructive pulmonary disease (491.xx, 492.xx), bronchiectasis (494.xx), chronic airway obstruction (not otherwise specified; 406.xx), cystic fibrosis (748.4), or bronchopulmonary dysplasia (770.7) on their problem list or in an encounter diagnosis. The study was approved with a waiver of patient consent by the Geisinger Health System institutional review board (Ref: 2010-0297).

Oral corticosteroid prescriptions analysis

After identifying all eligible asthma patients, we identified every oral corticosteroid prescription ordered for an asthma patient during the study period. Each order was classified on two dimensions: relation to asthma (yes or no) and pattern (acute or chronic). To determine whether an oral corticosteroid order was asthma-related, we relied on the diagnosis code assigned to the order by the provider. In collaboration with clinical experts, we classified ICD-9 codes 493.00 (extrinsic asthma, unspecified), 493.02 (extrinsic asthma with exacerbation), 493.90 (unspecified asthma), and 493.92 (unspecified asthma, with exacerbation) as asthma-related; all other codes were classified as non-asthma-related.

Whether the pattern of oral corticosteroid orders was acute or chronic was determined on the basis of the order information in the EHR (the details of which were described above). The definitions of acute and chronic use of oral corticosteroids were derived after investigator

review (FAR and LN) of a random sample of prescription orders. The initial definition was then applied to a subsequent sample of orders for validation. The final definition used for the analysis (described below) was endorsed through a third sample of orders reviewed alongside the proposed definition by a pulmonary physician with the Geisinger Health System. An acute order was defined as (1) an order with zero refills or (2) an order quantity <30. A chronic order was defined as an order quantity ≥30 with one or more refills. These resulting criteria were then applied to all oral corticosteroid orders for patients in the study population.

Data analysis

Because a single patient can have multiple prescription orders, separate descriptive analyses were conducted using, first, the patient, and second, the prescription order, as the unit of analysis. Patient-level analyses included: the number of patients with asthma, the number of asthma patients with asthma-related and non-asthma-related oral corticosteroid orders, and the number of asthma patients with patterns of oral corticosteroid orders consistent with acute versus chronic use. Prescription-level analyses included the total number of oral corticosteroid orders for asthma patients and the percentages of those orders written for asthma-related versus non-asthma-related conditions. Differences in acute and chronic order patterns along with diagnoses associated with OCS orders were examined for adolescents (ages 12–17 years), adults (18–44 and 45–64 years) and elderly patients (≥65 years).

Results

Characteristics of the asthma patient population

A total of 21,199 unique asthma patients were identified in the EHR database for the study period and met the study inclusion criteria (Figure 1; Table 1). The mean age was 39.5 years, and majorities of the patients were female (67.9%) and Caucasian (94.3%). The total average number of office visits per patient was 36.5, while the average number of asthma-related office visits was 8.3. Similarly, the average number of asthma-related emergency department visits and inpatient visits (1.6 and 1.5, respectively) was only a fraction of the total number of each type of visit (3.6 and 3.5, respectively). The most prevalent comorbidities, present in about half the study population, were acute sinusitis (58.6%), allergic rhinitis (56.1%), and acute bronchitis (48.8%).

Asthma patients with oral corticosteroid prescription orders

Of the 21,199 asthma patients, 15,017 (70.8%) had a prescription order for an oral corticosteroid. Among all patients with an oral corticosteroid prescription order,

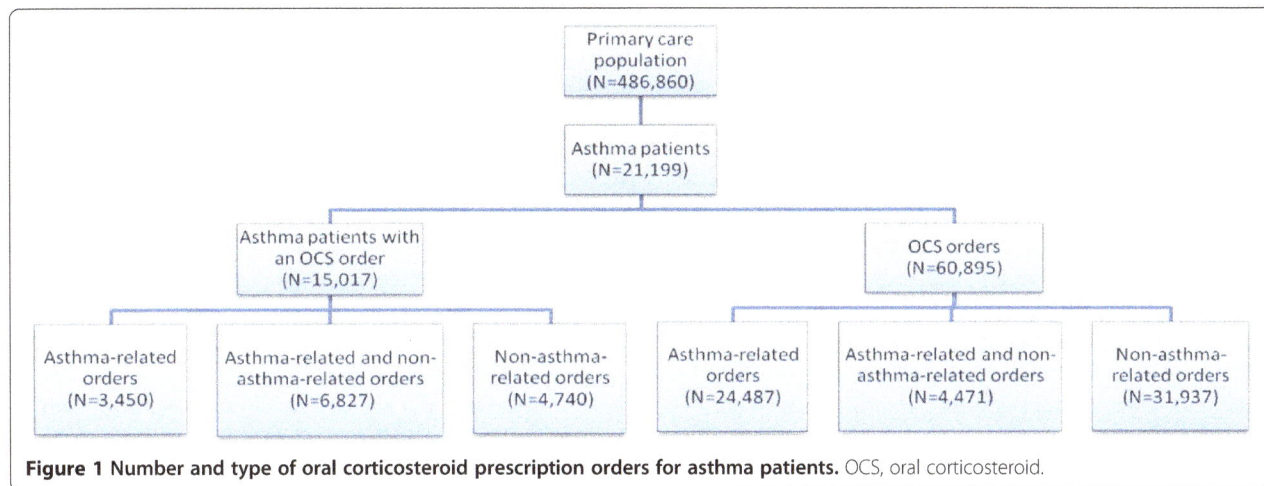

Figure 1 Number and type of oral corticosteroid prescription orders for asthma patients. OCS, oral corticosteroid.

3,450 (23.0%) had orders exclusively for an asthma-related condition, 4,740 (31.6%) had orders exclusively for a non-asthma-related condition, and 6,827 (45.5%) had orders for both asthma-related and non-asthma-related conditions. Most asthma patients (87.5%) were classified as acute users regardless of age (Table 2).

Oral corticosteroid prescription orders for asthma patients

A total of 60,355 oral corticosteroid prescription orders were placed for the asthma patients in this study— 24,487 (40.6%) for an asthma-related condition, 31,397 (52.0%) for non-asthma-related conditions, and 4,471 (7.4%) for both asthma-related and non-asthma-related

Table 1 Characteristics of the asthma patient population[a]

	Age 12–17		Age 18–64		Age ≥ 65		Total	
	N = 3,496		N = 15,352		N = 2,351		N = 21,199	
Age, years (mean, SD)	14.3	1.7	40.1	12.4	72.8	5.8	39.5	18.5
Female	1,879	54%	10,859	71%	1,650	70%	14,394	67.9%
Caucasian	3,181	91%	14,500	94%	2,304	98%	19,990	94.3%
Encounters, per patient (mean, SD)[b]								
Total office visits	27.6	23.1	36.6	31.7	48.6	35.4	36.5	31.4
Asthma-related office visits	6.3	5.4	8.5	8.0	10.3	9.8	8.3	7.9
Total ED visits	3.5	5.1	3.8	7.9	2.8	4.5	3.6	7.3
Asthma-related ED visits	1.7	1.1	1.5	1.4	1.4	1.1	1.6	1.6
Total inpatient visits	2.7	4.1	3.1	4.4	5.1	7.1	3.5	5.1
Asthma-related inpatient visits	1.5	1.3	1.5	1.4	1.4	1.1	1.5	1.4
Comorbidities								
Acute sinusitis	2,129	61%	9,353	61%	938	40%	12,420	58.6%
Allergic rhinitis	2,193	63%	8,733	57%	957	41%	11,883	56.1%
Acute bronchitis	1,167	33%	7,935	52%	1,248	53%	10,350	48.8%
Allergic rhinorrhea	1,719	49%	6,580	43%	666	28%	8,965	42.3%
Acute upper respiratory conditions	1,772	51%	5,700	37%	662	28%	8,134	38.4%
Gastroesophageal reflux disease	764	22%	6,159	40%	1,142	49%	8,065	38.0%
Chronic sinusitis	376	11%	2,458	16%	297	13%	3,131	14.8%
Chronic otitis media	755	22%	1,977	13%	131	6%	2,863	13.5%
Pneumonia	312	9%	1,523	10%	479	20%	2,314	10.9%
Current Smoker	515	15%	2,234	15%	52	2%	2,801	13.2%

ED emergency department, SD standard deviation.
[a]Data are presented as N (%) unless otherwise indicated.
[b]Office visits were calculated over the period 2001–2010, ED visits and inpatient visits were calculated over 2004–2010.

Table 2 Number of asthma patients with oral corticosteroid order patterns classified as acute or chronic

	Age 12–17 (N = 1,995)	Age 18–44 (N = 6,891)	Age 45–64 (N = 4,464)	Age ≥65 (N = 1,667)	Total (N = 15,017)
Acute	1,919 (96.2%)	6,249 (90.7%)	3,703 (83%)	1,263 (75.8%)	13,134 (87.5%)
Chronic	76 (3.8%)	642 (9.3%)	761 (17%)	404 (24.2%)	1,883 (12.5%)

conditions (Figure 1). Among patients with one or more prescriptions for oral corticosteroids, the median number (range) of oral corticosteroid prescription orders per patient was 2.0 (1–103) for asthma-related conditions and 2.0 (1–72) for conditions unrelated to asthma. The most common diagnoses associated with oral corticosteroid prescription orders among patients with asthma are listed in Table 3.

Discussion

In this population of primary care patients, over half (61.5%) of the oral corticosteroid prescriptions written for patients with asthma were prescribed for conditions unrelated to asthma (Table 3). This result suggests that, without an associated diagnosis, a prescription for an oral corticosteroid is not by itself an adequate marker for an asthma exacerbation in patients with asthma (but without other chronic respiratory diseases). This is consistent with evidence that a systemic corticosteroid prescription is poorly predictive of a diagnosis of asthma [17].

Oral corticosteroid use meets three of the four requirements for a core outcome measure in the NIH draft recommendations: it is clinically relevant, feasible,

and enables comparison across studies [15]. The fourth requirement, evidence of validity, requires further research. In particular, the factors that contribute to patient and clinician decisions to use oral corticosteroids need to be investigated [16]. This study is, to our knowledge, the first to report the frequency with which asthma patients receive oral corticosteroids for conditions unrelated to asthma.

Across all age groups in this sample, most asthma patients were acute users of oral corticosteroids. A minority (12.5% overall) were considered chronic users. However, frequent exacerbations are difficult to distinguish from poorly controlled persistent asthma. The chronic asthma-related use by some patients—the number of prescriptions ranged up to 103, i.e., 8 years of 30-day prescriptions—may represent poor control of persistent asthma due to inadequate use of long-term control medications (inhaled corticosteroids, etc.) rather than exacerbations. ('Chronic' use of systemic corticosteroids is an option to control severe asthma [1]). Thus, only the acute use (which was 87.5% of all use) can reliably be related to exacerbations.

The principal limitation of this analysis is uncertainty about the diagnosis associated with prescription orders.

Table 3 Diagnoses associated with oral corticosteroid orders for patients with asthma

Diagnosis category	Age 12-17 Count[a]	Age 12-17 Percent[b]	Age 18-44 Count[a]	Age 18-44 Percent[b]	Age 45-64 Count[a]	Age 45-64 Percent[b]	Age ≥65 Count[a]	Age ≥65 Percent[b]	Total Count[a]	Total Percent[b]
Asthma-related	3185	4.2%	13463	17.9%	9356	12.4%	2954	3.9%	28958	38.5%
Other[c]	661	0.9%	3987	5.3%	4251	5.6%	1509	2.0%	10408	13.8%
Other upper respiratory[d]	1008	1.3%	4522	6.0%	3130	4.2%	795	1.1%	9455	12.6%
Pain syndrome	316	0.4%	3505	4.7%	3196	4.2%	1100	1.5%	8117	10.8%
Missing	368	0.5%	2168	2.9%	1635	2.2%	867	1.2%	5038	6.7%
Allergic reaction	682	0.9%	2043	2.7%	1258	1.7%	364	0.5%	4347	5.8%
Systematic inflammatory	115	0.2%	1028	1.4%	1670	2.2%	1264	1.7%	4077	5.4%
Other lower respiratory	255	0.3%	775	1.0%	611	0.8%	271	0.4%	1912	2.5%
Other skin	177	0.2%	695	0.9%	453	0.6%	157	0.2%	1482	2.0%
Neoplasms	34	0.0%	194	0.3%	350	0.5%	220	0.3%	798	1.1%
Infection	18	0.0%	223	0.3%	277	0.4%	39	0.1%	557	0.7%
Unsure	11	0.0%	44	0.1%	34	0.0%	20	0.0%	109	0.1%
COPD	1	0.0%	6	0.0%	13	0.0%	14	0.0%	34	0.0%

[a]Column total does not equal the total number of distinct orders because each individual order can potentially have multiple diagnosis categories. Each diagnosis category represents a distinct count of orders.
[b]Percentages were calculated relative to the total number of prescription diagnoses (N = 75,292) associated with all OCS medication orders (N = 60,355) among asthma patients.
[c]Other includes included pain syndrome, endocrine, head and neck disorders, hematologic, infections and autoimmune conditions.
[d]Other upper respiratory includes rhinitis (allergic and chronic), chronic sinusitis, nasal polyps, tonsillitis and other conditions of the septum and larynx.

Physicians are required to enter a diagnosis code on each prescription order, but there is no quality check to ensure that the selected code is accurate. As a result, misclassification of asthma-related versus non-asthma-related prescription orders might occur. A small number (9.4%) of the oral corticosteroid orders in the EHR did not have an associated diagnosis, and these were categorized as being non-asthma-related in our analysis. Given the potential for orders classified as upper respiratory but not asthma-related to alter our results, we conducted a sensitivity analysis classifying bronchitis as an asthma-related condition. The resulting proportion of oral corticosteroid orders that were not asthma-related declined from 61.5% to 55.0%, which still supports our conclusions. In addition, the appearance of 'asthma' in a patient's problem list in an EHR has not been validated as a means of diagnosing asthma. Hence, it is possible that patients identified as having asthma solely on the basis of an entry in the patient's problem list did not actually have asthma. The validity of the use of health administrative databases to identify asthma patients, however, has been studied. In this study, patients were classified as having asthma if they had ≥2 office visits within a 12-month period with an associated ICD-9 code for asthma. Gershon et al. (2009) reported that a similar algorithm (≥2 ambulatory care visits and/or ≥1 hospitalization for asthma in a 2 year period) had a sensitivity and specificity of 83.8% and 76.5%, respectively, with expert chart review as the reference standard [18]. The positive predictive value was 61.5% (but 72.5% with the primary care physician chart diagnosis as reference standard) [18].

This analysis did not account for the chronology of the oral corticosteroid prescription with respect to exacerbations. Unless oral corticosteroid orders were recorded only *after* a diagnosis of asthma was entered into the EHR, it is possible that patients did not have asthma when the oral corticosteroid was prescribed. One way to improve this study design is to define the chronology of the prescription with respect to the asthma-related outpatient visit, as was done by Schatz et al., who noted that some oral corticosteroids may be prescribed prophylactically rather than for a current exacerbation [7]. Another way is to impose a limit on the time between an outpatient visit for asthma and a prescription order related to asthma (e.g., ≤5 days), as was done by Lee et al. [19]. A second level of stringency could include defining the days' supply of oral corticosteroid, as was done in two recent studies that defined exacerbations by oral corticosteroid prescriptions for <22 days' supply [13,14]. These approaches combined would ensure that the prescription was truly for an acute exacerbation and not the result of inadequate control of persistent asthma symptoms.

Conclusions

In this population of primary care patients, over half of the oral corticosteroid prescriptions for patients with asthma were for conditions unrelated to asthma. This finding has implications for how oral corticosteroid prescriptions should be interpreted in future observational research, particularly retrospective studies. In studies utilizing administrative claims data, a prescription for oral corticosteroids may be an unreliable marker of asthma exacerbations. Investigators should consider comorbid conditions for which oral corticosteroid use may also be indicated. The accuracy of an oral corticosteroid prescription as a marker of an exacerbation should be evaluated, and algorithms to identify oral corticosteroid prescriptions ordered for acute asthma episodes in administrative claims data should be developed and validated.

Abbreviations
ATS/ERS: American thoracic society and european respiratory society; EHR: Electronic health record; ICD: International classification of disease.

Competing interests
FAR and LN are employees of Merck & Co., Inc., which funded the study. JL, DM, HLK, and JBJ are employees of the Geisinger Clinic, whose electronic health record database was the source of the data for this study.

Authors' contributions
FAR and LN in conjunction with JBJ and HLK conceived of the study and participated in its design while DGM provided input and coordination. JL performed the statistical analysis. All authors participated in drafting the manuscript and have read and approved the final version.

Acknowledgments
Financial support for this work was provided by Merck & Co., Inc. Medical writing assistance was provided by SCRIBCO Pharmaceutical Writing. We thank Dr. Yasmine Wasfi, who provided background on clinical decisions related to prescribing of oral corticosteroids while employed by Merck & Co., Inc., and Drs. Paul Simonelli and Jonathan Darer of the Geisinger Clinic, both of whom assisted in the review of clinical diagnoses and prescription orders for oral corticosteroids in the Geisinger EHR.

Author details
[1]Merck & Co. Inc., West Point, PA 19486, USA. [2]Geisinger Clinic, Center for Health Research, Danville, PA 17822, USA. [3]Geisinger Clinic, Division of Medicine, Danville, PA 17822, USA.

References
1. National Asthma Education and Prevention Program Expert Panel: Guidelines for the diagnosis and management of asthma: full report. National heart, lung, and blood Institute. *J Allergy Clin Immunol.* 2007, 120(5 Suppl):S94–138.
2. Reddel HK, Taylor DR, Bateman ED, Boulet LP, Boushey HA, Busse WW, Casale TB, Chanez P, Enright PL, Gibson PG, *et al*: An official american thoracic society/european respiratory society statement: asthma control and exacerbations: standardizing endpoints for clinical asthma trials and clinical practice. *Am J Respir Crit Care Med* 2009, 180:59–99.
3. Travers J, Marsh S, Williams M, Weatherall M, Caldwell B, Shirtcliffe P, Aldington S, Beasley R: External validity of randomised controlled trials in asthma: to whom do the results of the trials apply? *Thorax* 2007, 62:219–223.

4.   Allen-Ramey FC, Duong PT, Riedel AA, Markson LE, Weiss KB: **Observational study of the effects of using montelukast vs fluticasone in patients matched at baseline.** *Ann Allergy Asthma Immunol* 2004, **93**:373–380.

5.   Schatz M, Nakahiro R, Jones CH, Roth RM, Joshua A, Petitti D: **Asthma population management: development and validation of a practical 3-level risk stratification scheme.** *Am J Manag Care* 2004, **10**:25–32.

6.   Bennett AV, Lozano P, Richardson LP, McCauley E, Katon WJ: **Identifying high-risk asthma with utilization data: a revised HEDIS definition.** *Am J Manag Care* 2008, **14**:450–456.

7.   Schatz M, Zeiger RS, Yang SJ, Chen W, Crawford WW, Sajjan SG, Allen-Ramey F: **Relationship of asthma control to asthma exacerbations using surrogate markers within a managed care database.** *Am J Manag Care* 2010, **16**:327–333.

8.   Sawicki GS, Vilk Y, Schatz M, Kleinman K, Abrams A, Madden J: **Uncontrolled asthma in a commercially insured population from 2002 to 2007: trends, predictors, and costs.** *J Asthma* 2010, **47**:574–580.

9.   Friedman HS, Navaratnam P, McLaughlin J: **Adherence and asthma control with mometasone furoate versus fluticasone propionate in adolescents and young adults with mild asthma.** *J Asthma* 2010, **47**:994–1000.

10. Fuhlbrigge A, Reed M, Stempel D, Ortega H, Fanning K, Stanford R: **The status of asthma control in the U.S. Adult population.** *Allergy Asthma Proc* 2009, **30**:529–533.

11. Finkelstein JA, Lozano P, Fuhlbrigge AL, Carey VJ, Inui TS, Soumerai SB, Sullivan SD, Wagner EH, Weiss ST, Weiss KB: **Practice-level effects of interventions to improve asthma care in primary care settings: the pediatric asthma care patient outcomes research team.** *Health Serv Res* 2005, **40**:1737–1757.

12. Friedman HS, Yawn BP: **Resource utilization in asthma: combined fluticasone propionate/salmeterol compared with inhaled corticosteroids.** *Curr Med Res Opin* 2007, **23**:427–434.

13. Stephenson JJ, Quimbo RA, Gutierrez B: **Subacute lack of asthma control as a predictor of subsequent acute asthma exacerbation in a managed care population.** *Am J Manag Care* 2010, **16**:108–114.

14. O'Connor RD, Bleecker ER, Long A, Tashkin D, Peters S, Klingman D, Gutierrez B: **Subacute lack of asthma control and acute asthma exacerbation history as predictors of subsequent acute asthma exacerbations: evidence from managed care data.** *J Asthma* 2010, **47**:422–428.

15. Busse WW, Morgan WJ, Taggart V, Togias A: **Asthma outcomes workshop: overview.** *J Allergy Clin Immunol* 2012, **129**:S1–S8.

16. Fuhlbrigge A, Peden D, Apter AJ, Boushey HA, Camargo CA Jr, Gern J, Heymann PW, Martinez FD, Mauger D, Teague WG, Blaisdell C: **Asthma outcomes: exacerbations.** *J Allergy Clin Immunol* 2012, **129**:S34–S48.

17. Himmel W, Hummers-Pradier E, Schumann H, Kochen MM: **The predictive value of asthma medications to identify individuals with asthma–a study in German general practices.** *Br J Gen Pract* 2001, **51**:879–883.

18. Gershon AS, Wang C, Guan J, Vasilevska-Ristovska J, Cicutto L, To T: **Identifying patients with physician-diagnosed asthma in health administrative databases.** *Can Respir J* 2009, **16**:183–188.

19. Lee TA, Chang CL, Stephenson JJ, Sajjan SG, Maiese EM, Everett S, Allen-Ramey F: **Impact of asthma controller medications on medical and economic resource utilization in adult asthma patients.** *Curr Med Res Opin* 2010, **26**:2851–2860.

4

Exploring the impact of elevated depressive symptoms on the ability of a tailored asthma intervention to improve medication adherence among urban adolescents with asthma

Lokesh Guglani[1*], Suzanne L Havstad[2], Dennis R Ownby[3], Jacquelyn Saltzgaber[2], Dayna A Johnson[2], Christine C Johnson[2] and Christine LM Joseph[2]

Abstract

Background: In patients with asthma, medication adherence is a voluntary behavior that can be affected by numerous factors. Depression is an important co-morbidity in adolescents with asthma that may significantly impact their controller medication adherence and other asthma-related outcomes. The modifying effect of depressive symptoms on an asthma intervention's ability to improve asthma controller medication adherence among urban adolescents with asthma has not yet been reported.

Objective: To assess self-reported symptoms of depression as an effect modifier of the relationship between randomization group and controller medication adherence at 6-month follow-up.

Methods: These analyses use data from a randomized controlled trial (RCT) conducted in Detroit high schools to evaluate a tailored asthma management program. The intervention included referrals to school or community resources for students reporting symptoms of depression and other issues. "Elevated depressive symptoms" was defined as a positive answer to ≥ 5 of 7 questions from a validated tool included on the baseline questionnaire. Self-reported adherence to controller medication was collected at intervention onset (session 1) and at 6-month follow up. Analyses were restricted to students with report of a controller medication at baseline. Logistic regression was used to assess elevated depressive symptoms as an effect modifier of the relationship between randomization group and 6-month adherence.

Results: Of the 422 students enrolled in the RCT, a controller medication was reported at intervention onset by n = 123 adolescents (29%). Analyzing this group, we observed an interaction between elevated depressive symptoms and adherence (p = 0.073). Stratified analysis showed better adherence in treatment group adolescents meeting criteria for elevated depressive symptoms at baseline as compared to the control group (adjusted Odds Ratio [aOR] = 9.50; p = 0.024). For adolescents without elevated depressive symptoms at baseline, differences in adherence by group assignment did not reach statistical significance (aOR 1.40, p = 0.49).

(Continued on next page)

* Correspondence: lguglani@med.wayne.edu
[1]Pediatric Pulmonary Division, Department of Pediatrics, Children's Hospital of Michigan, Wayne State University School of Medicine, 3901 Beaubien St, Detroit, MI 48201, USA
Full list of author information is available at the end of the article

(Continued from previous page)

Conclusions: In this sample of students reporting controller medications at baseline, report of elevated depressive symptoms at baseline and randomization to the intervention group was associated with significantly better adherence at 6-month follow up when compared to that of a control group. Larger studies are needed to evaluate the impact of depression on the relationship between adherence and asthma intervention effectiveness.

Keywords: Asthma, Depression, Medication adherence, Randomized controlled trial, Self-management, Adolescents, Urban

Background

There is a significantly higher prevalence of asthma in urban African American and Latino adolescents and these groups are known to have worse asthma-related outcomes than their White counterparts [1]. Asthma control is impacted by a number of factors, including adherence to prescribed regimens. Adherence, as per its definition, is an "active, voluntary and collaborative involvement of the patient in a mutually acceptable course of behavior to produce a therapeutic result". Adherence is influenced by a number of internal and external factors including patient beliefs and attitudes, disease and therapy-related factors, health system characteristics, and socioeconomic factors [2]. According to the literature, urban adolescents with asthma in general have poor adherence to asthma controller medications [3]. Studies using electronic monitoring of controller medication adherence in adolescents [4,5] have shown 40-50% adherence, with significantly lower rates of adherence in African American adolescents [6].

Depression is a known co-morbidity of asthma; however, few studies provide estimates of depression as co-morbidity in adolescents with asthma. Existing reports suggest the prevalence of depression among adolescents with asthma ranges from 7.2 to 16.3% [7-9]. Depression may impact quality of life in adolescents with asthma. In a previous analysis of Puff City data, we have shown that depressive symptoms significantly impact emotional quality of life [10]. Depression has been associated with medication adherence in adults and in diseases other than asthma [11-13], but the impact of depression on asthma intervention effectiveness with regard to controller medication adherence has not been explored in urban adolescents.

The present analyses explore the impact of elevated depressive symptoms at baseline on the ability of an asthma intervention to improve adherence to controller medications at 6-month follow-up, among urban teens with asthma. The intervention upon which these analyses are based is Puff City, a computer-tailored, web-based program for urban teens with asthma, originally developed and tested in 2001 [14]. An enhanced version was evaluated in Detroit high schools using a randomized controlled trial conducted from 2007–2011 [15]. The subgroup analyses reported here include urban teenagers that were enrolled in the 2007 – 2011 RCT of Puff City, and reported controller medication(s) at intervention onset.

Methods

The details of the Puff City randomized controlled trial have been published previously [14-16]. Briefly, to identify students with asthma or asthma symptoms, caregivers of all 9th through 12th grade students of six Detroit public high schools were notified by mail of a Lung Health Questionnaire (LHQ) to be administered during an English class. Parents could opt out of having their child complete the LHQ by signing and returning the letter to the school or by contacting the school. Eligibility to participate in the RCT was based on LHQ responses. To be eligible, the students had to have a physician diagnosis of asthma accompanied by one or more of the following: presence of daytime and/or nighttime symptoms in the last 30 days, medication use for asthma symptoms in the last 30 days, and ≥ 1 refill(s) of beta-agonists in the last 1 year. Adolescents without a physician diagnosis of asthma were also eligible to participate if they had positive responses to items selected from the International Study of Asthma and Allergies in Childhood (ISAAC) [17], and had symptom frequencies similar to those used in EPR 2 and 3 (e.g., for "mild persistent asthma" criteria from EPR3 include "symptoms ≥ 2 days/week, nighttime awakening $\geq$ 3-4x/month, and interference with normal activities = minor limitation") [18,19]. Students identified as eligible for the RCT based on the above criteria were mailed an invitation to participate in the RCT, along with forms for parental written consent and student written assent. Once consent and assent were obtained, a study ID was assigned and entered into the study database. In this way, no student data was shared with investigators until appropriate informed consent was obtained [15]. After a baseline assessment, consenting students were randomized into a treatment or control group (Figure 1). The treatment group underwent a total of 4 computer-based tailored online asthma management sessions that featured topics such as asthma management behaviors (including asthma medication use and adherence, having a rescue inhaler nearby, and smoking cessation and/or reduction), trigger avoidance

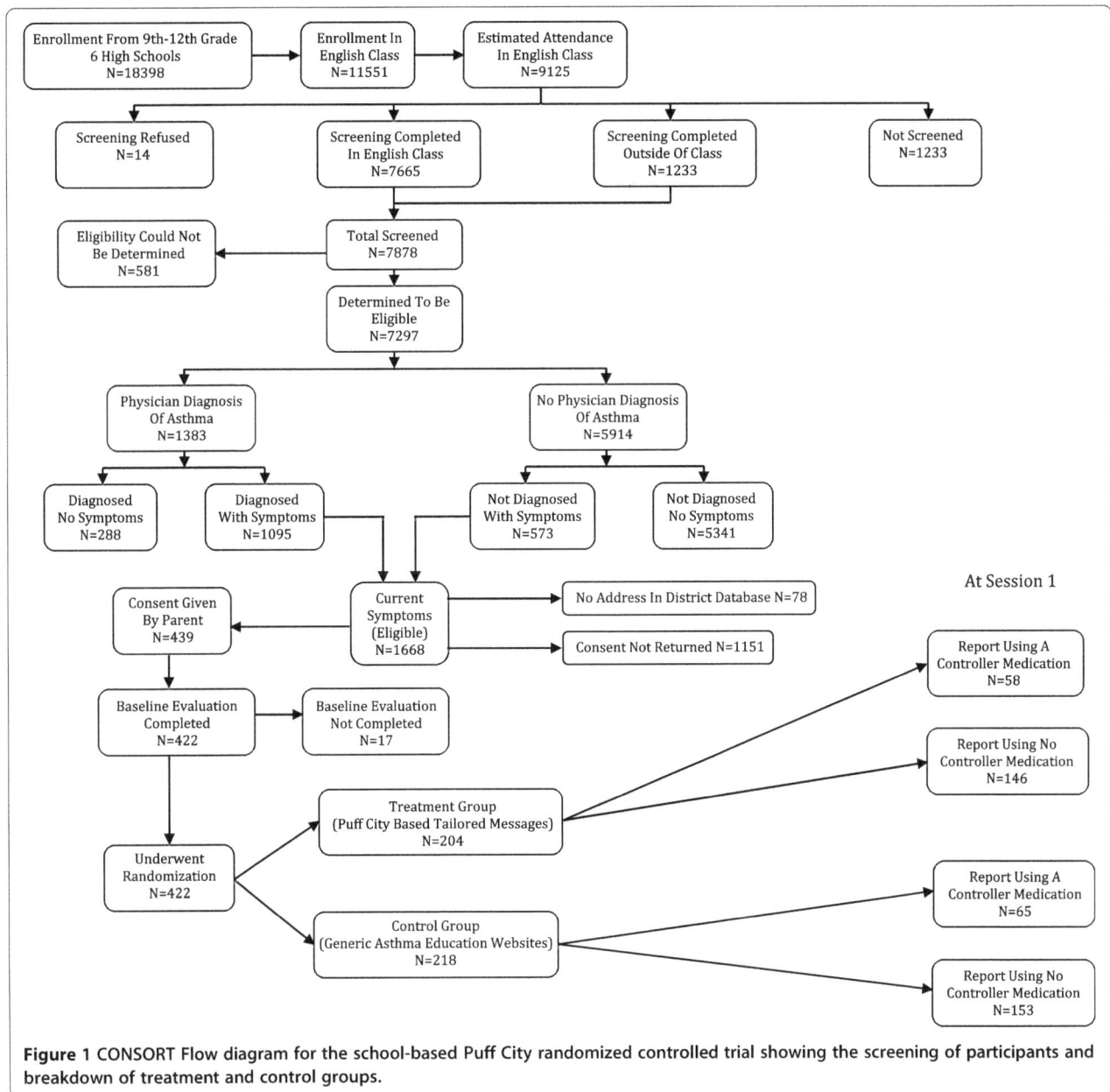

Figure 1 CONSORT Flow diagram for the school-based Puff City randomized controlled trial showing the screening of participants and breakdown of treatment and control groups.

and basic asthma physiology. The control group was provided access to existing, generic asthma education websites during 4 computer sessions of duration similar to that of the treatment group. Asthma controller medications that were prescribed by a physician were requested from both treatment and control group students at the onset of intervention session 1 using a medication selection module designed for this purpose. The module displayed pictures of medications listed in the Health plan Employer Data and Information Set (HEDIS) measure for asthma called Use of Appropriate Medications for People with Asthma [20], and included corticosteroids, inhaled steroid combinations, leukotriene receptor antagonists, mast cell stabilizers, and

antibody inhibitors. Participants were asked to select the asthma medications they were currently taking, if any. All medications reported by the participant were categorized as "controller" or "rescue".

A referral coordinator was also part of the intervention. The referral coordinator's task was to assess, refer, and follow-up with students in the intervention group identified to be at-risk of a serious event through a risk assessment report generated by the data management system [16]. Students were contacted if they reported sharing asthma medication, severe asthma symptoms, lack of physician or health insurance, and/or depressive symptoms. Treatment group students with depressive symptoms were usually referred to school-based resources (e.g., school counselor, school social worker, or school-based clinic); and to community-based resources when school resources were not available.

As part of the study protocol, participants received mail and telephone reminders to login to the program and complete a follow-up survey scheduled for 6-months post-baseline. Survey questions collected information on asthma outcomes (e.g., symptom-days, symptom-nights, days of restricted activity), as well as information on controller medication adherence. Follow-up questions were the same for treatment and control group students, although treatment group students could receive additional "booster" messages based on responses to the 6-month survey questions. This study was approved by the Institutional Review Boards of the participating institutions (IRB Protocol #4579) and by the Detroit Public Schools Office of Research, Evaluation and Assessment.

Study definitions
Depressive symptoms were reported at baseline using 7 questions from the Diagnostic Predictive Scale (DPS) that enquires about symptoms typically associated with depression in the preceding 6-months [21]. The DPS is a result of adaptations to the Diagnostic Interview Schedule for Children (DISC), which is a structured diagnostic instrument specifically designed for use by non-clinicians [22]. The fourth version (DISC-IV) was further adapted to create several shorter scales (including the Diagnostic Predictive Scale used in this study) for use as screening tools for various psychiatric diagnoses, including depression [21]. The DPS has been tested in various populations and has been reported to be an efficient and reliable screening tool [23,24] for children between the ages of 8 to 18 years. Using published cutoff scores established by Lucas et al. [21], elevated depressive symptoms was defined as a positive response to 5 or more questions on the DPS. Adherence to asthma controller medication was defined as self-reported use of the medication on 5 or more days out of last 7 days. Controller medication adherence collected at the 6-month follow-up was the primary outcome of these analyses.

Statistical analysis
Since the goal of these analyses was to assess the effect of depression on the ability of the intervention to improve

controller medication adherence, analyses were restricted to the group of adolescents reporting asthma controller medications at baseline. Logistic regression was used to assess elevated depressive symptoms as an effect modifier of the relationship between randomization group and controller medication adherence at 6-months using the p value of <0.10 as indicating the presence of effect modification and the need to present stratum-specific results [25]. Baseline controller medication adherence was included as a covariate in all logistic regression models. Adjusted odds ratios (aOR) and corresponding 95% confidence intervals were calculated to describe the association between randomization group and controller medication adherence at 6-months.

Results
The breakdown of the study population is shown in Figure 1. Baseline assessment was completed by 422 adolescents. A total of 58 adolescents in the treatment group (28.4%) and 65 in the control group (29.8%) reported a controller medication at the start of the intervention (Table 1). Among those reporting use of a controller medication at intervention onset, the percentage of adolescents in the treatment and control groups meeting criteria for elevated depressive symptoms was 20.7% (n = 12) and 24.6% (n = 16), respectively, p = 0.60. Controller medication adherence for treatment and control group students at intervention onset was 24.1% (n = 14) and 27.7% (n = 18) respectively.

At the 6-month follow up, after adjusting for baseline adherence, 22 adolescents in the treatment group (37.9%) reported controller medication adherence, as compared to 17 adolescents in the control group (26.2%) (Table 2). The relationship between elevated depressive symptoms at baseline and controller medication adherence met criterion for the presence of an interaction (p = 0.073) [16,25]. Stratified analysis is presented in Table 3. For adolescents that reported elevated depressive symptoms at baseline, 7/12 (58.3%) in the treatment group reported being adherent to their controller medication at the 6-month follow-up, while 2/16 (12.5%) were adherent in the control group, aOR = 9.5; p = 0.024. For adolescents that did not report depressive symptoms at baseline, medication adherence at 6-month follow-up was only slightly higher among students randomized to the treatment

Table 1 Prevalence of elevated depressive symptoms and controller medication adherence at intervention onset (Session 1) for teens in the treatment and control groups

	Treatment N = 58		Control N = 65		Odds ratio (95% CI)	p value
% of teens with elevated depressive symptoms at baseline (n)	20.7	(12)	24.6	(16)	0.80 (0.34, 1.87)	0.60
Core behavior and report of medication at session 1						
Controller medication, adherent ≥ 5 of last 7 days	24.1	(14)	27.7	(18)	0.83 (0.37, 1.87)	0.65
Controller medication, not adherent < 5 of last 7 days	75.9	(44)	72.3	(47)		

Table 2 Comparison of controller medication adherence at 6 month follow-up for by randomization group for students included in the analysis sample*

	Treatment N = 58		Control N = 65		Adjusted** odds ratio (95% CI)	p value
Core behavior at 6 months*						
Controller medication, adherent ≥ 5 of last 7 days	37.9	(22)	26.2	(17)	2.10 (0.89, 4.92)	0.089
Controller medication, not adherent < 5 of last 7 days	62.1	(36)	73.8	(48)		

*Students enrolled in Puff City and reporting a controller medication at baseline assessment. **Adjusted for controller medication adherence at start of intervention.*

group (32.6%) compared to the controls (30.6%) at the 6-month follow up, aOR = 1.4; p = 0.49.

Discussion

The Puff City program uses tailoring to promote positive behaviors such as regular use of controller medications by providing personalized health messages to help address the adolescents' beliefs, attitudes and barriers to behavior change in addition to referrals from an asthma referral coordinator. Results of these subgroup analyses suggest that the effectiveness of a program to improve adherence to controller medications in urban adolescents with asthma may be significantly impacted by the presence of depressive symptoms. For this reason, it may be worthwhile to address depressive symptoms when treating asthma in order to improve asthma-related outcomes. We did note a modicum of improvement in medication adherence among treatment group students who did not meet criteria for elevated depression at baseline, but a comparison to the control group did not reach statistical significance. Therefore, interventions to improve controller medication adherence in adolescents with and without depressive symptoms may still be needed. Our results may have important implications for designing future interventions specifically targeting improvements in controller medication adherence in urban adolescents with asthma.

Other investigators have also found depression to be a significant determinant of medication adherence in several disorders other than asthma. A recent meta-analysis of 31 studies (18,425 participants) of adults with various chronic conditions reported a 1.76 times greater odds

for non-adherence in depressed patients [26]. Another report suggests that approximately 20 to 30 percent of prescriptions are never filled (primary non-adherence) and 50% of medications prescribed for chronic diseases are not taken as prescribed [2]. Medication non-adherence is associated with higher downstream health care costs [27], and can be reduced by improved self-management of chronic disorders such as asthma. We are unaware of any other study that has reported the effectiveness of asthma interventions on controller medication adherence among adolescents with depressive symptoms.

Other co-morbidities have been observed in asthma. Besides depressive symptoms, adolescents with asthma have also been found to have a higher prevalence of anxiety disorder [28] and internalizing behaviors [29]. These are linked through several psychological and biological factors such as the stress of asthma management, medication regimens, and avoidance of allergic triggers; or through cognitive responses to asthma symptoms such as learned helplessness or fear of bodily sensations. In the case of adolescents, having asthma symptoms may induce social anxiety (due to concern for negative evaluation by peers) that can significantly impact asthma-related outcomes [30].

The overall rate of controller medication use in this study was low (29% at baseline) resulting in a small sample available for analyses. There are additional limitations to this study. First, we used self-reported measures of asthma controller medication adherence, which can have questionable validity and reliability [31,32]. We note that self-report of asthma controller medication adherence

Table 3 Comparison of controller medication adherence at 6 month follow-up by randomization group and by baseline elevated depressive symptoms, for students included in the analysis sample*

	Treatment		Control		Adjusted** odds ratio (95% CI)	p value
Meet criteria for elevated depressive symptoms at baseline:						
Core behavior at 6 months*						
Controller medication, adherent ≥ 5 of last 7 days	58.3	(7)	12.5	(2)	9.50 (1.35, 67.0)	0.024
Controller medication, not adherent < 5 of last 7 days	41.7	(5)	87.5	(14)		
Do not meet criteria for elevated depressive symptoms at baseline:						
Core behavior at 6 months*						
Controller medication, adherent ≥ 5 of last 7 days	32.6	(15)	30.6	(15)	1.40 (0.53, 3.67)	0.49
Controller medication, not adherent < 5 of last 7 days	67.4	(31)	69.4	(34)		

*Students enrolled in Puff City and reporting a controller medication at baseline assessment. **Adjusted for controller medication adherence at start of intervention.*

has been used in national surveys such as National Health and Nutrition Examination Survey (NHANES) [33], and National Asthma Survey (NAS) [34]. Second, we cannot determine which component of the intervention was instrumental in motivating participants to be more adherent, i.e., depressed students received tailored messages about controller medication through the online program in addition to referrals made by the asthma referral coordinator for their depressive symptoms. Moreover, we cannot confirm that students followed up on referrals from the asthma referral coordinator and cannot report on the therapies or advice these students may or may not have received from these referrals. Consequently, we cannot speculate on the *mechanism* by which controller medication adherence was improved among students reporting depressive symptoms at baseline. Third, a sustained intervention effect for controller medication adherence post 6-month follow-up is unknown. Finally, because this study was done in urban adolescents with asthma, the results may only be applicable to other populations with characteristics similar to that of our study population. Given the limitations of this study, additional analyses in larger study samples are needed.

Conclusions

In these subgroup analyses of data from a RCT to evaluate an online asthma management program for urban adolescents with asthma, students who were randomized to the treatment group and met criteria for elevated depressive symptoms had better controller medication adherence when compared to a control group at 6-month follow up. Adolescents without depressive symptoms at baseline did not show statistically significant improvement in controller medication adherence. Interventions aimed at improving controller medication adherence as part of asthma self-management programs may need to be tailored for adolescents with depressive symptoms.

Abbreviations

DPS: Diagnostic predictive scales; DISC: Diagnostic Interview Schedule for Children; aOR: adjusted odds ratio; ISAAC: International Study of Asthma and Allergies in Childhood; RCT: Randomized controlled trial; NHANES: National Health And Nutrition Examination Survey; NAS: National Asthma Survey; EPR: Expert panel report; HEDIS: Health plan Employer Data and Information Set; LHQ: Lung health questionnaire.

Competing interests

There is no personal or financial support or author involvement with organization(s) with financial interest in the subject matter.

Authors' contributions

LG participated in discussion of analysis approach, results and interpretation, and prepared the manuscript. SLH conducted statistical analysis, discussed results and interpretation of analysis; reviewed manuscript. CCJ, is a co-investigator with input on study design and implementation, reviewed manuscript. DRO is a co-investigator with input on study design and implementation; reviewed manuscript. CLMJ is the Principal Investigator, participated in discussion of analysis approach and interpretation of results, assisted in preparation of

manuscript and manuscript review. All the authors have read and approved the final manuscript.

Research support funding

This research was funded by the National Institutes of Health, National Heart, Lung, and Blood Institute. [Grant # R01 HL67462-01].

Author details

[1]Pediatric Pulmonary Division, Department of Pediatrics, Children's Hospital of Michigan, Wayne State University School of Medicine, 3901 Beaubien St, Detroit, MI 48201, USA. [2]Department of Public Health Sciences, Henry Ford Health System, Detroit, MI, USA. [3]Clinical Allergy and Immunology, Georgia Health Sciences University, Augusta, GA, USA.

References

1. Akinbami LJ MJ, Bailey C, Zahran HS, King M, Johnson CA, Liu X: **Trends in asthma prevalence, health care use, and mortality in the United States, 2001–2010.** In *NCHS Data Brief, vol. 94.* Hyattsville, MD: National Center for Health Statistics; 2012.
2. Sabate E: *(Ed): Adherence to long-term therapies: evidence for action.* Switzerland: World Health Organization; 2003.
3. Milgrom H, Bender B, Ackerson L, Bowry P, Smith B, Rand C: **Noncompliance and treatment failure in children with asthma.** *J Allergy Clin Immunol* 1996, **98:**1051–1057.
4. Bender B, Zhang L: **Negative affect, medication adherence, and asthma control in children.** *J Allergy Clin Immunol* 2008, **122:**490–495.
5. Naimi DR, Freedman TG, Ginsburg KR, Bogen D, Rand CS, Apter AJ: **Adolescents and asthma: why bother with our meds?** *J Allergy Clin Immunol* 2009, **123:**1335–1341.
6. Desai M, Oppenheimer JJ: **Medication adherence in the asthmatic child and adolescent.** *Curr Allergy Asthma Rep* 2011, **11:**454–464.
7. Katon W, Lozano P, Russo J, McCauley E, Richardson L, Bush T: **The prevalence of DSM-IV anxiety and depressive disorders in youth with asthma compared with controls.** *J Adolesc Health* 2007, **41:**455–463.
8. Ortega AN, McQuaid EL, Canino G, Goodwin RD, Fritz GK: **Comorbidity of asthma and anxiety and depression in Puerto Rican children.** *Psychosomatics* 2004, **45:**93–99.
9. Goodwin RD, Fergusson DM, Horwood LJ: **Asthma and depressive and anxiety disorders among young persons in the community.** *Psychol Med* 2004, **34:**1465–1474.
10. Guglani L, Havstad SL, Johnson CC, Ownby DR, Joseph CL: **Effect of depressive symptoms on asthma intervention in urban teens.** *Ann Allergy Asthma Immunol* 2012, **109:**237–242. e232.
11. Dempe C, Junger J, Hoppe S, Katzenberger ML, Moltner A, Ladwig KH, Herzog W, Schultz JH: **Association of anxious and depressive symptoms with medication nonadherence in patients with stable coronary artery disease.** *J Psychosom Res* 2013, **74:**122–127.
12. Sjosten N, Nabi H, Westerlund H, Salo P, Oksanen T, Pentti J, Virtanen M, Kivimaki M, Vahtera J: **Effect of depression onset on adherence to medication among hypertensive patients: a longitudinal modelling study.** *J Hypertens* 2013, **31:**1477–1484.
13. Tang HY, Sayers SL, Weissinger G, Riegel B: **The role of depression in medication adherence among heart failure patients.** *Clin Nurs Res* 2013. Epub ahead of print: April 2, 2013, doi: 10.1177/1054773813481801.
14. Joseph CL, Peterson E, Havstad S, Johnson CC, Hoerauf S, Stringer S, Gibson-Scipio W, Ownby DR, Elston-Lafata J, Pallonen U, et al: **A web-based, tailored asthma management program for urban African-American high school students.** *Am J Respir Crit Care Med* 2007, **175:**888–895.
15. Joseph CL, Ownby DR, Havstad SL, Saltzgaber J, Considine S, Johnson D, Peterson E, Alexander G, Lu M, Gibson-Scipio W, et al: **Evaluation of a web-based asthma management intervention program for urban teenagers: reaching the hard to reach.** *J Adolesc Health* 2013, **52:**419–426.
16. Joseph CL, Baptist AP, Stringer S, Havstad S, Ownby DR, Johnson CC, Williams LK, Peterson EL: **Identifying students with self-report of asthma and respiratory symptoms in an urban, high school setting.** *J Urban Health* 2007, **84:**60–69.

17. Weiland SK, Bjorksten B, Brunekreef B, Cookson WO, von Mutius E, Strachan DP: Phase II of the international study of asthma and allergies in childhood (ISAAC II): rationale and methods. *Eur Respir J* 2004, **24:**406–412.

18. NIH: *Expert Panel Report 2: Guidelines for the Diagnosis and Management of Asthma.* Bethesda: National Institutes of Health; 1997. NIH Publication No. 97–4051: NHLBI.

19. National Institutes of Health: *Expert Panel Report 3: Guidelines for the Diagnosis and Management of Asthma.* Washington DC: National Institute of Health; 2007. NHLBI ed., vol. NIH Publication No. 07–4051.

20. National Committee for Quality Assurance: *Use of Appropriate Medications for People with Asthma: HEDIS 2002, Technical Specifications, Volume 2.* Washington, DC: National Committee for Quality Assurance; 2001.

21. Lucas CP, Zhang H, Fisher PW, Shaffer D, Regier DA, Narrow WE, Bourdon K, Dulcan MK, Canino G, Rubio-Stipec M, *et al:* The DISC Predictive Scales (DPS): efficiently screening for diagnoses. *J Am Acad Child Adolesc Psychiatry* 2001, **40:**443–449.

22. Shaffer D, Fisher P, Lucas CP, Dulcan MK, Schwab-Stone ME: NIMH diagnostic interview schedule for children version IV (NIMH DISC-IV): description, differences from previous versions, and reliability of some common diagnoses. *J Am Acad Child Adolesc Psychiatry* 2000, **39:**28–38.

23. Cubo E, Velasco SS, Benito VD, Villaverde VA, Galin JM, Santidrian AM, Vicente JM, Guevara JC, Louis ED, Leon JB: Psychometric attributes of the DISC predictive scales. *Clin Pract Epidemiol Ment Health* 2010, **6:**86–93.

24. Leung PW, Lucas CP, Hung SF, Kwong SL, Tang CP, Lee CC, Ho TP, Lieh-Mak F, Shaffer D: The test-retest reliability and screening efficiency of DISC predictive scales-version 4.32 (DPS-4.32) With chinese children/youths. *Eur Child Adolesc Psychiatry* 2005, **14:**461–465.

25. Hosmer DW, Lemeshow S: *Applied Logistic Regression.* 2nd edition. New York: John Wiley and Sons; 2000.

26. Grenard JL, Munjas BA, Adams JL, Suttorp M, Maglione M, McGlynn EA, Gellad WF: Depression and medication adherence in the treatment of chronic diseases in the United States: a meta-analysis. *J Gen Intern Med* 2011, **26:**1175–1182.

27. Bender BG, Rand C: Medication non-adherence and asthma treatment cost. *Curr Opin Allergy Clin Immunol* 2004, **4:**191–195.

28. Goodwin RD: Asthma and anxiety disorders. *Adv Psychosom Med* 2003, **24:**51–71.

29. Feldman JM, Ortega AN, McQuaid EL, Canino G: Comorbidity between asthma attacks and internalizing disorders among Puerto Rican children at one-year follow-up. *Psychosomatics* 2006, **47:**333–339.

30. Bruzzese JM, Fisher PH, Lemp N, Warner CM: Asthma and social anxiety in adolescents. *J Pediatr* 2009, **155:**398–403.

31. Jerant A, DiMatteo R, Arnsten J, Moore-Hill M, Franks P: Self-report adherence measures in chronic illness: retest reliability and predictive validity. *Med Care* 2008, **46:**1134–1139.

32. Garfield S, Clifford S, Eliasson L, Barber N, Willson A: Suitability of measures of self-reported medication adherence for routine clinical use: a systematic review. *BMC Med Res Methodol* 2011, **11:**149.

33. Kit BK, Simon AE, Ogden CL, Akinbami LJ: Trends in preventive asthma medication use among children and adolescents, 1988–2008. *Pediatrics* 2012, **129:**62–69.

34. Crocker D, Brown C, Moolenaar R, Moorman J, Bailey C, Mannino D, Holguin F: Racial and ethnic disparities in asthma medication usage and health-care utilization: data from the national asthma survey. *Chest* 2009, **136:**1063–1071.

5

Reduction in oral corticosteroid use in patients receiving omalizumab for allergic asthma in the real-world setting

Gert-Jan Braunstahl[1*], Jan Chlumský[2], Guy Peachey[3] and Chien-Wei Chen[4]

Abstract

Background: Oral corticosteroids (OCS) are commonly administered in patients with severe persistent allergic asthma. Despite their efficacy, they are associated with a wide variety of adverse events. The eXpeRience registry was set up to investigate real-world outcomes among patients receiving omalizumab for the treatment of uncontrolled allergic asthma. Here, we present the effect of omalizumab treatment on OCS use.

Methods: eXpeRience was a 2-year, multinational, non-interventional, observational registry of patients receiving omalizumab for uncontrolled allergic asthma. OCS use (proportion of patients on maintenance OCS, mean total daily OCS dose and change in status of OCS therapy) was assessed at baseline, 16 weeks, and 8, 12, 18, and 24 months after the initiation of omalizumab. Response to omalizumab was assessed using the physician's Global Evaluation of Treatment Effectiveness (GETE) at approximately Week 16. Safety data were also recorded.

Results: A total of 943 patients (mean age, 45 years; female, 64.9%) were enrolled in the registry, 263 of whom were receiving maintenance OCS at baseline. The proportion of patients taking maintenance OCS was markedly lower at Months 12 (16.1%) and 24 (14.2%) than at baseline (28.6%; intent-to-treat population). GETE status was determined in 915 patients receiving omalizumab: 64.2% were responders (excellent or good response), 30.7% were non-responders (moderate, poor or worsening response); 5.1% had no assessment. The frequency of serious adverse events was comparable to that seen in controlled trials of omalizumab.

Conclusions: Omalizumab use is associated with an OCS-sparing effect in patients with uncontrolled persistent allergic asthma in the real-world setting.

Keywords: Anti-immunoglobulin E, Oral corticosteroid use, Omalizumab, Registry, Uncontrolled persistent allergic asthma

Background

Patients with allergic asthma are often inadequately controlled despite treatment with high-dose inhaled corticosteroids (ICS) and long-acting β_2-agonists (LABA) [1,2]. Oral corticosteroids (OCS) are commonly administered to suppress airway inflammation and improve asthma control in these patients; however, their long-term use is associated with significant adverse effects, such as diabetes, osteoporosis and cataract formation, placing a major burden on patients and healthcare resources [3-6].

Interventions that allow OCS treatment to be reduced or withdrawn completely are likely to benefit patients receiving these agents for the treatment of asthma.

Omalizumab, a humanized anti-immunoglobulin E (IgE) monoclonal antibody, is approved for the treatment of patients with uncontrolled moderate-to-severe (US) or severe (EU) persistent allergic (IgE-mediated) asthma [7,8]. Omalizumab has been shown to reduce asthma exacerbations and hospital visits, as well as corticosteroid use, in patients with allergic asthma [9-11]. Omalizumab has also been shown to have a direct OCS-sparing effect in a 32-week randomized, open-label study in adolescents and adults (12–75 years) with severe asthma [12], as well as in

* Correspondence: g.braunstahl@sfg.nl
[1]Department of Pulmonary Medicine, Sint Franciscus Gasthuis, Kleiweg 500, 3045 PM, Rotterdam, The Netherlands
Full list of author information is available at the end of the article

a 16-week uncontrolled therapeutic trial in children (median age 12 years) [13].

eXpeRience was an international registry initiated to evaluate outcomes in patients receiving omalizumab for uncontrolled persistent allergic asthma in 'real-world' clinical practice. The primary results, published previously [14,15], showed that omalizumab was associated with improvements in clinical outcomes such as asthma exacerbations and objective measures of asthma control. Here, we evaluate the real-world effect of omalizumab treatment on the use of OCS over a 2-year period.

Methods

eXpeRience was a multinational, non-interventional, observational registry established to collect data on the real-world effectiveness and safety of omalizumab therapy during routine clinical practice in patients with uncontrolled persistent allergic (IgE-mediated) asthma. The registry design has been published previously [15].

Briefly, the registry included male and female patients with uncontrolled persistent allergic asthma who had commenced omalizumab treatment within the previous 15 weeks. Patients from 14 countries in Europe, America and Asia were enrolled, and were followed for up to 2 years after initiation of omalizumab. After entry into the registry, data were collected prospectively at approximately 16 weeks and at 8, 12, 18 and 24 months after initiation of omalizumab treatment, with a minimum requirement of two data collections per year.

Treatment and follow-up of patients was at the discretion of the treating physician, according to local medical practice and label/reimbursement guidelines. The registry design and amendments were reviewed by independent ethics committees or institutional review boards at each participating centre, as required.

Registry assessments

Data on OCS use were collected at each pre-determined time-point. The variables evaluated included: proportion of patients receiving OCS as maintenance therapy; total daily OCS dose; change from baseline in OCS dose; number of patients in whom OCS therapy was stopped, reduced (without stopping), or increased as compared with baseline; time to reduction in OCS dose or stopping OCS therapy. Data on ICS use were also collected at each time-point, including: total daily ICS dose; change from baseline in ICS dose; number of patients in whom ICS therapy was stopped, reduced (without stopping), or increased as compared with baseline.

Response to omalizumab was assessed using the physician's Global Evaluation of Treatment Effectiveness (GETE) at approximately Week 16 after the initiation of treatment. OCS use among omalizumab responders (i.e. those with an "excellent" or "good" response by GETE) and

non-responders (i.e. "moderate" or "poor" response, or "worsening" asthma) was evaluated. OCS doses were converted to prednisolone equivalents (1 mg prednisone = 1 mg prednisolone; 1 mg methylprednisolone = 1.25 mg prednisolone).

Safety was assessed by recording the nature and frequency of serious adverse events (SAEs) that occurred during the registry, which were followed until resolution.

Statistical analysis

All efficacy analyses reported are based on the intent-to-treat (ITT) population, consisting of all randomized patients who had at least one post-baseline efficacy assessment. All safety analyses are based on the safety population, which included all patients who received at least one dose of omalizumab and had at least one post-baseline safety assessment.

Statistical analyses were mainly descriptive. Summary statistics describing change from baseline in OCS dose, reduction or cessation of OCS treatment, and time to reduction were calculated for all patients receiving maintenance OCS therapy at baseline, and for GETE-defined responders and non-responders.

Results

Patient disposition and baseline characteristics

A total of 943 patients were included in the eXpeRience registry. Of these patients, 694 (73.6%) completed the registry and 157 (16.6%) discontinued; status was unknown for 92 (9.8%). The most common reasons for discontinuation were loss to follow-up (n = 52; 5.5%) and withdrawal of consent (n = 27; 2.9%) [14]. Demographic and clinical characteristics of the patients receiving OCS at baseline were comparable with the overall population (Table 1; [14]). The ITT population included 916 patients and the safety population included 925 patients. Of the 263 patients receiving OCS at baseline, the ITT population included 246 patients and the safety population included 263 patients.

OCS use

The most commonly used OCS was prednisone (n = 131 at baseline; 49.8% of all patients receiving OCS). The proportion of patients receiving OCS was lower at Months 12 (16.1%) and 24 (14.2%) than at baseline (28.6%) (Figure 1). The mean total daily OCS dose (prednisolone equivalent) decreased between baseline (15.5 mg) and Month 12 (7.7 mg), and continued to decrease between Months 12 and 24 (5.8 mg) (Figure 2).

Among patients receiving OCS at baseline, there was a reduction in or discontinuation of OCS treatment in 57.1% and 69.0% of patients at Months 12 and 24, respectively (Figure 3). The mean (SD) time to reduction or discontinuation of OCS was 198.5 (114.29) days and 291.2 (210.86)

Table 1 Baseline demographics and clinical characteristics of patients in the eXpeRience registry (safety population)

Variable	Patients on OCS at baseline (n = 263)	Overall population (n = 925)
Mean age, years (SD)	46.0 (13.3)	45.0 (15.0)
Female, n (%)	169 (64.3)	600 (64.9)
Race, n (%)		
Caucasian	246 (93.5)	855 (92.4)
Others	17 (6.5)	70 (7.6)
Mean duration of allergic asthma, years (**SD**)	20.3 (13.6) [n = 261]	19.4 (13.6)
Positive skin-prick test/RAST for perennial aeroallergens, n (%)	232 (88.2)	816 (88.2)[†]
History of seasonal allergy, n (%)	177 (67.3)	587 (63.5)[†]
Smoking history, n (%)		
Never smoked	202 (76.8)	719 (77.7)[‡]
Ex-smoker	52 (19.8)	173 (18.7)
Current smoker	9 (3.4)	30 (3.2)
Asthma clinical symptoms, n (%)		
Daytime asthma symptoms	245 (93.2)	838 (90.6)
Limitations of activities	239 (90.9)	795 (85.9)
Nocturnal symptoms/awakenings	218 (82.9)	737 (79.7)
Asthma control (investigator assessment), n (%)		
Controlled	3 (1.1)	13 (1.4)[†]
Partly controlled	42 (16.0)	215 (23.2)
Uncontrolled	218 (82.9)	693 (74.9)

[†]Data missing for one patient; [‡]Data missing for three patients.
RAST, radioallergosorbent test; SD, standard deviation.

days, assessed at Months 12 and 24, respectively. Five patients (2.6%) at Month 12 and four patients (2.4%) at Month 24 had an increase in OCS dose.

OCS use according to response

Of the 915 patients assessed using the GETE, 64.2% were responders (excellent, 11.4%; good, 52.8%) and 30.7% were non-responders (moderate, 23.4%; poor, 6.8%; worsening of asthma, 0.5%) based on GETE status; 5.1% had no assessment. Following the GETE assessment, the vast majority of responders (98.1%) and 'moderate' non-responders (96.3%) continued with treatment.

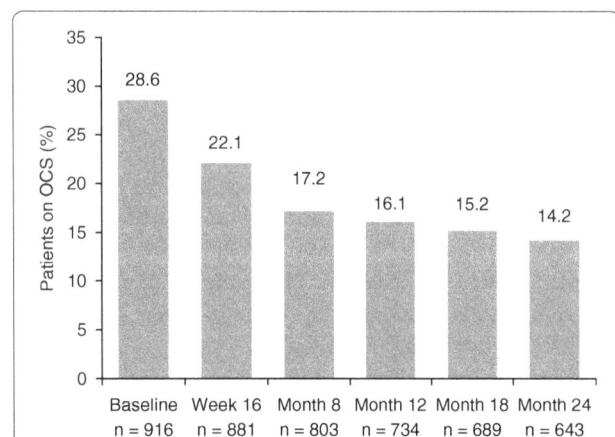

Figure 1 Proportion of patients on maintenance OCS. n = Number of evaluable patients at each time point. OCS, oral corticosteroids.

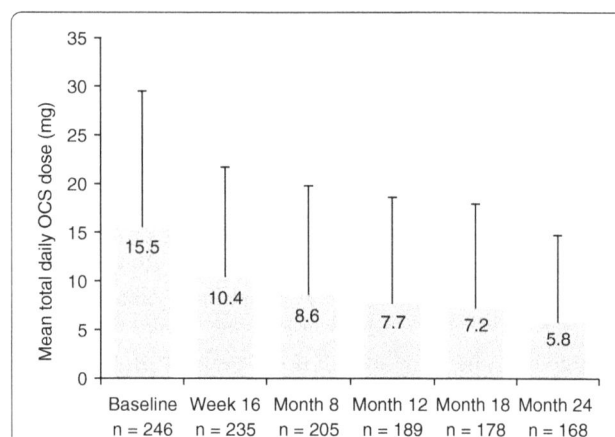

Figure 2 Mean total daily OCS dose (prednisolone equivalent) (ITT population). n = number of evaluable patients at each time-point. OCS, oral corticosteroids; SD, standard deviation; ITT, intent-to-treat. Error bars represent SD. Post-baseline data include doses of zero for patients no longer receiving OCS.

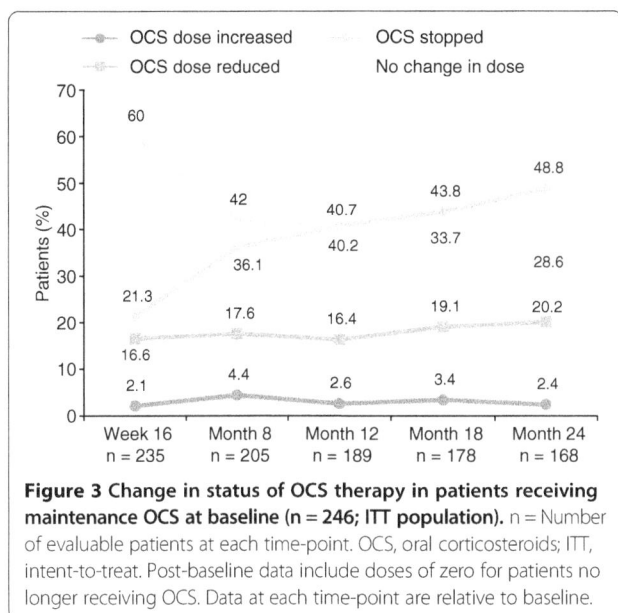

Figure 3 Change in status of OCS therapy in patients receiving maintenance OCS at baseline (n = 246; ITT population). n = Number of evaluable patients at each time-point. OCS, oral corticosteroids; ITT, intent-to-treat. Post-baseline data include doses of zero for patients no longer receiving OCS. Data at each time-point are relative to baseline.

Among responders, the proportion of patients on maintenance OCS treatment decreased from 28.1% at baseline to 13.8% at Month 12 and 12.1% at Month 24. Mean (SD) total daily dose (prednisolone equivalent) decreased from 15.5 (14.63) mg at baseline to 6.5 (10.13) mg at Month 12, and 5.1 (8.94) mg at Month 24.

Among GETE non-responders, the proportion of patients on maintenance OCS treatment decreased from 28.5% at baseline to 20.9% at Month 12 and 17.9% at Month 24. Mean (SD) total daily dose (prednisolone equivalent) decreased from 14.7 (10.92) mg at baseline to 11.3 (12.85) mg at Month 12, and 8.1 (8.99) mg at Month 24.

ICS use

At baseline, 895 of 916 patients (98%) were receiving ICS maintenance therapy. Among patients who provided ICS information, 173 of 705 (24.5%) and 182 of 613 (29.7%) had stopped or reduced ICS use at Months 12 and 24, respectively. The majority of patients did not change their ICS dose (495 [70.2%] at Month 12 and 389 [63.5%] at Month 24), while 37 patients (5.2%) and 42 patients (6.9%) had an increase in dose at Months 12 and 24, respectively. Mean (SD) total daily ICS doses (beclomethasone equivalent) decreased from 1675 (947) µg at baseline to 1461 (950) at Month 12 and 1381 (961) at Month 24. Mean (SD) percentage reductions in ICS dose from baseline were 9.6% (49.8) at Month 12 and 11.8% (57.1) at Month 24.

ICS use according to response

Among GETE responders, the mean (SD) ICS dose decreased from baseline by 266 (759) µg at Month 12 and

313 (819) µg at Month 24, with mean (SD) percentage reductions of 12.9 (41.8) and 14.8 (47.4), respectively. Among the responders, 133 of 487 (27.3%) and 137 of 435 (31.5%) had stopped or reduced ICS use at Months 12 and 24, respectively.

Among GETE non-responders, the mean (SD) ICS dose decreased from baseline by 134 (847) µg at Month 12 and 246 (1122) µg at Month 24, with mean (SD) percentage reductions of 2.8 (65.9) and 4.8 (77.9), respectively. Among the non-responders, 40 of 200 (20.0%) and 44 of 164 (26.8%) had stopped or reduced ICS use at Months 12 and 24, respectively.

Safety

Detailed safety findings from the registry have been published previously [14]. Briefly, a total of 64 patients (6.9%) reported 150 SAEs. Of these, 25 SAEs (16.7%) were suspected to be related to omalizumab. The most common SAE was asthma (n = 32, 3.5%), followed by dyspnoea and pneumonia (both n = 7, 0.8%). Nine deaths occurred during the registry; none were suspected to be related to omalizumab (causes of death have been described previously [14]).

Discussion

In this registry, omalizumab was associated with a reduction in maintenance OCS use in patients with uncontrolled persistent allergic asthma over a 2-year treatment period in a real-world setting. Approximately half of the patients on maintenance OCS at baseline were able to stop or reduce their OCS dose. In addition, there were also reductions in maintenance ICS use over the 2 years of the study. We believe that the observed reductions in OCS and ICS use reflect improved asthma control during treatment with omalizumab, and are likely to be associated with a reduction in the risk of steroid-related adverse effects. Reductions in OCS use and mean total daily OCS dose were greater in patients classified as responders to omalizumab treatment than in non-responders. Nevertheless, a reduction in OCS use and mean total daily OCS dose was seen in non-responders, possibly due to the fact that the definition of non-responders included patients with a moderate response to omalizumab (as well as those with a poor or worsening response). This is highlighted by the vast majority of moderate 'non-responders' continuing with treatment, following the GETE assessment.

Corticosteroids are widely prescribed to treat inflammatory conditions, including asthma, for which they are often the mainstay of treatment [5]. Patients with uncontrolled severe asthma may require long-term maintenance therapy with OCS. However, such use is associated with serious long-term adverse effects such as hypothalamic-pituitary-adrenal axis suppression, impaired glucose tolerance and diabetes, osteoporosis, hypertension, and cataract formation. There is therefore a need for therapies that improve outcomes, have acceptable safety and tolerability profiles, while allowing reductions in OCS use [12].

Despite the observed reductions in OCS use, patients enrolled in the eXpeRience registry had fewer clinically significant asthma exacerbations after 12 or 24 months' treatment with omalizumab (annualized mean 1.0 and 0.6, respectively) compared with pre-treatment values (annualized mean 4.9) [14]. Relatedly, omalizumab was also associated with reductions in healthcare utilization (hospitalizations, emergency room visits and unscheduled doctor visits), from 6.2 during the 12-month pre-treatment period to 1.0 per year at Month 12 and 0.5 per year at Month 24 [14]. Annualized numbers of days of absence from work and school due to asthma were also lower at Month 12 (3.5 and 1.6 days, respectively) and Month 24 (1.0 and 1.9 days, respectively) than during the 12-month pre-treatment period (26.4 and 20.7 days, respectively) [14].

Our findings are in agreement with those of other real-life studies of omalizumab. A pooled analysis of data from French and German patients (n = 346) with severe persistent allergic asthma showed that omalizumab treatment for at least 16 weeks was associated with a reduction or discontinuation of OCS in 50% of patients receiving OCS at baseline (n = 84/166) [16]. The mean reduction in daily OCS dose from baseline was 74.3% [16]. An additional French historic-prospective study showed that 48.1% of patients reduced or discontinued maintenance OCS over a period of ≥5 months of omalizumab treatment [17].

Decreased use of OCS subsequent to treatment with omalizumab has also been shown in observational studies conducted in Italy [18], Belgium [19], Israel [20] and the United Kingdom [21]. These studies enrolled between 22 and 142 patients, who were followed up for between 16 and 52 weeks. Between 20% and 70% of patients taking OCS at baseline were able to stop or reduce treatment, and showed meaningful reductions in exacerbations rates.

The results of this analysis indicate that a significant proportion of patients on omalizumab therapy were classed as responders by physician's GETE at Week 16. These results are consistent with omalizumab clinical trials. In an early randomized controlled study, 53% of omalizumab-treated patients had an excellent/good response to omalizumab, compared with 33% for placebo [22]; in a more recent study, 72.8% in the omalizumab plus optimized asthma therapy (OAT) group responded, compared to 31.2% for OAT alone [23]. However, not all responses to omalizumab are achieved within the first 16 weeks of therapy, with some patients taking longer to respond [23].

Bousquet et al. demonstrated that the physician's GETE at Week 16 is an effective predictor of longer-term outcomes, including exacerbation rates, overall asthma control and unscheduled medical interventions [24]. Subsequently, Bousquet et al. also showed that the majority of patients classified as responders or non-responders at Week 16 have the same classification at Week 32 [23]. Consistent with the findings of Bousquet et al. [23,24], the present study also indicated that asthma control (as reflected in OCS use) is improved to a greater extent among responders to omalizumab, compared with non-responders, and that these improvements (and the differences between responders and non-responders) persist between Week 16 and 2 years.

Most of the observational studies conducted with omalizumab support a reduction in maintenance OCS dose to improve asthma management. However, in rare cases, patients receiving omalizumab may present with systemic hypereosinophilic syndrome or allergic eosinophilic granulomatous vasculitis (Churg-Strauss syndrome) [25], and these events are usually, but not always, associated with a reduction in OCS dose. We did not observe any cases of either hypereosinophilic syndrome or Churg-Strauss syndrome in the eXpeRience registry, but we believe that clinicians attempting OCS reduction or withdrawal in patients with allergic asthma should be aware of this.

Despite our positive findings, it is important to recognize the limitations of observational studies, namely the lack of a control group and the open-label design.

Conclusions

In conclusion, this 2-year, international and observational registry, conducted in a real-life setting, confirms that omalizumab is associated with OCS-sparing effects in patients with uncontrolled persistent allergic (IgE-mediated) asthma.

Abbreviations

OCS: Oral corticosteroids; GETE: Global Evaluation of Treatment Effectiveness; ICS: Inhaled corticosteroids; LABA: Long-acting β_2-agonists; IgE: Immunoglobulin E; SAEs: Serious adverse events; ITT: Intent-to-treat; OAT: Optimized asthma therapy.

Competing interests

G-JB has received grant/research support for consultations and/or speaking at conferences from Novartis, GSK, AstraZeneca, and MSD. JC has received lecture fees from Novartis, and has been an investigator in studies sponsored by several other pharmaceutical companies. C-WC and GP are Novartis employees.

Authors' contributions

G-JB has contributed to the enrolment of patients, data capture and processing and has reviewed and commented various drafts of the manuscript. JC has contributed to enrolment of patients and has reviewed and commented various drafts of the manuscript. GP is a clinical lead accountable for the conduct and reporting of the registry; oversight of all operational aspects of the registry (e.g. patient enrolment; document management, etc.); scientific review of registry data, and lead author of the clinical study reports (interim and final). C-WC has contributed to data analysis. All authors read and approved the final manuscript.

Acknowledgements
The registry was sponsored by Novartis Pharma AG. The authors were assisted in the preparation of the manuscript by Dr. Madhavi Dokku (Novartis). Writing support was funded by the registry sponsor.

List of Independent Ethics Committees or Institutional Review Boards
• Argentina, Buenos Aires: Comite Independiente De Etics Para Ensayos En Farmacologia Clinica• Bulgaria, Sofia: Ethics Committee for Multicenter Trials• Canada, Alberta: University of Calgary Conjoint Health Research Ethics Board• Canada, British Columbia: University of British Columbia, Office of Research Ethics• Canada, Nova Scotia: Capital Health Research Ethics Board; University Health Network• Canada, Ontario: IRB Services• Canada, Québec: Centre de Recherche du CHUM; Comité d'éthique du Centre de santé et de services sociauc du Nord de Lansudière; Research Ethics Board Montreal Children's Hospital; Centre de santé et de services sociaux de Laval, Cité de la Santé de Laval• Cyprus, Nicosia: Cyprus National Bioethics Committee• Czech Republic, Prague: Ethics Committee of the AIFP• Hungary, Budapest: Egészségügyi Tudományos Tanács Tudományos és Kutatásetikai Bizottság• Netherlands: N/A (EC approval not required in Netherlands)• Philippines, Manila: Our Lady of Lourdes Hospital Ethics and Review Committee • Portugal, Almada: Comissão de ética do Hospital Garcia de Orta• Portugal, Amadora: Comissão de ética do Hospital Fernando Fonseca• Portugal, Coimbra: Comissão de ética do CHC• Portugal, Colvilhã: Comissão de ética do Centro Hospitalar Cova da Beira• Portugal, Évora: Comissão de ética do HESE• Portugal, Faro: Comissão de ética Hospital de Faro• Portugal, Guarda: Comissão de ética da Unidade Local de Saúde da Guarda• Portugal, Lisboa: Comissão de ética do Centro Hospitalar Lisboa Norte; Comissão de ética do Centro Hospitalar de Lisboa Ocidental• Portugal, Penafiel: Comissão de ética do Centro Hospitalar do Tâmega e Sousa• Portugal, Portalegre: Comissão de ética da Unidade Local de Saúde do Norte Alentejano• Portugal, Porto: Comissão de ética do Hospital São João• Portugal, Santarém: Comissão de ética Hospital Distrital de Santarém• Portugal, Torres Vedras: Comissão de ética do Centro Hospitalar de Torres Vedras• Portugal, Vila Nova de Gaia: Comissão de ética do Centro Hospitalar Gaia-Espinho• Russia: N/A (EC approval not required in Russia)• Slovakia, Bratislava: Bratislavsky Samosprávny Kraj• Slovenia, Ljubljana: Komisija Republike Slovenije za Medicinsko Etiko• Spain, Córdoba: Comite Etico de Investigación Clinica• Spain, Mallorca: Comite Etico de Investigacion Clinica de las Illes Baleares, Coselleria de Salut y Consum• Spain, San Bartolomé-Orihuela: Comite Etico de Investigación Clínica• Spain, Santiago de Compostela: Comite Etico de Investigacion Clinica de Galicia• Spain, Sevilla: CAEC- Comite Coordinador de Etica de la Investigacion Biomedica de Andalucia• Spain, Valencia: Dirección general de Farmacia y Productos Sanitarios; Conselleria de Sanitat, Dirección general de Farmacia y Productos Sanitarios• Spain, Vitoria-Gasteiz: Comite Etico de Investigacion Clinica- hospital Virgen de las Nieves; CEIC-E, Direccion de Farmacia del Departamento de Sanidad del Gobierno Vasco• Taiwan, Taichung: National Cheng Kung University Hospital Institutional Review Board • Taiwan, Tainan City: Taichung Veterans General Hospital Institutional Review Board • Taiwan, Taipei: National Taiwan University Hospital Research Ethics Committee; Chang Gung Memorial Hospital Institutional Review Board.

Author details
[1]Department of Pulmonary Medicine, Sint Franciscus Gasthuis, Kleiweg 500, 3045 PM, Rotterdam, The Netherlands. [2]Department of Pulmonary Disease, Thomayer Hospital, Charles University, Prague, Czech Republic. [3]Novartis Pharmaceuticals UK Limited, Horsham, West Sussex, UK. [4]Novartis Pharmaceuticals Corporation, East Hanover, NJ, USA.

References
1. Hanania NA, Alpan O, Hamilos DL, Condemi JJ, Reyes-Rivera I, Zhu J, Rosen KE, Eisner MD, Wong DA, Busse W: Omalizumab in severe allergic asthma inadequately controlled with standard therapy: a randomized trial. Ann Intern Med 2011, 154:573–582.

2. Humbert M, Beasley R, Ayres J, Slavin R, Hébert J, Bousquet J, Beeh KM, Ramos S, Canonica GW, Hedgecock S, Fox H, Blogg M, Surrey K: Benefits of omalizumab as add-on therapy in patients with severe persistent asthma who are inadequately controlled despite best available therapy (GINA 2002 step 4 treatment): INNOVATE. Allergy 2005, 60:309–316.

3. Curtis JR, Westfall AO, Allison J, Bijlsma JW, Freeman A, George V, Kovac SH, Spettell CM, Saag KG: Population-based assessment of adverse events associated with long-term glucocorticoid use. Arthritis Rheum 2006, 55:420–426.

4. Fardet L, Flahault A, Kettaneh A, Tiev KP, Généreau T, Tolédano C, Lebbé C, Cabane J: Corticosteroid-induced clinical adverse events: frequency, risk factors and patient's opinion. Br J Dermatol 2007, 157:142–148.

5. Manson SC, Brown RE, Cerulli A, Vidaurre CF: The cumulative burden of oral corticosteroid side effects and the economic implications of steroid use. Respir Med 2009, 103:975–994.

6. Walsh LJ, Wong CA, Oborne J, Cooper S, Lewis SA, Pringle M, Hubbard R, Tattersfield AE: Adverse effects of oral corticosteroids in relation to dose in patients with lung disease. Thorax 2001, 56:279–284.

7. EMA Xolair SmPC. http://www.ema.europa.eu/docs/en_GB/document_library/EPAR__Product_Information/human/000606/WC500057298.pdf.

8. US Food and Drug Administration: Omalizumab (Xolair®) prescribing information. http://www.fda.gov/Drugs/DrugSafety/PostmarketDrugSafetyInformationfor PatientsandProviders/ucm126456.htm.

9. Holgate ST, Chuchalin AG, Hebert J, Lötvall J, Persson GB, Chung KF, Bousquet J, Kerstjens HA, Fox H, Thirlwell J, Cioppa GD: Omalizumab 011 International Study Group: efficacy and safety of a recombinant anti-immunoglobulin E antibody (omalizumab) in severe allergic asthma. Clin Exp Allergy 2004, 34:632–638.

10. Lafeuille MH, Dean J, Zhang J, Duh MS, Gorsh B, Lefebvre P: Impact of omalizumab on emergency-department visits, hospitalizations, and corticosteroid use among patients with uncontrolled asthma. Ann Allergy Asthma Immunol 2012, 109:59–64.

11. Solèr M, Matz J, Townley R, Buhl R, O'Brien J, Fox H, Thirlwell J, Gupta N, Della Cioppa G: The anti-IgE antibody omalizumab reduces exacerbations and steroid requirement in allergic asthmatics. Eur Respir J 2001, 18:254–261.

12. Siergiejko Z, Świebocka E, Smith N, Peckitt C, Leo J, Peachey G, Maykut R: Oral corticosteroid sparing with omalizumab in severe allergic (IgE-mediated) asthma patients. Curr Med Res Opin 2011, 27:2223–2228.

13. Brodlie M, McKean MC, Moss S, Spencer DA: The oral corticosteroid-sparing effect of omalizumab in children with severe asthma. Arch Dis Child 2012, 97:604–609.

14. Braunstahl G-J, Chen C-W, Maykut R, Georgiou P, Peachey G, Bruce J: The eXpeRience registry: the 'real-world' effectiveness of omalizumab in allergic asthma. Resp Med 2013, 107:1141–1151.

15. Braunstahl G-J, Leo J, Thirlwell J, Peachey G, Maykut R: Uncontrolled persistent allergic asthma in practice: eXpeRience registry baseline characteristics. Curr Med Res Opin 2011, 27:761–767.

16. Molimard M, Buhl R, Niven R, Le Gros V, Thielen A, Thirlwell J, Maykut R, Peachey G: Omalizumab reduces oral corticosteroid use in patients with severe allergic asthma: real-life data. Respir Med 2010, 104:1381–1385.

17. Molimard M, de Blay F, Didier A, Le Gros V: Effectiveness of omalizumab (Xolair) in the first patients treated in real-life practice in France. Respir Med 2008, 102:71–76.

18. Cazzola M, Camiciottoli G, Bonavia M, Gulotta C, Ravazzi A, Alessandrini A, Caiaffa MF, Berra A, Schino P, Di Napoli PL, Maselli R, Pelaia G, Bucchioni E, Paggiaro PL, Macchia L: Italian real-life experience of omalizumab. Respir Med 2010, 104:1410–1416.

19. Brusselle G, Michils A, Louis R, Dupont L, Van de Maele B, Delobbe A, Pilette C, Lee CS, Gurdain S, Vancayzeele S, Lecomte P, Hermans C, MacDonald K, Song M, Abraham I: "Real-life" effectiveness of omalizumab in patients with severe persistent allergic asthma: The PERSIST study. Respir Med 2009, 103:1633–1642.

20. Rottem M: Omalizumab reduces corticosteroid use in patients with severe allergic asthma: real-life experience in Israel. J Asthma 2012, 49:78–82.

21. Niven R: A UK survey of oral corticosteroid use in patients treated with omalizumab [abstract]. Thorax 2007, 62(3):A98. P91.

22. Busse W, Corren J, Lanier BQ, McAlary M, Fowler-Taylor A, Cioppa GD, van As A, Gupta N: Omalizumab, anti-IgE recombinant humanized monoclonal antibody, for the treatment of severe allergic asthma. J Allergy Clin Immunol 2001, 108:184–190.

23. Bousquet J, Siergiejko Z, Świebocka E, Humbert M, Rabe KF, Smith N, Leo J, Peckitt C, Maykut R, Peachey G: **Persistency of response to omalizumab therapy in severe allergic (IgE-mediated) asthma.** *Allergy* 2011, **66:**671–678.
24. Bousquet J, Rabe K, Humbert M, Chung KF, Berger W, Fox H, Ayre G, Chen H, Thomas K, Blogg M, Holgate S: **Predicting and evaluating response to omalizumab in patients with severe allergic asthma.** *Respir Med* 2007, **101:**1483–1492.
25. Wechsler ME, Wong DA, Miller MK, Lawrence-Miyasaki L: **Churg-strauss syndrome in patients treated with omalizumab.** *Chest* 2009, **136:**507–518.

6

Confounding with familial determinants affects the association between mode of delivery and childhood asthma medication – a national cohort study

Lennart Bråbäck[1,2,8]*, Cecilia Ekéus[3], Adrian J Lowe[1,4,5] and Anders Hjern[6,7]

Abstract

Background: Mode of delivery may affect the risk of asthma but the findings have not been consistent and factors shared by siblings may confound the associations in previous studies.

Methods: The association between mode of delivery and dispensed inhaled corticosteroid (ICS) (a marker of asthma) was examined in a register based national cohort (n=199 837). A cohort analysis of all first born children aged 2-5 and 6-9 years was performed. An age-matched sibling-pair analysis was also performed to account for shared genetic and environmental risk factors.

Results: Analyses of first-borns demonstrated that elective caesarean section was associated with an increased risk of dispensed ICS in both 2-5 (adjusted odds ratio (aOR)=1.19, 95% confidence interval (CI) 1.09-1.29) and 6-9 (aOR=1.21, 1.09-1.34) age groups. In the sibling-pair analysis, the increased risk associated with elective caesarean section was confirmed in 2-5 year olds (aOR=1.22, 1.05-1.43) but not in 6-9 year olds (aOR=1.06, 0.78-1.44). Emergency caesarean section and vacuum extraction had some association with dispensed ICS in the analyses of first-borns but these associations were not confirmed in the sibling-pair analyses.

Conclusions: Confounding by familial factors affects the association between mode of delivery and dispensed ICS. Despite this confounding, there was some evidence that elective caesarean section contributed to a modestly increased risk of dispensed ICS but only up to five years of age.

Keywords: Asthma, Caesarean section, Child, Epidemiology, Inhaled corticosteroids, Sib pair analysis

Introduction

A moderate (20%) increase in asthma prevalence has been described in children delivered by caesarean section [1,2]. A number of studies have also suggested that instrumental vaginal delivery (vacuum extraction and forceps) may contribute to the development of asthma [3-5]. This represents a major public health concern, as there has been a substantial increase in deliveries by caesarean sections and vacuum extractions in high and middle-income countries all over the world [6].

Most previous studies have used a simple dichotomised categorisation of deliveries as being vaginal or caesarean, not taking into account the important differences between elective and emergency caesarean sections, and unaided and assisted vaginal deliveries. It has been hypothesed that the increased risk of asthma in children born by caesarean section is due to a lack of microbial exposure during labour, via the vagina, resulting in delayed and altered colonization of the infant gut [7,8]. Altered microbial colonization may be more pronounced in children born by elective caesarean sections, where rupture of the membranes prior to delivery is rare. Children delivered by elective caesarean section may also be at increased risk of neonatal respiratory morbidity [9] and asthma later in childhood [10], as they do not experience the stress of

* Correspondence: lennart.braback@lvn.se
[1]Occupational & Environmental Medicine, Department of Public Health and Clinical Medicine, Umeå University, Umeå, Sweden
[2]Department of Research and Development, Västernorrland County Council, Sundsvall, Sweden
Full list of author information is available at the end of the article

labour, which helps initiate the infant lungs to switch from secretion to absorption [9,11]. There is also some evidence that instrumental vaginal delivery contributes to an increased risk of asthma [3-5], possibly because of the prolonged maternal stress associated with these deliveries [4]. However, instrumental vaginal deliveries, and emergency caesarean sections, may be markers for complications in pregnancy, and it may be these complications, rather than mode of delivery, that confers the increased risk of asthma.

Some of the inconsistencies in previous studies may be due to insufficient control of confounding, differences in study size, age at outcome assessment and outcome measures.

In this study, we used a Swedish national cohort to overcome some of these obstacles to determine if mode of delivery affects the risk of dispensed ICS, as an indicator of asthma, whilst taking into account relevant sociodemographic and perinatal confounders. The large study population has enabled us to both detect very small differences, and to examine these effects in an aged-matched sibling pair analysis, to account for shared genetic and environmental exposures in the family. A recent and similar Swedish registry-based study did not detect any association between elective caesarean section and asthma in sibling-pairs aged 9 and 12 years. In contrast, association by indication seemed to explain an increased risk for asthma related to emergency caesarean section [12]. The aim of our study was to assess whether elective caesarean section had any association with asthma medication in children born at term and aged less than 9 years and whether the association between mode of delivery and asthma was affected by familial determinants. A potential effect from mode of delivery on the risk of asthma could be transient and only observed in the youngest age groups. We have therefore assessed whether the associations between mode of delivery and asthma medication differed between children aged 2-5 years and 6-9 years.

Methods

This study was based on information from the national health data bases held by the Swedish National Board of Health and Welfare and Statistics Sweden. Cross-linkage between registers was performed using each individual's unique personal identification number. This study was approved by the regional ethics committee in Stockholm.

The catchment population for this study were all full term (gestational week 37-<42), singleton children born in Sweden between 1/1/1999 and 31/12/2006, according to the Swedish Medical Birth Register. From this population we selected children who were residents in Sweden on December 2009 (according to the Register of the Total Population), were offspring of two native Swedish parents, had no major malformations reported at birth

by the attending paediatrician or cerebral palsy according to the Hospital Discharge Register. Children with improbable combinations of birth weight and gestational age (<-6SD and >3SD) were excluded, as were children with both instrumental vaginal delivery and caesarean section delivery recorded.

Information about parity, maternal age (at childbirth), measured maternal BMI in early pregnancy, mode of delivery, smoking habits in early pregnancy, maternal diseases and pregnancy complications was collected from Swedish Medical Birth Register. From the same register, perinatal data about sex, gestational age, birth weight, and low Apgar scores (<7 at five minutes) of the offspring were collected. Birth weight and gestational age were used to create the indicator of small -for-gestation-age (SGA, <2 SD) and large-for-gestational-age (LGA, >2 SD) [13]. Mode of delivery was categorised into; non-assisted vaginal delivery, emergency caesarean section, elective caesarean section and vacuum extraction. Classification of the caesarean section as emergency or elective is often missing in the register. However, information concerning onset of labour is rarely missing. Therefore, caesarean section was defined as emergency if the operation was made after the onset of labor and otherwise considered as elective. Maternal diseases and pregnancy complications were coded according to the International Classification of Diseases, tenth revisions.

Data on parental education was defined as the highest formal education attained. Educational level was categorised by years of education into <10 years, 10-12 years, 13-14 years and >14 years. Social welfare benefits received were collected from the Income and Enumeration survey for 2008 and dichotomised into any versus none.

We created three proxy indicators for asthma based on data of retrieved prescriptions from the Swedish Prescribed Drug Register, which contains all drugs prescribed and dispensed in Swedish pharmacies, excluding drug treatment in hospital care. The indicators "dispensed inhaled corticosteroid (ICS)" was defined as the purchase of at least one prescription of inhaled steroids, either by itself (Anatomical Therapeutic Chemical [ATC]-code starting with R03BA) or in combination with other agents (ATC codes R03AK06 or R03AK07) while dispensed ICS at least twice was defined as purchase of at least two prescriptions during the same calendar year with these definitions.. Finally, an indicator labeled "any asthma medication" was defined as the purchase of at least one prescription during a calendar year with an ATC-code that starts with R03 (any medication for obstructive lung disease).

In the cohort of firstborns, ICS during 2009 was used as our primary outcome variable, while dispensed ICS from all four years (2006 to 2009) was used to create age-equalised comparisons for the sibling-pair analysis.

Parental ICS was defined as receipt of an ICS during 2009 for all analyses and was used as a proxy for parental asthma.

There were considerable regional differences in the purchase of asthma medications reflecting regional differences in prevalence of asthma as well as differences in access to care and prescription patterns. A four-category *county* variable with different levels of retrieval of prescribed ICS was created to adjust the analysis to these regional differences.

Statistical analysis

Two related forms of analysis were performed. In the first, all first born children were included, and unconditional logistic regression models were used to assess the relationship between the different modes of delivery and risk of dispensed ICS by the child during 2009. Model 1 was adjusted for year of birth and sex only, in Model 2 we added other socio-demographic confounders (including smoking and maternal age) and parental dispensed ICS, in Model 3 we added perinatal risk factors associated with mode of delivery.

In a second analysis, the effect of mode of delivery was assessed within sibling pairs discordant for mode of delivery and asthma medication, using conditional logistic regression (children grouped according to sharing the same mother). In this analysis we have adjusted for the potential confounders that might vary between the two pregnancies, but not for confounders that vary between mothers only. Model 1 was adjusted for sex, in Model 2 we added maternal age and parity and Model 3 was also adjusted for SGA, LGA, preeclampsia, maternal body mass index, maternal diabetes and gestational diabetes and neonatal respiratory distress, Sibling-pairs were selected on the basis of having the widest age gap possible, whilst still being able to match siblings on age. In this analysis sib age was equalised by taking ICS dispensing at the age of the youngest sib in the analysis in 2009 from the calendar year 2006 to 2008.

For all forms of analysis, potential non-linear effects of maternal BMI were assessed using the "fracpoly" command within Stata (release 10.1, College Station, Texas). Effect modification, by gender, parity, maternal smoking, parental asthma (dispensed ICS) was assessed using Wald tests. As the nature of wheeze changes with age, the exposure to asthma medications was classified into two discrete age groups, 2-5 and 6-9 years of age.

Results

Altogether 13 179 (12.7%) boys and 9934 (9.2%) girls in the age two to nine years had purchased any asthma medication in 2009, and of these 7180 (6.9%) boys and 4722 (4.6%) girls had retrieved at least one prescription of ICS.

Dispensed asthma medication increased gradually with increasing maternal BMI (Table 1). Children whose mother had a pre-existing condition or a pregnancy complication were more likely to receive asthma medication. In addition, being born in gestational week 37-38 had higher rates of medication than those born in week 39-41. Having had neonatal respiratory problems was also associated with a higher risk of asthma medication

Table 2 shows that mothers giving birth by caesarean section or vacuum extraction were more likely than those born by non-assisted vaginal delivery to be older and to have chronic disorders, pregnancy complications and asthma medications. Maternal overweight or obesity was more common among children delivered by caesarean section but not among those born by vacuum extraction deliveries. Furthermore, newborns delivered instrumentally (both caesarean section and vacuum extraction) more often had respiratory distress, low Apgar scores, meconium aspiration and were classified as SGA or LGA. Some maternal complications, *e.g.* hypertension and diabetes were more common in those who were delivered by elective caesarean section compared with those who were delivered by emergency caesarean section. In contrast, low Apgar was overrepresented after emergency caesarean section and vacuum extraction.

Children delivered by non-instrumental vaginal delivery had the lowest rates of asthma medication in all age groups (Figure 1). Children delivered by elective caesarean section had the highest rates in all age groups except the 4-5 year olds while emergency caesarean section and vacuum extraction had a similar rate in all age groups.

When compared to vaginal delivery without assistance, both elective and emergency caesarean sections were associated with a modest increase in risk of any dispensed ICS (at least one prescription) in the 2-5 year olds after adjustment for socio-demographic confounders (Table 3, model 2),. Adjusting for perinatal risk factors attenuated these risks slightly (model 3). In the 6-9 year olds, children delivered by elective caesarean section had an increased risk (adjusted odds ratios (aOR) 1.21, 95% confidence interval (CI) 1.09-1.34 for model 3). The association with emergency caesarean section delivery and dispensed ICS was weaker, and no evidence of an association remained after adjustments for the confounding and mediating variables (aOR 1.05, 95% CI 0.93-1.17 for model 3).

Delivery by vacuum extraction was associated with a slightly increased risk of dispensed ICS, in the 6-9-years olds (aOR 1.15, 95% CI 1.05-1.25), after adjustment for confounders and a borderline increased risk in the 2-5 year olds (aOR 1.07, 95% CI 0.99-1.15). Interaction analyses showed that the effect of mode of delivery was similar in boys and girls.

We have also assessed the associations between mode of delivery and at least two dispensed prescriptions of

Table 1 Asthma medication by socio-demographic and neonatal indicators (%) in 2-9 year olds

N=199 837

		N	Any ICS %	ICS twice %	Any asthma medication %
Sex	Boys	100 688	7.1	3.6	10.9
	Girls	99 149	4.6	2.4	7.6
Age (in years)	2-3	53 346	7.1	3.9	12.8
	4-5	52 411	5.8	3.0	9.0
	6-7	49 214	5.2	2.5	7.5
	8-9	44 866	5.2	2.5	7.5
Maternal age at delivery (years)	−24	43 079	5.6	2.6	9.1
	25-34	138 135	5.9	9.3	9.3
	>34	18 623	6.2	10.0	10.0
Maternal body mass index	Underweight	4311	5.1	2.3	8.4
	Normal	117 552	5.5	2.9	8.8
	Overweight	38 443	6.4	3.4	10.1
	Obese 1	10 955	7.1	4.0	11.0
	Obese2	4104	7.9	3.1	12.4
	Missing	24 472	5.9	3.0	9.4
Gestational age (weeks)	39-41	159 368	5.7	2.9	9.0
	37-38	40 469	6.7	3.5	10.3
Hypertension	Preeclampsia	2457	7.5	3.7	11.5
	Pregestational	7409	6.4	3.5	9.8
Diabetes type 1	Yes	708	5.6	3.5	9.6
Gestational diabetes	Yes	1163	7.6	4.4	11.4
Oligohydramniom	Yes	2094	6.8	3.6	11.0
Premature ruptures ruptures of membranes	Yes	750	5.9	2.9	9.5
Low apgar score	Yes	1980	6.7	3.5	9.6
Small for gestational age (SGA)	Yes	4388	7.1	3.9	11.2
Large for gestational age (LGA)	Yes	3840	6.7	3.6	10.2
Any neonatal respiratory complication	Yes	4237	6.6	3.7	10.4
Maternal smoking	10+	3508	6.3	3.0	10.2
	1-9	13 693	5.9	2.8	9.8
	0	169 700	5.8	3.0	9.2
	Missing data	12 936	6.6	3.4	10.2
Maternal asthma medication	Yes	5916	15.2	8.8	20.4
Paternal asthma medication	Yes	5491	11.1	6.3	15.9
Maternal education (years)	<=9	12 461	5.9	2.7	9.7
	10-12	86 807	5.9	2.9	9.5
	13-14	28355	5.9	3.0	9.2
	15+	71 808	5.8	3.2	9.0
County category	1	48 002	6.4	3.2	10.4
	2	36 950	6.0	3.1	9.3
	3	76 915	5.6	3.1	8.9
	4	37 970	5.5	2.7	8.6
All		199 837	5.9	3.0	9.3

Table 2 Asthma medication, socio-demographic and neonatal indicators by mode of delivery in 2-9 year olds

N=199 837

		Vaginal N=143 347 %	Elective CS N=16 050 %	Emergency CS N=13 875 %	Vacuum extraction N=26 565 %
Any asthma medication (child)	Yes	8.9	11.3	10.2	9.8
ICS (child)	Yes	5.6	7.1	6.5	6.4
ICS at least twice (child)	Yes	2.8	3.8	3.6	3.4
ICS (mother)	Yes	2.7	4.2	3.5	3.1
ICS (father)	Yes	2.6	3.7	3.0	2.8
Maternal age at delivery (years)	11-24	24.1	13.6	14.4	16.3
	25-34	68.5	67.1	71.6	72.3
	>34	7.4	19.3	14.0	11.4
Maternal body mass index	Underweight	2.3	1.8	1.3	2.0
	Normal	60.5	52.4	49.7	58.5
	Overweight	18.4	21.5	23.7	20.1
	Obese1	5.0	7.6	8.4	5.2
	Obese2	1.8	3.6	3.5	1.9
	Missing	12.0	13.1	13.4	12.3
Gestational age (weeks)	37-38	18.1	53.8	16.7	13.3
Hypertension	Preeclampsia	1.1	2.1	1.2	1.3
	Pregestational	3.0	11.2	2.7	3.6
Diabetes type 1	Yes	0.2	1.6	0.6	0.5
Gestational diabetes	Yes	0.5	1.3	0.7	0.5
Low Apgar score	Yes	0.5	1.3	2.4	2.6
SGA	Yes	1.8	4.6	3.2	2.2
LGA	Yes	1.4	4.1	4.2	2.2
Any neonatal respiratory complication	Yes	1.6	3.1	3.9	3.3
Maternal smoking	Yes	8.7	9.4	8.6	7.4
Social welfare	Yes	2.5	2.0	1.8	1.6
Maternal education	<10 years	6.6	6.2	5.5	4.9
	10-12	43.4	44.0	44.6	43.2
	13-14	14.0	15.1	15.2	14.5
	>14	36.0	34.6	34.7	37.3
County category	1	22.6	29.2	26.6	27.2
	2	19.2	17.2	17.8	15.8
	3	39.4	35.5	36.8	36.2
	4	18.8	18.1	18.8	20.9

Abbreviations: CS, caesarean section; ICS, inhaled corticosteroid use; LGA, large for gestational age; SGA, small for gestational age.

ICS as the outcome. The findings differed only slightly from the analyses based on at least one dispensed prescription of ICS (Additional file 1: Table S1)

Sibling pair analysis

In the sibling pair analysis, of the 30 515 sibling pairs aged 6-9 years, 2290 were discordant for ICS use, and of these 569 were also discordant for mode of delivery (Additional file 2: Table S2). In this age group, all effects were marginal with wide confidence intervals when compared to the unconditional analysis (Table 4). Of the 80 140 sib pairs aged 2-5 years, 1 965 were discordant for both ICS use and mode of delivery. In this age group children delivered by elective caesarean section had an

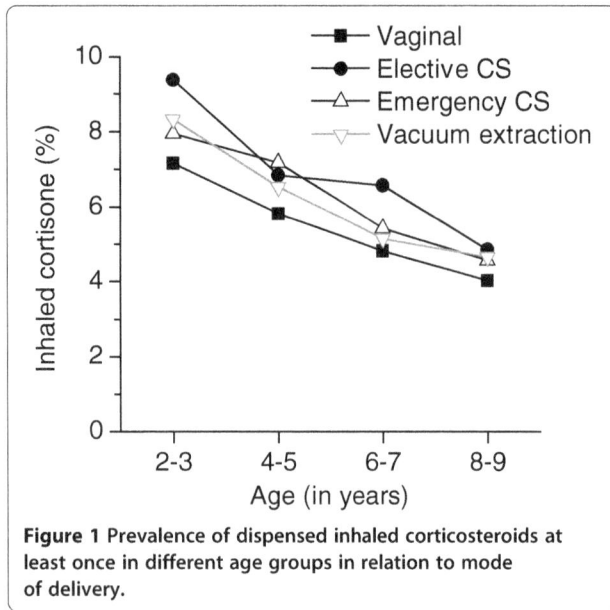

Figure 1 Prevalence of dispensed inhaled corticosteroids at least once in different age groups in relation to mode of delivery.

increased risk of asthma medication use, when compared to their age matched sibling (crude OR 1.21, 95% CI 1.05-1.41 and aOR 1.19, 95% CI 1.09-1.29).

Discussion

Our analyses of first-borns demonstrated that elective caesarean sections were associated with modestly increased risk of dispensed ICS, a marker of asthma. The sibling-pair analysis, which inherently adjusts for shared environmental and genetic factors, confirmed this association in elective caesarean in the two to five year olds, but not in the older children. The associations between

emergency caesarean section and vacuum extraction and risk of dispensed ICS observed in the analyses of first-borns where not confirmed in the sibling-pair analyses, suggesting these effects are due to residual confounding.

Several large cohort studies from Scandinavian countries have suggested that emergency as well as elective section could affect the risk of asthma [5,14] or asthma hospitalisation in young children [3]. The conventional, unconditional logistic regression, analysis in our study indicated that emergency caesarean sections and vacuum extraction were associated with an increased risk of asthma medication but these associations disappeared completely in the sibling pair analyses suggesting that these effects in the unconditional logistics regression were due to residual confounding by familial risk factors. It remains unclear what these unmeasured confounding factors in the conventional analysis could be. We have adjusted for a range of potential confounders, including socio-economic status, parental asthma, and pregnancy and neonatal complications. Adjustment for these factors did not greatly alter the observed associations. Maternal anxiety is associated with an increased risk of pregnancy complications [15] and emergency caesarean sections [16] and maternal stress during pregnancy could contribute to an increased risk of childhood asthma [17]. Although we did adjust our analysis for proxy indicators for parental asthma (dispensed ICS), there may well be residual genetic confounding that connects perinatal complications with asthma later in life.

The current study underlines the difficulties to control for confounding in conventional analyses of mode of delivery and asthma. It is based on register data covering

Table 3 The association between mode of delivery and dispense of at least one prescription of inhaled cortisone[1]

Mode of delivery	Inhaled corticosteroid use			Unadjusted		Model 1		Model 2		Model 3	
	No of cases	Total No	%	OR	95% CI	aOR	95% CI	aOR	95% CI	aOR	95% CI
2-5 years											
Vaginal[2]	4597	74694	6.2	1.0	1.0	1.0	1.0	1.0	1.0	1.0	1.0
Elective CS	698	9061	7.7	1.27	1.17, 1.38	1.26	1.16, 1.37	1.22	1.12, 1.33	1.19	1.09, 1.29
Emergency CS	546	7478	7.3	1.20	1.10, 1.32	1.18	1.08, 1.29	1.17	1.06, 1.28	1.14	1.04, 1.25
Vacuum extraction	981	14524	6.8	1.10	1.03, 1.19	1.08	1.00, 1.16	1.07	1.00, 1.15	1.07	0.99, 1.15
6-9 years											
Vaginal[2]	3391	68653	4.9	1.0	1.0	1.0	1.0	1.0	1.0	1.0	1.0
Elective CS	442	6989	6.3	1.30	1.17, 1.44	1.29	1.17, 1.43	1.24	1.12, 1.38	1.21	1.09, 1.34
Emergency CS	358	6397	5.6	1.14	1.02, 1.28	1.11	1.00, 1.25	1.08	0.78, 1.21	1.05	0.93, 1.17
Vacuum extraction	711	12041	5.9	1.21	1.01, 1.31	1.17	1.07, 1.27	1.16	1.06, 1.26	1.15	1.05, 1.25

Crude and adjusted odds ratios after non-conditional logistic regression.
Abbreviations: CI, confidence interval; aOR, adjusted odds ratio; OR, odds ratio.
Model 1 is adjusted for year of birth and sex. **Model 2**: also adding: maternal and paternal asthma medication. socioeconomic indicators (maternal education. social welfare) maternal age, maternal smoking, urban/rural living, county. **Model 3** also adding factors that may increase the risk of caesarean section: maternal history of diabetes and hypertension, premature rupture of the membranes, preeclampsia, gestational diabetes, gestational hypertension, maternal body mass index, small for gestational age, large for gestational age, maternal fever during labour,. chorioamnionitis, meconium aspiration, neonatal respiratory distress, transient tachypnoea.
[1]Only first born children included, [2]Non-instrumental vaginal delivery.

Table 4 Conditional logistic regression models for the association between mode of delivery and dispense of at least one prescription of inhaled cortisone at least once in discordant sibling-pairs

Mode of delivery	Unadjusted		Model 1		Model 2		Model 3	
	OR	95% CI	aOR	95% CI	aOR	95% CI	aOR	95% CI
2-5 years (n= 7 688 contrasting sib pairs)								
Vaginal[1]	1.0	1.0	1.0	1.0	1.0	1.0	1.0	1.0
Elective CS	1.21	1.05, 1.41	1.19	1.03, 1.39	1.22	1.05, 1.42	1.23	1.05, 1.43
Emergency CS	0.88	0.74, 1.06	0.84	0.70, 1.02	0.95	0.79, 1.15	0.95	0.78, 1.14
Vacuum extraction	0.94	0.83, 1.06	0.89	0.79, 1.01	1.06	0.92, 1.21	1.05	0.92, 1.20
6-9 years (n=2 290 contrasting sib pairs)								
Vaginal[1]	1.0	1.0	1.0	1.0	1.0	1.0	1.0	1.0
Elective CS	1.05	0.79, 1.40	1.08	0.80, 1.46	1.09	0.81, 1.47	1.06	0.78, 1.44
Emergency CS	1.05	0.75, 1.46	1.00	0.71, 1.42	1.03	0.73, 1.46	1.02	0.72, 1.44
Vacuum extraction	0.93	0.74, 1.17	0.89	0.70, 1.12	0.91	0.71, 1.17	0.92	0.72, 1.18

Odds ratios in relation to the reference, Non-instrumental vaginal delivery in different age groups.
Abbreviations: CI, confidence interval; aOR, adjusted odds ratio; OR, odds ratio.
Model 1 – adjusted for infant gender, **Model 2** – also adjusted for maternal age and parity, **Model 3** – also adjusted for small for gestational age, large for gestational age, preeclampsia, maternal body mass index, maternal diabetes and gestational diabetes and neonatal respiratory distress.
[1]Non-instrumental vaginal delivery.

the whole Swedish population. There is no recall or selection bias. However, some of the indicators in the registers are crude proxies for the true exposures [18]. It is particulary difficult to cover life style factors, and the specific indications for elective caesareans. These factors may affect mode of delivery [19,20] as well as the risk of asthma [21], use of medication and access to health care [22].

Studies with a sibling design are a powerful tool to control for familial confounding due to genetic or environmental factors [23]. With the exception of the recent study by Almqvist et al [12], this design has not been used in epidemiological studies of mode of delivery and asthma. A prerequisite is a sufficient number of discordant sibling pairs. Our study is based on all ethnic Swedish children born term between 1992 and 2008 with data available on over 110 000 sibling pairs. Despite these quite impressive sibling populations, only 1965 sibling pairs at age 2-5 and 569 at age 6-9 were discordant for both mode of delivery and asthma medication use, and thus were informative for this analysis. These sample sizes were insufficient to obtain precise estimates of these comparatively small effects, thus requiring cautious interpretation. In comparison, Almqvist et al. had 1005 informative sibling pairs available in their study. Although the majority of our findings are consistent with those of Almqvist et al. they observed an association between emergency caesarean section and increased risk of asthma [12], while we did not. This may be due to multiple differences in the design of these two studies. Specifically, we excluded all children born pre-term, and those who had malformations or cerebral palsy. These conditions may result in delivery by emergency caesearan

section and increased risk of developing various respiratory illnesses including asthma.

Childhood asthma is a heterogenous disease and a number of phenotypes with partly different risk factors have been identified [24]. Almqvist et al did not observe any association between elective caesarean section and an increased risk of asthma in sibling-pairs aged 9 and 12 years [12]. Our study suggests that elective caesarean section could be associated with a slightly increased risk of transient wheeze up to five years of age. Maternal complications during pregnancy have previously been linked to an increased risk of childhood wheeze [25]. Hypertension and diabetes were more likely in women who were delivered by elective caesarean section but the increased risk for asthma medication persisted also after adjustment for these factors. However, we cannot exclude that other undetected complications contributed to the increased risk of asthma medication in preschoolers.

This study has a number of limitations. Defining asthma within epidemiological studies is a challenge. We have chosen to use prescription of inhaled corticosteroids (ICS) to define current symptoms of asthma. We have previously used a similar definition [26] as has a similar study from Finland [5] A number of studies have assessed the validity of prescription registry based information on asthma medicine use against parent report of asthma [27], standardised questionnaire based definitions of asthma [28], and doctor diagnosis [29] in similar settings to the current study. These studies generally find that prescription registry data provides a reasonably valid definition of asthma. We have elected to exclude use of beta-agonists from our primary definition of the outcome, as these are a less specific marker for asthma.

However, dispensed medication as a proxy for asthma is affected by a number of factors at different levels such as awareness of the symptoms by the child and the parents, severity of asthma, health seeking behavior, diagnostic criteria by the doctor, attitude to medication and its related costs. If one sibling has asthma, other siblings are more likely to be diagnosed and get a prescription for an asthma medication than children in families where the symptoms of asthma are less familiar. Sharing of medication may occur in families where several members suffer from asthma. When asthma is diagnosed compliance with medication probably differ in different families, and this will have an effect on subsequent prescriptions. Many of these family effects could contribute to a negative outcome and some of these such as sharing of medication could weaken the associations also in the sibling analyses. Using purchase of ICS may imply that we have missed individuals (parents or children) with undiagnosed or mild asthma. Therefore, residual confounding may explain some of the reduced effect sizes in the sibling analysis.

In young children, dispensed ICS is a proxy for respiratory illness, but not always for asthma. as diagnosis of asthma is very difficult in preschool children. By the age of 6 years, the prevalence of transient viral wheeze has largely passed, and a diagnosis of asthma is much easier to confirm, making this a reasonable time point to divide the cohort of children. Variability in prescription pattern could dilute the association between asthma medication and mode of delivery in young children [30]. For this reason, we have also excluded children aged less than two years, and used ICS rather than all asthma medication as our main outcome. Children with nonspecific clinical symptoms sometimes get one prescription of ICS as a test for asthma. One may therefore ague that at least two prescriptions of ICS would have been a better proxy for asthma in our study but we have tested analyses based on at least two prescriptions of ICS and the findings were fairly similar.

An association between caesarean section and asthma could also be weakened or even missed, if potential effects are restricted to specific genetic variants or subgroups of asthma. We do not have direct measures for atopy in this study. Therefore, we cannot exclude that mode of delivery could affect allergic induced symptoms. Moreover, we have no information in the registers concerning postnatal exposures. However, a recent birth cohort study failed to identify modification of the association of between mode of delivery and childhood asthma by a range of key postnatal exposures, including breast-feeding behavior and age at day care entry [14].

We cannot exclude the risk of some misclassification of the caesarean sections. "Elective" caesarean sections were not necessarily optional. We considered a caesarean section to be emergent if the operation was made after the onset of labour. Therefore, caesarean sections due to emergencies such as fetal distress or a severe maternal complication were defined as elective if the caesarean sections were performed without preceding labour. Although this would have resulted in some misclassification between emergency and elective caesarean sections, as this reason for cesarean section is relatively uncommon, we consider it to be an unlikely source of a major bias in this study. The major indications in Sweden for elective caesarean sections after 36 weeks are breech presentation, previous caesarean section, cephalopelvic disproportion and psychosocial factors. They accounted for more than 80% of all elective caesarean sections between 1996 and 2007 [31].

To conclude, elective caesarean section contributes to a modestly increased risk of asthma medication, but only up to five years of age. The associations between emergency caesarean section or vacuum extraction and asthma medication seen in the firstborns appear to be due to residual confounding by familial factors.

Competing interests

All authors declare that they have no competing interests.

Authors' contributions

LB contributed to the design of the study, conducted the literature review, prepared the first draft and revised the final version of the manuscript. CE contributed to the design of the study, conducted the data analyses and revised the final version of the manuscript. AL designed the study's analytic strategy, performed the sibling analyses and revised the manuscript. AH designed the study and the analytic strategy, performed register linkages, created the dataset, performed some statistical analyses, directed the implementation including quality assurance and control and contributed to all parts of the manuscript. All authors read and approved the final manuscript.

Acknowledgements

This project was supported by the Swedish Research Council, through Swedish Initiative for Research on Microdata in the Social And Medical Sciences (SIMSAM) network, Umeå University (http://www.org.umu.se/simsam/english/), who provided financial support (grant no. 2008-7491) to A. L. and L.B. to undertake this project. Also, A.L. was supported by the Australian National Health and Medical Research Council and CE was supported by grants from the Swedish Research Council.

Author details

[1]Occupational & Environmental Medicine, Department of Public Health and Clinical Medicine, Umeå University, Umeå, Sweden. [2]Department of Research and Development, Västernorrland County Council, Sundsvall, Sweden. [3]Department of Women's and Children's Health, Division of Reproductive and Perinatal Health, Karolinska Institutet, Stockholm, Sweden. [4]Murdoch Childrens Research Institute, Melbourne, Australia. [5]Centre for MEGA Epidemiology , School of Population Health, The University of Melbourne,

Melbourne, Australia. [6]Centre for Health Equity Studies (CHESS), Karolinska Institutet/Stockholm University, Stockholm, Sweden. [7]Clinical Epidemiology, Department of Medicine, Karolinska Institutet, Stockholm, Sweden. [8]Department of Research and Development, Sundsvalls sjukhus, Sundsvall SE 85186, Sweden.

References

1. Bager P, Wohlfahrt J, Westergaard T: Caesarean delivery and risk of atopy and allergic disease: meta-analyses. Clin Exp Allergy 2008, 38:634–642.
2. Thavagnanam S, Fleming J, Bromley A, Shields MD, Cardwell CR: A meta-analysis of the association between Caesarean section and childhood asthma. Clin Exp Allergy 2008, 38:629–633.
3. Håkansson S, Källén K: Caesarean section increases the risk of hospital care in childhood for asthma and gastroenteritis. Clin Exp Allergy 2003, 33:757–764.
4. Keski-Nisula L, Harju M, Järvelin MR, Pekkanen J: Vacuum-assisted delivery is associated with late-onset asthma. Allergy 2009, 64:1530–1538.
5. Metsälä J, Kilkkinen A, Kaila M, Tapanainen H, Klaukka T, Gissler M, Virtanen SM: Perinatal factors and the risk of asthma in childhood--a population-based register study in Finland. Am J Epidemiol 2008, 168:170–178.
6. Shorten A: Maternal and neonatal effects of caesarean section. BMJ 2007, 335:1003–1004.
7. Björkstén B: Effects of intestinal microflora and the environment on the development of asthma and allergy. Springer Semin Immunopathol 2004, 25:257–270.
8. Guarner F, Malagelada JR: Gut flora in health and disease. Lancet 2003, 361:512–519.
9. Borgwardt L, Bach D, Nickelsen C, Gutte H, Boerch K: Elective caesarean section increases the risk of respiratory morbidity of the newborn. Acta Paediatr 2009, 98:187–189.
10. Liem JJ, Huq SI, Ekuma O, Becker AB, Kozyrskyj AL: Transient tachypnea of the newborn may be an early clinical manifestation of wheezing symptoms. J Pediatr 2007, 151:29–33.
11. Olver R, Walters D: Why babies don't drown at birth? Acta Paediatr 2008, 97:1324–1326.
12. Almqvist C, Cnattingius S, Lichtenstein P, Lundholm C: The impact of birth mode of delivery on childhood asthma and allergic diseases – a sibling study. Clin Exp Allergy 2012, 42:1369–76.
13. Marsal K, Persson PH, Larsen T, Lilja H, Selbing A, Sultan B: Intrauterine growth curves based on ultrasonically estimated foetal weights. Acta Paediatr 1996, 85:843–848.
14. Magnus MC, Håberg SE, Stigum H, Nafstad P, London SJ, Vangen S, Nystad W: Delivery by cesarean section and early childhood respiratory symptoms and disorders: the norwegian mother and child cohort study. Am J Epidemiol 2011, 174:1275–1285.
15. Mulder EJ, Robles De Medina PG, Huizink AC, Van den Bergh BR, Buitelaar JK, Visser GH: Prenatal maternal stress: effects on pregnancy and the (unborn) child. Early Hum Dev 2002, 70(1-2):3–14.
16. Wangel AM, Molin J, Östman M, Jernström H: Emergency cesarean sections can be predicted by markers for stress, worry and sleep disturbances in first-time mothers. Acta Obstet Gynecol Scand 2011, 90:238–244.
17. Cookson H, Granell R, Joinson C, Ben-Shlomo Y, Henderson AJ: Mothers' anxiety during pregnancy is associated with asthma in their children. J Allergy Clin Immunol 2009, 123:847–853 e811.
18. Olsen J: Register-based research: some methodological considerations. Scand J Public Health 2011, 39:225–229.
19. Cesaroni G, Forastiere F, Perucci CA: Are cesarean deliveries more likely for poorly educated parents? a brief report from italy. Birth 2008, 35:241–244.
20. Fairley L, Dundas R, Leyland AH: The influence of both individual and area based socioeconomic status on temporal trends in Caesarean sections in Scotland 1980-2000. BMC Publ Health 2011, 11:330.
21. Almqvist C, Pershagen G, Wickman M: Low socioeconomic status as a risk factor for asthma, rhinitis and sensitization at 4 years in a birth cohort. Clin Exp Allergy 2005, 35:612–618.
22. Piper CN, Glover S, Elder K, Baek JD, Wilkinson L: Disparities in access to care among asthmatic children in relation to race and socioeconomic status. J Child Health Care 2010, 14:271–279.
23. Susser E, Eide MG, Begg M: Invited commentary: the use of sibship studies to detect familial confounding. Am J Epidemiol 2010, 172:537–539.
24. Siroux V, Garcia-Aymerich J: The investigation of asthma phenotypes. Curr Opin Allergy Clin Immunol 2011, 11:393–399.
25. Rusconi F, Galassi C, Forastiere F, Bellasio M, De Sario M, Ciccone G, Brunetti L, Chellini E, Corbo G, La Grutta S, Lombardi E, Piffer S, Talassi F, Biggeri A, Pearce N: Maternal complications and procedures in pregnancy and at birth and wheezing phenotypes in children. Am J Respir Crit Care Med 2007, 175:16–21.
26. Lowe A, Bråbäck L, Ekeus C, Hjern A, Forsberg B: Maternal obesity during pregnancy as a risk for early-life asthma. J Allergy Clin Immunol 2011, 128:1107–1109.
27. Furu K, Karlstad O, Skurtveit S, Håberg SE, Nafstad P, London SE, Nystad W: High validity of mother-reported use of antiasthmatics among children: a comparison with a population-based prescription database. J Clin Epidemiol 2011, 64:878–884.
28. Nwaru BI, Lumia M, Kaila M, Luukkainen P, Tapanainen H, Erkkola M, Ahonen S, Pekkanen J, Klaukka T, Veijola R, Simell O, Knip M, Virtanen SM: Validation of the Finnish ISAAC questionnaire on asthma against anti-asthmatic medication reimbursement database in 5-year-old children. Clin Respir J 2011, 4:211–218.
29. Moth G, Vedsted P, Schiotz P: Identification of asthmatic children using prescription data and diagnosis. Eur J Clin Pharmacol 2007, 63:605–611.
30. Zuidgeest MG, Van Dijk L, Spreeuwenberg P, Smit HA, Brunekreef B, Arets HG, Bracke M, Leufkens HG: What drives prescribing of asthma medication to children? a multilevel population-based study. Ann Fam Med 2009, 7:32–40.
31. Källén K: Increasing prevalence of caesarean sections and its causes (in Swedish). In Caesarean section: Swedish Society for Obstetrics and Gynecology. Edited by Andolf E, Bottinga R, Larsson C, Lilja H. Stockholm: Libris; 2010:11–18.

7

Birth weight, gestational age, fetal growth and childhood asthma hospitalization

Xiaoqin Liu[1,2]*, Jørn Olsen[1,3], Esben Agerbo[4,5], Wei Yuan[2], Sven Cnattingius[6], Mika Gissler[7,8] and Jiong Li[1]

Abstract

Background: Childhood asthma may have a fetal origin through fetal growth and development of the immunocompetence or respiratory organs.

Objective: We examined to which extent short gestational age, low birth weight and fetal growth restriction were associated with an increased risk of asthma hospitalization in childhood.

Methods: We undertook a cohort study based on several national registers in Denmark, Sweden and Finland. We included all live singleton born children in Denmark during 1979-2005 (N = 1,538,093), in Sweden during 1973-2004 (N = 3,067,670), and a 90% random sample of singleton children born in Finland during 1987-2004 (N = 1,050,744). The children were followed from three years of age to first hospitalization for asthma, emigration, death, their 18th birthday, or the end of study (the end of 2008 in Denmark, and the end of 2007 in Sweden or Finland), whichever came first. We computed the pseudo-values for each observation and used them in a generalized estimating equation to estimate relative risks (RR) for asthma hospitalization.

Results: A total of 131,783 children were hospitalized for asthma during follow-up. The risk for asthma hospitalization consistently increased with lower birth weight and shorter gestational age. A 1000-g decrease in birth weight corresponded to a RR of 1.17 (95% confidence interval (CI) 1.15-1.18). A one-week decrease in gestational age corresponded to a RR of 1.05 (95% CI 1.04-1.06). Small for gestational age was associated with an increased risk of asthma hospitalization in term but not in preterm born children.

Conclusions: Fetal growth and gestational age may play a direct or indirect causal role in the development of childhood asthma.

Keywords: Asthma, Birth weight, Gestational age, Hospitalization, Small for gestational age

Introduction

Asthma is a significant health problem for families and society [1]. More than 50% of children with asthma develop symptoms before their fifth birthday [2], indicating that pre- or perinatal factors may play a causal role.

Preterm birth, low birth weight and fetal growth restriction may be associated with disturbed immunocompetence and restrict normal lung growth and development [3-6], thereby predispose children to asthma later in life

* Correspondence: lxq@soci.au.dk
[1]Section for Epidemiology, Department of Public Health, Aarhus University, Aarhus, Denmark
[2]Department of Epidemiology and Social Science on Reproductive Health, Shanghai Institute of Planned Parenthood Research, WHO Collaborating Center for Research in Human Reproduction, National Population & Family Planning Key Laboratory of Contraceptive Drugs and Devices, Shanghai, China
Full list of author information is available at the end of the article

[4,7]. However, epidemiologic findings linking gestational age, birth weight, fetal growth and childhood asthma are inconsistent. Gestational age has been associated with asthma in some studies [8-17] but not in others [18-23]. Previous studies on birth weight and asthma are also contradictory with both inverse [8,9,13,14,21,23-26], direct [18,27], as well as null results [19,20,28,29]. As gestational age and birth weight are strongly correlated, small for gestational age (SGA) is commonly used as a proxy for fetal growth restriction [30]. Findings on asthma and SGA have also been inconclusive. While some indicated an association between SGA and increased risk of asthma [15,31], others found no association [9,32,33], or even an inverse association [34,35]. Comparison of these studies is hampered by differences in defining the study populations and their size, e.g. children born with different gestational age

and different follow-up time periods. Results from twin studies may not reflect associations for singletons [19,23-25]. Studies that found no association were often based on smaller sample sizes [18,20,33]. And there has currently been no "gold standard" for diagnosis of asthma and it remains unclear how the condition should be defined and measured in epidemiological studies. Self-reported asthma may be subject to recall bias and subjective interpretation of disease status [19-22,25,29,33]. Asthma diagnosis is considered less accurate in young children due to its clinical instability in early years of life [33,36,37]. In addition, different reference curves for birth weight for gestational age have been used to estimate fetal growth [38]. Further, these curves are usually based on the distribution of live births and do not necessarily reflect normal fetal growth. Preterm born infants are smaller than fetuses of the same gestational age due to the fact that fetal growth restriction is a risk factor for both medically indicated and spontaneous preterm birth [39].

Large population-based studies using the register systems in three Nordic countries allowed a detailed analysis of the association between gestational age, birth weight, fetal growth and risk of childhood asthma. We included information on a number of social demographic variables and explored the risk for asthma hospitalization as a function of gestational age, birth weight, and fetal growth in a cohort of children followed until they reached 18 years of age.

Methods
Study population
We used a cohort study based on linkage between several national registers in Denmark, Sweden and Finland. All live-born children and new residents in the three Nordic countries are assigned a unique personal identification number, which can be used to link information at the individual level in all national registers. We first identified all singleton live births during 1979-2005 recorded in the Danish Medical Birth Registry (DMBR) and during 1973-2004 in the Swedish Medical Birth Register (SMBR). In Finland, we were only allowed to include a 90% random sample of singleton children born during 1987-2004 in the Finnish Medical Birth Registry (FMBR). The DMBR has been computerized since 1973 and includes data on gestational age from 1978. The SMBR was established in 1973, and the FMBR was established in 1987. The DMBR was linked to the Danish Civil Registration System, the Danish National Patient Register [40], and the Danish Integrated Database for Longitudinal Labor Market Research. The SMBR was linked to the Swedish Multi-generation Register, the Swedish Patient Register [41], and the Swedish Education Register. The FMBR was linked to the Finnish Hospital Discharge Register [42] and the Population Register at Statistics

Finland. A total of 5,928,759 births were recorded during the study period in the birth registries. We excluded 198,733 (3.3%) infants who had missing or unrealistic gestational age or birth weight data (gestational age < 154 or > 315 days and birth weight < 300 or > 6400 grams), 44 infants whose mothers' data on parity were missing, 30,424 deceased infants and 43,051 infants who emigrated under three years of age. Seven infants were reported to die from asthma before three years of age. Of remaining 5,656,507 children, 1,538,093 were born in Denmark (27.2%), 3,067,670 in Sweden (54.2%), and 1,050,744 in Finland (18.6%).

Exposures
We used three different indicators of fetal development and growth: gestational age, birth weight, and SGA. Information on birth weight and gestational age were obtained from the DMBR, SMBR and FMBR. Gestational age in the DMBR was previously based on the date of last menstrual period (LMP), but in the recent 20 years, ultrasound measurements have been increasingly used to correct LMP if needed. In Sweden, early second trimester ultrasonography to estimate gestational age is routinely offered since 1990, and 95% of women accept this offer, otherwise the date of the LMP is used. Gestational age in the FMBR was estimated from the date of the LMP, unless there was a discrepancy with the first-or second-trimester ultrasonography measurements of more than seven or 14 days, respectively, in which case the latter measurements were used. We categorized gestational age at birth into six groups: 22-28 weeks, 29-32 weeks, 33-36 weeks, 37-38 weeks, 39-41 weeks, and 42-45 weeks. We categorized birth weight into 10 groups: <1000 g, 1000-1499 g, 1500-1999 g, 2000-2499 g, 2500-2999 g, 3000-3499 g, 3500-3999 g, 4000-4499 g, 4500-4999 g, and ≥5000 g. Expected birth weight was calculated using the sex-specific fetal growth curves for gestational age by Marsal et al. [43]. SGA was defined as a birth weight < –2 SD of expected birth weight, large for gestational age (LGA) as >2 SD of expected birth weight [43], and appropriate for gestational age (AGA) as ≥ –2 SD and ≤2 SD of expected birth weight. Z-scores were calculated using the following formula: Z-score = (birth weight-expected birth weight according to gestational age and sex)/SD of expected birth weight according to gestational age and sex.

Outcome
Diagnosis of asthma in young children aged 0-3 years is difficult because asthma symptoms are often non-specific [44]. Self-reported asthma cannot be validated against a medical diagnosis because of recall bias and individual differences in symptom perception [45]. Using population-based register data to obtain information

about asthma can be useful as they do not depend on recall but upon routinely medically diagnosed asthma cases. For that reason, we used hospitalization for asthma after three years of age, as recorded in the Danish National Hospital Register, the Swedish Patient Register, and the Finnish Hospital Discharge Register. The Danish National Patient Registry includes inpatient diagnosis on all hospitalizations in the country since 1977; outpatient diagnoses were included from 1995 onwards [40]. The Swedish Patient Register has collected information on inpatient care since 1964/1965 and reached nation-wide coverage in 1987 [41]. The Finnish Hospital Discharge Register contains nationwide linkable data on all inpatient hospital discharges since 1969 and all outpatient visits to public hospitals since 1998 [42]. Asthma was identified based on the following International Classification of Diseases (ICD) codes: 493 (ICD-8 and ICD-9); and J45, J46 (ICD-10). The first hospitalization for asthma was defined as the date of first admission in the registers for those who had one of the above mentioned ICD codes.

Follow-up

The children were followed from three years of age to hospitalization for asthma, emigration, death, their 18th birthday, or the end of follow up (the end of 2008 in Denmark, and the end of 2007 in Sweden or Finland), whichever came first.

Statistical analysis

We measured the cumulative risk for asthma hospitalization, using STATA (version 11.2). A method based on pseudo-values has been proposed for direct regression modeling of cumulative incidence function with right censored data at a fixed point in time [46], which was 18 years of age in our study. The pseudo-values were calculated for each individual and generated once. We computed the pseudo-values for each observation based on the difference between the complete sample and the leave-one-out estimators of relevant survival quantities. All computations were performed in STATA using the stpsurv command for generating the pseudo-observations for the failure function [46]. We used these pseudo-values in a generalized estimating equation (GEE) to model the effects of fetal development on asthma hospitalization with a log link function. The relative risk (RR) for asthma hospitalization was estimated with 95% confidence interval (CI). All multivariable models were adjusted for potential confounders, including country of residence (Denmark, Sweden, and Finland), maternal age at delivery (15-26 years, 27-30 years, ≥ 31 years), parity (1st, 2nd, 3rd and higher), mode of delivery (delivered vaginally, delivered by cesarean section), maternal social status at birth (not in labor market, unskilled workers, skilled workers and white collar workers, top level status), family

history of asthma (in father, mother or sibling), sex of the children, and calendar year of birth (1973-1977, 1978-1982, 1983-1987, 1988-1992, 1993-1997, 1998-2002, 2003-2005).

We explored the association between gestational age, birth weight, SGA and asthma hospitalization separately. When we focused on predictors as recorded at birth, we did the analysis by including gestational age and birth weight in the same model. In order to explore whether the association between fetal growth and asthma hospitalization changed with gestational age, we also performed the analysis stratified by gestational age. The association between birth weight and asthma risk was explored using 3500-3999 g as a reference. We used full term (39-41 weeks) children as the reference group when analyzing the association between gestational age and hospitalization for asthma. The association between estimated fetal growth and asthma risk was explored using AGA children as reference.

As cesarean section has been proposed to affect immune system development [47], we did a sub-analysis stratified on mode of delivery. In order to find whether fetal development acts on asthma hospitalization through complications of preterm birth, we did a sub-analysis using Danish and Finnish registers by further adjustment for complications of preterm birth (bronchopulmonary dysplasia and respiratory distress syndrome). We also did a subgroup analysis to estimate residual confounding by linking to the Danish National Birth Cohort [48]. In addition to aforementioned potential confounders, the confounding effect of weight before pregnancy, maternal asthma during pregnancy, maternal smoking during pregnancy, breastfeeding duration, environmental tobacco smoke (ETS) exposure, contact with pets in childhood, mother's marital status, and cohabit status was estimated in this subsample.

To examine whether associations between fetal development and onset of asthma were dependent on the asthma definition, we also replicated our analyses by identifying asthma on the basis of asthma medications in live singleton births during 1993-2005 recorded in the DMBR. Information on asthma medication was obtained from the Danish National Prescription Registry [49]. The anatomical therapeutical chemical (ATC) codes for inhaled asthma drugs were: inhaled β_2-agonists (R03AC02, R03AC03, R03AC04, R03AC12 and R03AC13), inhaled glucocorticoids (R03BA01, R03BA02 and R03BA05), fixed-dose combination of inhaled β_2-agonists and glucocorticoids (R03AK06 and R03AK07), and leukotriene receptor antagonists (R03DC03). We defined asthma according to at least two prescriptions of asthma drugs after three years of age. Medications prescribed on the same day were considered to represent one prescription. The first asthma occurrence was defined as the date of first anti-asthmatic drugs redeemed.

Table 1 Characteristics of study population according to estimated fetal growth

Characteristics	N	SGA	AGA	LGA
Gestational age				
22-28 weeks	10,632	21.5	72.5	6.0
29-32 weeks	31,964	22.0	72.4	5.6
33-36 weeks	218,432	8.5	85.4	6.1
37-38 weeks	934,450	3.1	91.3	5.6
39-41 weeks	4,010,066	2.3	94.7	3.0
42-45 weeks	450,963	4.4	94.2	1.4
Birth weight				
<1000 g	7,633	54.3	44.9	0.8
1000-1499 g	17,555	49.3	50.1	0.6
1500-1999 g	36,768	45.9	53.7	0.4
2000-2499 g	123,725	42.2	57.5	0.3
2500-2999 g	598,400	13.5	86.3	0.2
3000-3499 g	1,828,077	0.3	99.5	0.2
3500-3999 g	1,995,356	0	99.2	0.8
4000-4499 g	855,601	0	91.8	8.2
4500-4999 g	170,630	0	50.7	49.3
≥5000 g	22,762	0	4.1	95.9
Country of residence				
Denmark	1,538,093	3.5	93.0	3.5
Sweden	3,067,670	3.0	93.8	3.2
Finland	1,050,744	2.2	93.6	4.2
Maternal age at delivery				
15-26 years	2,089,571	3.4	94.1	2.5
27-30 years	1,604,838	2.7	93.9	3.4
≥31 years	1,961,791	2.7	92.7	4.6
Unknown	307	5.9	91.2	2.9
Maternal social status				
Not in labor market	836,704	3.3	93.3	3.4
Unskilled workers	1,131,613	3.0	93.5	3.5
Skilled workers and white collar workers	1,591,435	2.8	93.7	3.5
Top level status	778,580	2.8	93.6	3.6
Unknown	1,318,175	3.0	93.5	3.5
Parity				
1	2,332,141	4.1	93.9	2.0
2	2,018,981	2.2	93.9	3.9
≥3	1,305,385	2.2	92.3	5.5
Mode of delivery				
Delivered vaginally	5,020,529	2.5	94.3	3.2
Delivered by cesarean section	635,077	6.7	87.4	5.9
Unknown	901	3.6	92.2	4.2

Table 1 Characteristics of study population according to estimated fetal growth (Continued)

Sex of the child				
Boy	2,902,138	2.9	93.5	3.6
Girl	2,754,369	3.0	93.6	3.4
Calendar year of birth				
1973-1977	493,193	4.5	93.0	2.5
1978-1982	629,589	3.8	93.6	2.6
1983-1987	777,959	3.3	93.7	3.0
1988-1992	1,178,159	2.8	93.6	3.6
1993-1997	1,106,229	2.5	93.5	4.0
1998-2002	995,480	2.5	93.6	3.9
2003-2005	475,898	2.4	93.7	3.9
Family history of asthma				
Yes	416,278	3.7	92.8	3.5
No	5,240,229	2.9	93.6	3.5

Ethics

The study was approved by Danish Data Protection Agency and Scientific Ethics Committee of Central Region Jutland in Denmark and Research Ethics Committee (EPN) at Karolinska Institute in Sweden, Statistics Finland and National Institute for Health and Welfare (THL) in Finland. No informed consent is needed for register-based study based on encrypted data according to the legislation in Denmark, Sweden, and Finland.

Results

The mean follow-up time was 10.6 years (95% CI 1.1-15.0), altogether 6.0×10^7 person-years. A total of 131,783 children were hospitalized at least once for asthma during the study period. Table 1 shows the characteristics of the study population.

The risk of hospitalization for asthma increased with lower birth weight and shorter gestational age. The highest cumulative incidence was found in children born with a birth weight of < 1000 g and extremely preterm births (children born at 22-28 weeks) (Figures 1 and 2). A 1000-g decrease in birth weight corresponded to a RR of 1.17 (95% CI 1.15-1.18). Compared with full term (39-41 weeks) children, the adjusted RR of asthma hospitalization born at 22-28 weeks was 2.26 (95% CI 2.10-2.43). Even early term (37-38 weeks) children had a higher risk of hospitalization for asthma than full term children (RR 1.10, 95% CI 1.09-1.12). A one-week decrease in gestational age corresponded to a RR of 1.05 (95% CI 1.04-1.06). Children born SGA were associated with a moderately increased risk of asthma hospitalization (RR 1.20, 95% CI 1.16-1.24). Risk for asthma increased steadily with decreasing Z-score for children (RR 1.03, 95% CI 1.02-1.04) (Table 2). When analyzing predictors

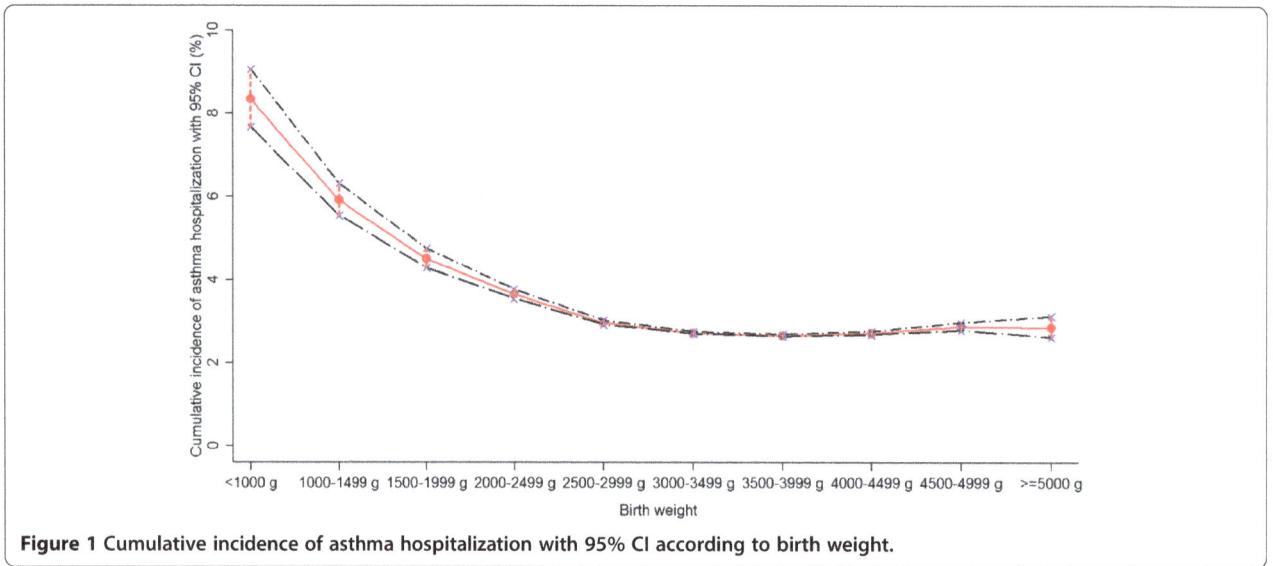

Figure 1 Cumulative incidence of asthma hospitalization with 95% CI according to birth weight.

for asthma hospitalization, we included gestational age and birth weight in the same model. The RR was 1.08 (95% CI 1.06-1.09) for a 1000-g decrease in birth weight and 1.04 (95% CI 1.03 -1.05) for a one-week decrease in gestational age.

We estimated the association between fetal growth and asthma hospitalization stratified by gestational age. There was a significant association between SGA and increased risk of asthma in term but not in preterm born (<37 weeks) children. However, with the exception of extremely preterm born children (22–28 weeks) and children born after 42 gestational weeks, the risk of asthma

increased with decreasing Z-sore in all preterm and term gestational age groups. In extremely and moderately preterm born children (22-32 weeks), LGA children had a decreased risk of asthma hospitalization (Table 3).

The associations were similar in children who were delivered vaginally and by cesarean section (data not shown). The associations between low birth weight, short gestational age, SGA, and risk of asthma hospitalization attenuated slightly by further adjustment for complications of preterm birth but remained statistically significant (data not shown). In sub-analysis, after further adjustment for weight before pregnancy, maternal asthma

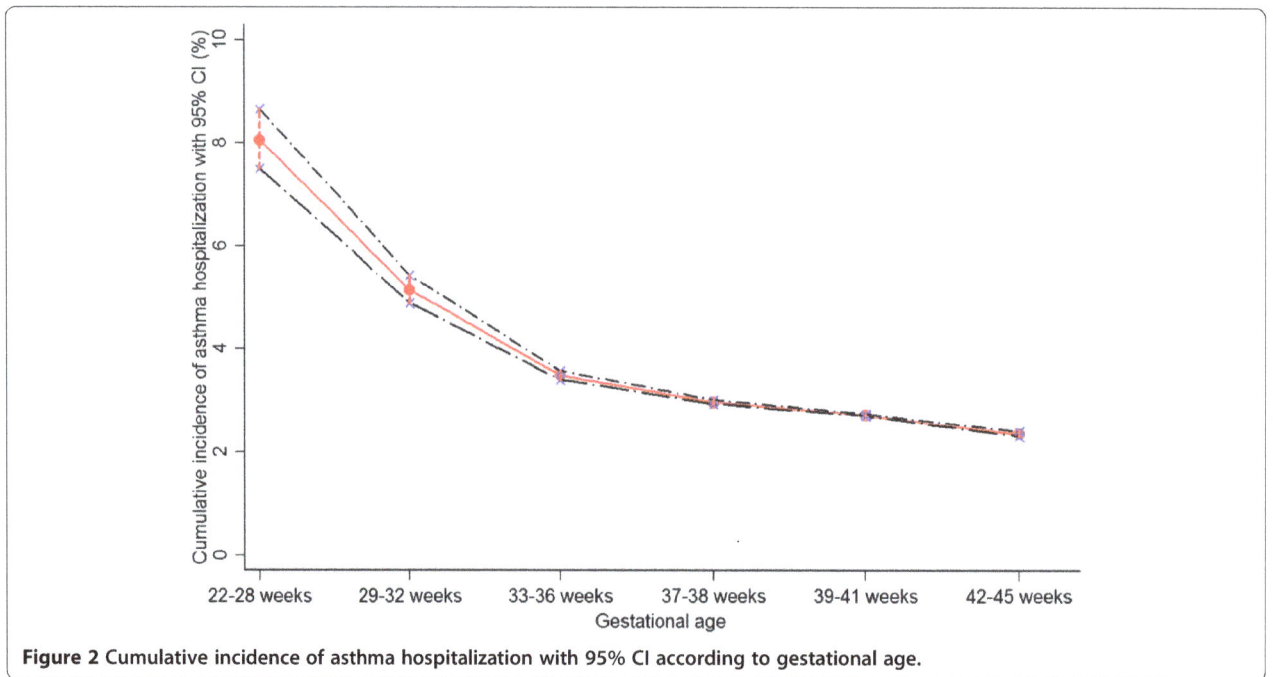

Figure 2 Cumulative incidence of asthma hospitalization with 95% CI according to gestational age.

Table 2 RR for asthma hospitalization in childhood according to birth weight, gestational age, and fetal growth

Fetal development variables	Cases	Cumulative incidence (%)	Crude RR	Adjusted RR* (95% CI)
Birth weight				
<1000 g	542	8.35	3.03	2.33 (2.14-2.53)
1000-1499 g	897	5.93	2.21	1.81 (1.68-1.95)
1500-1999 g	1,423	4.51	1.69	1.48 (1.40-1.57)
2000-2499 g	3,823	3.67	1.38	1.33 (1.28-1.38)
2500-2999 g	14,992	2.98	1.12	1.15 (1.12-1.17)
3000-3499 g	41,716	2.73	1.02	1.05 (1.04-1.07)
3500-3999 g	44,451	2.67	1	1 (ref)
4000-4499 g	19,371	2.73	1.02	0.99 (0.97-1.01)
4500-4999 g	4,037	2.89	1.08	1.03 (0.99-1.06)
≥5000 g	531	2.87	1.08	1.01 (0.92-1.11)
Birth weight per 1000-g decrease	-	-	1.18	1.17 (1.15-1.18)
Gestational age				
22-28 weeks	737	8.07	2.89	2.26 (2.10-2.43)
29-32 weeks	1,416	5.16	1.88	1.63 (1.54-1.73)
33-36 weeks	6,471	3.50	1.28	1.26 (1.22-1.29)
37-38 weeks	23,062	2.98	1.09	1.10 (1.09-1.12)
39-41 weeks	91,055	2.73	1	1 (ref)
42-45 weeks	9,042	2.37	0.86	0.98 (0.95-1.00)
GA per reduced week	-	-	1.07	1.05 (1.04-1.06)
Fetal growth				
SGA	4,878	3.38	1.23	1.20 (1.16-1.24)
AGA	121,741	2.76	1	1 (ref)
LGA	5,164	3.18	1.15	1.05 (1.02-1.09)
Z-score per decreased of SD	-	-	1.00	1.03 (1.02-1.04)

*Adjusted for country of residence, maternal age at delivery, maternal social status, parity, mode of delivery, sex of the child, calendar year of birth and family history of asthma.

Table 3 RR for asthma hospitalization in childhood according to gestational age and estimated fetal growth

Fetal development variables	Cases	Cumulative incidence (%)	Crude RR	Adjusted RR* (95% CI)
22-28 weeks				
SGA	180	9.09	1.14	1.02 (0.86-1.21)
AGA	527	7.96	1	1 (ref)
LGA	30	5.43	0.71	0.71 (0.46-1.11)
Z-score per decreased of SD	-	-	1.04	1.02 (0.99-1.04)
29-32 weeks				
SGA	359	6.15	1.20	1.07 (0.94-1.22)
AGA	1,010	5.05	1	1 (ref)
LGA	47	2.96	0.58	0.60 (0.43-0.85)
Z-score per decreased of SD	-	-	1.06	1.04 (1.02-1.07)
33-36 weeks				
SGA	675	4.27	1.26	1.06 (0.97-1.17)
AGA	5,409	3.43	1	1 (ref)
LGA	387	3.41	0.99	0.94 (0.84-1.05)
Z-score per decreased of SD	-	-	1.05	1.03 (1.01-1.04)
37-38 weeks				
SGA	860	3.56	1.22	1.15 (1.07-1.24)
AGA	20,735	2.93	1	1 (ref)
LGA	1,467	3.43	1.17	1.03 (0.97-1.09)
Z-score per decreased of SD	-	-	0.99	1.02 (1.01-1.03)
39-41 weeks				
SGA	2,349	3.01	1.12	1.12 (1.07-1.17)
AGA	85,611	2.71	1	1 (ref)
LGA	3,095	3.06	1.13	1.06 (1.02-1.10)
Z-score per decreased of SD	-	-	0.99	1.02 (1.01-1.03)
42-45 weeks				
SGA	455	2.51	1.07	1.11 (0.98-1.25)
AGA	8,449	2.36	1	1 (ref)
LGA	138	2.83	1.20	1.15 (0.95-1.40)
Z-score per decreased of SD	-	-	1.00	1.02 (0.99-1.05)

*Adjusted for country of residence, maternal age at delivery, maternal social status, parity, mode of delivery, sex of the child, calendar year of birth and family history of asthma.

during pregnancy, maternal smoking during pregnancy, breastfeeding duration, ETS exposure, contact with pets, mother's marital status, and cohabit status, the estimated RRs were similar to those obtained without adjustment for these potential confounders (data not shown).

When the outcome was asthma medication, the aforementioned associations remained statistically significant although the magnitude of associations decreased slightly (Table 4).

Discussion

Our results indicated that risk for asthma hospitalization increased with lower birth weight and shorter gestational age. Even early term (37-38 weeks) children had a higher risk of hospitalization for asthma than full term

(39-41 weeks) children. SGA was associated with a slightly increased risk of hospitalization for asthma in term but not in preterm born children. LGA was associated with a decreased risk of asthma hospitalization in extremely and moderately preterm born children.

The inverse association we found between birth weight and asthma hospitalization concurs with most previous

Table 4 RR for asthma hospitalization and medication in childhood according to birth weight, gestational age and fetal growth in Denmark, 1993-2005

Fetal development variables	Asthma hospitalization				Asthma medication			
	Cases	Cumulative incidence (%)	Crude RR	Adjusted RR* (95% CI)	Cases	Cumulative incidence (%)	Crude RR	Adjusted RR* (95% CI)
Birth weight								
<1000 g	94	13.58	2.64	2.82 (2.12-3.74)	306	34.06	2.00	1.94 (1.75-2.15)
1000-1499 g	184	9.01	1.91	1.71 (1.42-2.06)	624	27.12	1.63	1.51 (1.39-1.65)
1500-1999 g	318	7.76	1.64	1.41 (1.21-1.64)	1,107	24.23	1.45	1.37 (1.28-1.47)
2000-2499 g	812	6.87	1.46	1.30 (1.17-1.44)	2,950	22.30	1.34	1.29 (1.22-1.36)
2500-2999 g	2,919	5.29	1.12	1.10 (1.03-1.18)	11,142	18.79	1.13	1.11 (1.07-1.16)
3000-3499 g	8,099	5.01	1.06	1.07 (1.02-1.13)	30,145	16.89	1.02	1.01 (0.98-1.04)
3500-3999 g	8,500	4.72	1	1 (ref)	32,242	16.43	1	1 (ref)
4000-4499 g	4,045	4.89	1.04	1.01 (0.95-1.08)	14,984	16.55	1.00	0.99 (0.95-1.02)
4500-4999 g	869	4.74	1.01	1.02 (0.92-1.12)	3,165	16.59	1.00	1.00 (0.95-1.05)
≥5000 g	135	5.56	1.18	1.15 (0.91-1.45)	463	16.48	1.01	0.99 (0.89-1.08)
Birth weight per 1000-g decrease	-	-	1.17	1.15 (1.11-1.19)	-	-	1.13	1.11 (1.10-1.13)
Gestational age								
22-28 weeks	129	11.72	2.34	2.37 (1.87-2.99)	412	30.69	1.86	1.78 (1.64-1.94)
29-32 weeks	301	8.65	1.79	1.49 (1.29-1.72)	1,084	25.67	1.56	1.45 (1.36-1.54)
33-36 weeks	1,318	6.36	1.32	1.20 (1.10-1.30)	5,021	21.90	1.33	1.26 (1.22-1.30)
37-38 weeks	4,464	5.67	1.17	1.14 (1.08-1.21)	16,967	18.69	1.13	1.10 (1.08-1.13)
39-41 weeks	17,616	4.79	1	1 (ref)	65,682	16.44	1	1 (ref)
42-45 weeks	2,147	4.61	0.96	0.94 (0.88-1.01)	7,962	17.40	1.05	1.05 (0.95-1.16)
GA per reduced week	-	-	1.06	1.05 (1.04-1.06)	-	-	1.04	1.04 (1.03-1.05)
Birth weight for gestational age								
SGA	1,055	6.36	1.29	1.20 (1.10-1.31)	3,776	21.15	1.25	1.19 (1.14-1.24)
AGA	23,784	4.94	1	1 (ref)	89,263	17.02	1	1 (ref)
LGA	1,136	5.32	1.07	1.11 (0.99-1.24)	4,089	17.34	1.02	1.04 (0.99-1.09)
Z-score per decreased of SD	-	-	1.03	1.01 (0.99-1.03)	-	-	1.03	1.02 (1.01-1.03)

*Adjusted for maternal age at delivery, maternal social status, parity, mode of delivery, sex of the child, calendar year of birth and family history of asthma.

cohort studies [8,9,14,21,23-26]. Low birth weight often results from fetal growth restriction, preterm birth or both. Low birth weight may act as a mediating factor between the determinants of low birth weight and asthma hospitalization. Thus, these associations may reflect unknown causes of asthma also influencing fetal growth and/or length of gestation.

In the present study, an increased risk of hospitalization for asthma was associated with decreasing gestational age. The finding is consistent with most [8-17], although not all [18-22], previous cohort studies, which may reflect instable results due to small sample sizes [18-22]. Wheezing symptoms in children under three years are common and often transient [50], and including children with transient wheezes in the asthma group may dilute possible associations specific to asthma [51]. The inconsistent finding may reflect that the association we found is mainly seen for severe cases. The preterm birth may be related to a

deficit in the structure and function of the lung at birth [3], which may increase the risk of subsequent asthma development. It is also possible that preterm birth and asthma share common genetic determinants or environmental exposures. For instance, studies have indicated that maternal asthma is associated with both preterm birth and childhood asthma [9,52].

We also found that early term children had a higher risk of hospitalization for asthma compared with full term children [17]. Although the relative risk of hospitalization for asthma for early term children is lower than for preterm children, the larger number of children born at early term may present a greater disease burden in the population.

Evidence linking fetal growth restriction to childhood asthma is limited. In the present study, SGA was associated with a slightly increased risk of hospitalization for asthma. Our findings are in concordance with two of three cohort studies [15,24], but not with an early study [9]. Several studies have limited power to detect the modest association we observed [32,33,53,54]. And cross-sectional studies may be vulnerable to recall bias [14,16,17]. As preterm born infants are smaller than fetuses of the same gestational age [39], studies, categorizing SGA based on the distributions of live births [32,33,53] may misclassify SGA as AGA, and thereby dilute a possible association. Two previous studies explored the association between fetal growth and asthma using measured fetal growth as a predictor for asthma [9,54], with null findings. One study had limited power to detect the modest association we observed due to smaller sample size [54]. Use of a broader asthma definition may lead to more non-differential misclassification and therefore dilute the association [9]. The conflicting findings may also suggest that the association between fetal growth and hospitalization for asthma is weak, or is caused by factors that correlate with fetal growth. Normal lung development depends on the presence of appropriate oxygen tension and nutrition. Children born with fetal growth restriction have a greater risk of developing brochopulmonary dysplasia [4], which is associated with childhood asthma [55], providing a potential mechanism by which fetal growth restriction may increase the risk of asthma. However, this probably does not fully explain the association we observed as the association attenuated after further adjustment for the respiratory complications of preterm birth but remained statistically significant. Factors responsible for fetal growth restriction may also lead to "programming" of the respiratory or immune systems [56], predisposing children to the development of asthma. The association between SGA and hospitalization for asthma was observed in term but not in preterm born children. The underlying mechanism is not clear. Further studies elucidating the mechanisms are warranted.

A novel finding in our study was LGA was associated with a deceased risk for asthma hospitalization in extremely and moderately preterm born children. Our result is consistent with one previous study showing the association of high birth weight for gestational age and a decreased risk of asthma in preterm children [24]. Our data support the previous study that has found a reduced risk of chronic lung disease in children born large for gestational age and preterm, compared with children born appropriate for gestational age and preterm [4].

Our study is the largest study so far on this topic. The large sample size allowed us to analyze the association between birth characteristics and child hospitalization for asthma with almost complete follow-up.

Our study also has limitations. We did not investigate confounding from familial lifestyle and environmental factors, including housing status, early exposure to allergens, diet and nutrition. We used first hospital discharge diagnosis after three years of age as the outcome, and therefore, our findings addressed severe asthma or factors that may lower the threshold for asthma hospitalization. Although we did a sub-analysis with asthma medication and got similar findings, we did not include all patients with mild symptoms who did not seek medical help. Therefore, our findings cannot be generalized to those children as well as children with transient asthma. Second, children born with low gestational age or fetal growth restriction may have more opportunities to have asthma diagnosed because they are hospitalized more frequently due to co-morbidity [57]. Our findings were similar to those reported in other large cohort studies using different definitions of asthma [15, 24]. In a sub-analysis, we compared findings using two different criteria to identify cases: prescription data and hospitalization data. We found that short gestational age and fetal growth restriction increased the risk of asthma regardless of data source. Third, our study focused on the Nordic populations, which have comprehensive and mainly publicly financed health care systems. In addition, asthma is a heterogeneous disease and the distribution of asthma subtypes is dependent upon the interaction of genetic characteristics and environmental factors. Thereby, our findings may not be generalized to other population.

Conclusions

Fetal growth and gestational age may play a direct or indirect causal role in the development of childhood asthma.

Abbreviations
AGA: Appropriate for gestational age; CI: Confidence interval; DMBR: The Danish Medical Birth Registry; ETS: Environmental tobacco smoke; FMBR: The Finnish Medical Birth Register; GA: Gestational age; ICD: The International Classification of Diseases; LGA: Large for gestational age; LMP: Last menstrual period; RR: Relative risk; SGA: Small for gestational age; SMBR: The Swedish Medical Birth Register.

Competing interests
All authors declare that they have no competing interests.

Authors' contributions
XL contributed to data preparation, analysis and interpretation of data, and drafted the manuscript. JO contributed to study design, data analysis, interpretation of the results, and revised the manuscript. EA contributed to study design, data analysis, interpretation of the results, and revised the manuscript. WY contributed to study design, data analysis, the interpretation of the results, and revised the manuscript. SC contributed to study design, data analysis, the interpretation of the results, and revised the manuscript. MG contributed to study design, data analysis, the interpretation of the results, and revised the manuscript. JL contributed to the conception and the design of the study, to data acquisition, data analysis, the interpretation of the results, and revised the manuscript. All authors approved the final manuscript as submitted.

Acknowledgements
The study was supported by the European Research Council (ERC-2010-StG-260242-PROGEURO), the Danish Medical Research Council (project no. 09-072986), and the Swedish Council for Working Life and Social Research (Grant no. 2010-0092). XL is also supported by Mobility PhD fellowship from Aarhus University.

Author details

[1]Section for Epidemiology, Department of Public Health, Aarhus University, Aarhus, Denmark. [2]Department of Epidemiology and Social Science on Reproductive Health, Shanghai Institute of Planned Parenthood Research, WHO Collaborating Center for Research in Human Reproduction, National Population & Family Planning Key Laboratory of Contraceptive Drugs and Devices, Shanghai, China. [3]Department of Epidemiology, Fielding School of Public Health, University of California, Los Angeles, CA, USA. [4]National Centre for Register-Based Research, Aarhus University, Aarhus, Denmark. [5]CIRRAU-Centre for Integrated Register-based Research, Aarhus University, Aarhus, Denmark. [6]Clinical Epidemiology Unit, Department of Medicin Solna, Karolinska University Hospital, Karolinska Institute, Stockholm, Sweden. [7]Information Department, THL National Institute for Health and Welfare, Helsinki, Finland. [8]NHV Nordic School of Public Health, Gothenburg, Sweden.

References

1. Karaca-Mandic P, Jena AB, Joyce GF, Goldman DP: Out-of-pocket medication costs and use of medications and health care services among children with asthma. *JAMA* 2012, **307**(12):1284–1291.
2. National Institutes of Health: National Heart, Lung, and Blood Institute: *National Asthma Education and Prevention Program Expert Panel Report 3: Guidelines for the Diagnosis and Management of Asthma. NIH Publication No. 07-4051.* Bethesda, MD: National Heart, Lung, and Blood Institute; 2007.
3. Moss TJ: Respiratory consequences of preterm birth. *Clin Exp Pharmacol Physiol* 2006, **33**(3):280–284.
4. Lal MK, Manktelow BN, Draper ES, Field DJ: Chronic lung disease of prematurity and intrauterine growth retardation: a population-based study. *Pediatrics* 2003, **111**(3):483–487.
5. Canoy D, Pekkanen J, Elliott P, Pouta A, Laitinen J, Hartikainen AL, Zitting P, Patel S, Little MP, Jarvelin MR: Early growth and adult respiratory function in men and women followed from the fetal period to adulthood. *Thorax* 2007, **62**(5):396–402.
6. McDade TW, Beck MA, Kuzawa C, Adair LS: Prenatal undernutrition, postnatal environments, and antibody response to vaccination in adolescence. *Am J Clin Nutr* 2001, **74**(4):543–548.
7. Haland G, Carlsen KC, Sandvik L, Devulapalli CS, Munthe-Kaas MC, Pettersen M, Carlsen KH: Reduced lung function at birth and the risk of asthma at 10 years of age. *N Engl J Med* 2006, **355**(16):1682–1689.
8. Metsala J, Kilkkinen A, Kaila M, Tapanainen H, Klaukka T, Gissler M, Virtanen SM: Perinatal factors and the risk of asthma in childhood–a population-based register study in Finland. *Am J Epidemiol* 2008, **168**(2):170–178.
9. Jaakkola JJ, Gissler M: Maternal smoking in pregnancy, fetal development, and childhood asthma. *Am J Public Health* 2004, **94**(1):136–140.
10. Kelly YJ, Brabin BJ, Milligan P, Heaf DP, Reid J, Pearson MG: Maternal asthma, premature birth, and the risk of respiratory morbidity in schoolchildren in Merseyside. *Thorax* 1995, **50**(5):525–530.
11. Miller JE: Predictors of asthma in young children: does reporting source affect our conclusions? *Am J Epidemiol* 2001, **154**(3):245–250.
12. Yuan W, Fonager K, Olsen J, Sorensen HT: Prenatal factors and use of anti-asthma medications in early childhood: a population-based Danish birth cohort study. *Eur J Epidemiol* 2003, **18**(8):763–768.
13. Dik N, Tate RB, Manfreda J, Anthonisen NR: Risk of physician-diagnosed asthma in the first 6 years of life. *Chest* 2004, **126**(4):1147–1153.
14. Davidson R, Roberts SE, Wotton CJ, Goldacre MJ: Influence of maternal and perinatal factors on subsequent hospitalisation for asthma in children: evidence from the Oxford record linkage study. *BMC Pulm Med* 2010, **10**:14.
15. Kallen B, Finnstrom O, Nygren KG, Otterblad Olausson P: Association between preterm birth and intrauterine growth retardation and child asthma. *Eur Respir J* 2013, **41**(3):671–676.
16. Goyal NK, Fiks AG, Lorch SA: Association of late-preterm birth with asthma in young children: practice-based study. *Pediatrics* 2011, **128**(4):e830–e838.
17. Boyle EM, Poulsen G, Field DJ, Kurinczuk JJ, Wolke D, Alfirevic Z, Quigley MA: Effects of gestational age at birth on health outcomes at 3 and 5 years of age: population based cohort study. *BMJ (Clin Res Ed)* 2012, **344**:e896.
18. Leadbitter P, Pearce N, Cheng S, Sears MR, Holdaway MD, Flannery EM, Herbison GP, Beasley R: Relationship between fetal growth and the

19. Rasanen M, Kaprio J, Laitinen T, Winter T, Koskenvuo M, Laitinen LA: Perinatal risk factors for asthma in Finnish adolescent twins. *Thorax* 2000, **55**(1):25–31.
20. Steffensen FH, Sorensen HT, Gillman MW, Rothman KJ, Sabroe S, Fischer P, Olsen J: Low birth weight and preterm delivery as risk factors for asthma and atopic dermatitis in young adult males. *Epidemiol (Cambridge, Mass)* 2000, **11**(2):185–188.
21. Annesi-Maesano I, Moreau D, Strachan D: In utero and perinatal complications preceding asthma. *Allergy* 2001, **56**(6):491–497.
22. Katz KA, Pocock SJ, Strachan DP: Neonatal head circumference, neonatal weight, and risk of hayfever, asthma and eczema in a large cohort of adolescents from Sheffield, England. *Clin Exp Allergy* 2003, **33**(6):737–745.
23. Villamor E, Iliadou A, Cnattingius S: Is the association between low birth weight and asthma independent of genetic and shared environmental factors? *Am J Epidemiol* 2009, **169**(11):1337–1343.
24. Ortqvist AK, Lundholm C, Carlstrom E, Lichtenstein P, Cnattingius S, Almqvist C: Familial factors do not confound the association between birth weight and childhood asthma. *Pediatrics* 2009, **124**(4):e737–e743.
25. Kindlund K, Thomsen SF, Stensballe LG, Skytthe A, Kyvik KO, Backer V, Bisgaard H: Birth weight and risk of asthma in 3-9-year-old twins: exploring the fetal origins hypothesis. *Thorax* 2010, **65**(2):146–149.
26. Rautava L, Hakkinen U, Korvenranta E, Andersson S, Gissler M, Hallman M, Korvenranta H, Leipala J, Peltola M, Tammela O, Lehtonen L: Health and the use of health care services in 5-year-old very-low-birth-weight infants. *Acta Paediatr* 2010, **99**(7):1073–1079.
27. Sin DD, Spier S, Svenson LW, Schopflocher DP, Senthilselvan A, Cowie RL, Man SF: The relationship between birth weight and childhood asthma: a population-based cohort study. *Arch Pediatr Adolesc Med* 2004, **158**(1):60–64.
28. Caudri D, Wijga A, Gehring U, Smit HA, Brunekreef B, Kerkhof M, Hoekstra M, Gerritsen J, de Jongste JC: Respiratory symptoms in the first 7 years of life and birth weight at term: the PIAMA Birth Cohort. *Am J Respir Crit Care Med* 2007, **175**(10):1078–1085.
29. Rusconi F, Galassi C, Forastiere F, Bellasio M, De Sario M, Ciccone G, Brunetti L, Chellini E, Corbo G, La Grutta S, Lombardi E, Piffer S, Talassi F, Biggeri A, Pearce N: Maternal complications and procedures in pregnancy and at birth and wheezing phenotypes in children. *Am J Respir Crit Care Med* 2007, **175**(1):16–21.
30. Gardosi J: Customized fetal growth standards: rationale and clinical application. *Semin Perinatol* 2004, **28**(1):33–40.
31. Wang WH, Chen PC, Hsieh WS, Lee YL: Joint effects of birth outcomes and childhood body mass index on respiratory symptoms. *Eur Respir J* 2012, **39**(5):1213–1219.
32. Protudjer JL, Dwarkanath P, Kozyrskyj AL, Srinivasan K, Kurpad A, Becker AB: Subsequent childhood asthma and wheeze amongst small-for-gestational-age infants in Manitoba and India: an international partnership initiative. *Allergy Asthma Clin Immunol* 2010, **6**(Suppl 3):P36–P36.
33. Miyake Y, Tanaka K: Lack of relationship between birth conditions and allergic disorders in Japanese children aged 3 years. *J Asthma* 2013, **50**(6):555–559.
34. Grischkan J, Storfer-Isser A, Rosen CL, Larkin EK, Kirchner HL, South A, Wilson-Costello DC, Martin RJ, Redline S: Variation in childhood asthma among former preterm infants. *J Pediatr* 2004, **144**(3):321–326.
35. Koshy G, Akrouf KA, Kelly Y, Delpisheh A, Brabin BJ: Asthma in children in relation to pre-term birth and fetal growth restriction. *Matern Child Health J* 2012, **17**(6):1119–1129.
36. To T, Guan J, Wang C, Radhakrishnan D, McLimont S, Latycheva O, Gershon AS: Is large birth weight associated with asthma risk in early childhood? *Arch Dis Child* 2012, **97**(2):169–171.
37. Taveras EM, Camargo CA Jr, Rifas-Shiman SL, Oken E, Gold DR, Weiss ST, Gillman MW: Association of birth weight with asthma-related outcomes at age 2 years. *Pediatr Pulmonol* 2006, **41**(7):643–648.
38. Thomson AM, Billewicz WZ, Hytten FE: The assessment of fetal growth. *J Obstet Gynaec Brit Cwlth* 1968, **75**:903–916.
39. Morken NH, Kallen K, Jacobsson B: Fetal growth and onset of delivery: a nationwide population-based study of preterm infants. *Am J Obstet Gynecol* 2006, **195**(1):154–161.
40. Andersen TF, Madsen M, Jorgensen J, Mellemkjoer L, Olsen JH: The Danish national hospital register: a valuable source of data for modern health sciences. *Dan Med Bull* 1999, **46**(3):263–268.

41. Kvalitet och innehåll i patientregistret: *Utskrivningar från sluttenvården 1964-2007 och besök i specialiserad öppenvård (exclusive primärvårdsbesök) 1997-2007*. [http://www.socialstyrelsen.se/Lists/Artikelkatalog/Attachments/8306/2009-125-15_200912515_rev2.pdf]

42. Sund R: **Quality of the Finnish hospital discharge register: a systematic review.** *Scand J Public Health* 2012, **40**(6):505–515.

43. Marsal K, Persson PH, Larsen T, Lilja H, Selbing A, Sultan B: **Intrauterine growth curves based on ultrasonically estimated foetal weights.** *Acta Paediatr* 1996, **85**(7):843–848.

44. Martinez FD, Wright AL, Taussig LM, Holberg CJ, Halonen M, Morgan WJ: **Asthma and wheezing in the first six years of life: the group health medical associates.** *N Engl J Med* 1995, **332**(3):133–138.

45. Peat JK, Toelle BG, Marks GB, Mellis CM: **Continuing the debate about measuring asthma in population studies.** *Thorax* 2001, **56**(5):406–411.

46. Parner ET, Andersen PK: **Regression analysis of censored data using pseudo-observations.** *Stata J* 2010, **10**(3):408–422.

47. Biasucci G, Benenati B, Morelli L, Bessi E, Boehm G: **Cesarean delivery may affect the early biodiversity of intestinal bacteria.** *J Nutr* 2008, **138**(9):1796S–1800S.

48. Olsen J, Melbye M, Olsen SF, Sorensen TI, Aaby P, Andersen AM, Taxbol D, Hansen KD, Juhl M, Schow TB, Sørensen HT, Andresen J, Mortensen EL, Olesen AW, Søndergaard C: **The Danish national birth cohort–its background, structure and aim.** *Scand J Public Health* 2001, **29**(4):300–307.

49. Kildemoes HW, Sorensen HT, Hallas J: **The Danish national prescription registry.** *Scand J Public Health* 2011, **39**(7 Suppl):38–41.

50. Zuidgeest MG, van Dijk L, Smit HA, van der Wouden JC, Brunekreef B, Leufkens HG, Bracke M: **Prescription of respiratory medication without an asthma diagnosis in children: a population based study.** *BMC Health Serv Res* 2008, **8**:16.

51. Hansen S, Strom M, Maslova E, Mortensen EL, Granstrom C, Olsen SF: **A comparison of three methods to measure asthma in epidemiologic studies: results from the Danish national birth cohort.** *PLoS One* 2012, **7**(5):e36328.

52. Firoozi F, Lemiere C, Beauchesne MF, Perreault S, Forget A, Blais L: **Impact of maternal asthma on perinatal outcomes: a two-stage sampling cohort study.** *Eur J Epidemiol* 2012, **27**(3):205–214.

53. Gessner BD, Chimonas MA: **Asthma is associated with preterm birth but not with small for gestational age status among a population-based cohort of medicaid-enrolled children <10 years of age.** *Thorax* 2007, **62**(3):231–236.

54. Bardin C, Piuze G, Papageorgiou A: **Outcome at 5 years of age of SGA and AGA infants born less than 28 weeks of gestation.** *Semin Perinatol* 2004, **28**(4):288–294.

55. Palta M, Sadek-Badawi M, Sheehy M, Albanese A, Weinstein M, McGuinness G, Peters ME: **Respiratory symptoms at age 8 years in a cohort of very low birth weight children.** *Am J Epidemiol* 2001, **154**(6):521–529.

56. Moore SE: **Nutrition, immunity and the fetal and infant origins of disease hypothesis in developing countries.** *Proc Nutr Soc* 1998, **57**(2):241–247.

57. Selling KE, Carstensen J, Finnstrom O, Josefsson A, Sydsjo G: **Hospitalizations in adolescence and early adulthood among Swedish men and women born preterm or small for gestational age.** *Epidemiol (Cambridge, Mass)* 2008, **19**(1):63–70.

8

Vitamin C and common cold-induced asthma

Harri Hemilä

Abstract

Background: Asthma exacerbations are often induced by the common cold, which, in turn, can be alleviated by vitamin C.

Objective: To investigate whether vitamin C administration influences common cold-induced asthma.

Methods: Systematic review and statistical analysis of the identified trials. Medline, Scopus and Cochrane Central were searched for studies that give information on the effects of vitamin C on common cold-induced asthma. All clinically relevant outcomes related to asthma were included in this review. The estimates of vitamin C effect and their confidence intervals [CI] were calculated for the included studies.

Results: Three studies that were relevant for examining the role of vitamin C on common cold-induced asthma were identified. The three studies had a total of 79 participants. Two studies were randomized double-blind placebo-controlled trials. A study in Nigeria on asthmatics whose asthma attacks were precipitated by respiratory infections found that 1 g/day vitamin C decreased the occurrence of asthma attacks by 78% (95% CI: 19% to 94%). A cross-over study in former East-Germany on patients who had infection-related asthma found that 5 g/day vitamin C decreased the proportion of participants who had bronchial hypersensitivity to histamine by 52 percentage points (95% CI: 25 to 71). The third study did not use a placebo. Administration of a single dose of 1 gram of vitamin C to Italian non-asthmatic common cold patients increased the provocative concentration of histamine (PC_{20}) 3.2-fold (95% CI: 2.0 to 5.1), but the vitamin C effect was significantly less when the same participants did not suffer from the common cold.

Conclusions: The three reviewed studies differed substantially in their methods, settings and outcomes. Each of them found benefits from the administration of vitamin C; either against asthma attacks or against bronchial hypersensitivity, the latter of which is a characteristic of asthma. Given the evidence suggesting that vitamin C alleviates common cold symptoms and the findings of this systematic review, it may be reasonable for asthmatic patients to test vitamin C on an individual basis, if they have exacerbations of asthma caused by respiratory infections. More research on the role of vitamin C on common cold-induced asthma is needed.

Keywords: Anti-asthmatic agents, Ascorbic acid, Asthma, Bronchial provocation tests, Bronchoconstriction, Common cold, Forced expiratory flow rates, Histamine, Rhinovirus, Upper respiratory tract infections

Introduction

Moses Maimonides, a 12th-century physician, wrote about asthma: "I conclude that this disorder starts with a common cold, especially in the rainy season..." [1]. Consistent with this statement, recent prospective studies have detected respiratory viruses in up to 80% of asthma exacerbations of children and adults [1-5]. The severity of the cold in asthmatics within its first two days predicted the subsequent severity of the asthma exacerbation [6]. The common cold may lead to a transient bronchial hypersensitivity, which is one characteristic of asthma [7-12]. Hypothetically, preventing or alleviating common cold symptoms might reduce the incidence and severity of asthma exacerbations caused by respiratory viruses.

Vitamin C was identified in the early 1900s, in the search for the etiology of scurvy [13]. After its identification, there was much interest in the effects of vitamin C

Correspondence: harri.hemila@helsinki.fi
Department of Public Health, POB 41, University of Helsinki, Mannerheimintie 172, FIN-00014 Helsinki, Finland

on diseases unrelated to scurvy, but its role against other diseases is still undetermined. In placebo-controlled trials 1 g/day or more of vitamin C shortened the duration of colds in adults by 8% and in children by 18% [14-17]. The common cold studies did not examine the effect of vitamin C on pulmonary functions, but two trials found a greater effect on lower respiratory symptoms than on upper respiratory symptoms. Elwood et al. found that vitamin C significantly decreased the incidence of "chest colds" (−18%; cough or other chest symptoms) but not of "simple colds" (+1%; runny nose or sneezing) [18,19]. Anderson et al. found that vitamin C significantly decreased the incidence of "throat colds" (−21%) but not of "nose colds" (−2%) [18,20]. Furthermore, vitamin C prevented pneumonia in three controlled trials with participants under special conditions [17,21].

The use of vitamin C for treating asthma dates back to the 1940s. A few physicians reported that vitamin C seemed beneficial for some of their asthma patients, but other physicians found no such improvements in their asthma patients [22,23]. A recent meta-analysis of three randomized trials on vitamin C and exercise-induced bronchoconstriction found that vitamin C halved the post-exercise decline of forced expiratory volume in 1 second (FEV_1), which indicates that vitamin C has effects on some phenotypes of asthma [24].

This study was motivated by the findings that asthma exacerbations are often induced by the common cold, which in turn is alleviated by vitamin C. The objective of this systematic review was to summarize the evidence on the possible role of vitamin C administration on common cold-induced asthma.

Methods
Types of studies
Intervention studies, randomised and non-randomised, and placebo-controlled and non-placebo-controlled, that give information on the effect of vitamin C on common cold-induced asthma and/or bronchial hypersensitivity were included in this systematic review.

Types of participants
Studies on children and adults of either sex at any age were eligible.

Types of interventions
The interventions considered were the oral or intravenous administration of vitamin C (ascorbic acid or its salts) as a single dose or as multiple doses for a period.

Outcomes
All clinically relevant outcomes related to asthma such as the number of asthma exacerbations, the severity of

asthma, airway hypersensitivity and pulmonary functions were included in this review.

Literature searches
Medline (OVID) was searched using terms: (exp Ascorbic acid/ or ascorb*.mp) and (exp Asthma/ or asthma*.mp or bronch*.mp) and (exp Common cold/ or exp Respiratory Tract Infections/ or respiratory infect*.mp). Similar searches were carried out via Scopus and the Cochrane Central Register of Controlled Trials. No language restrictions were used. The databases were searched from their inception to September 2013. Studies that fulfilled the selection criteria were included. The reference lists of the identified studies and relevant review articles were screened for additional references. Finally, a cited article search of the Web of Science database was carried out to search for papers that cited the trials identified in the primary search. See Additional file 1 for the flow diagram of the literature search.

Selection of studies and data extraction
Three studies that were relevant to the investigation of the role of vitamin C on common cold-induced asthma were identified (Tables 1 and 2). The data of the three included trials were extracted and analyzed by this author (see below and Additional files 2 and 3). Dr. Bucca was contacted for the original data, but she no longer retained those data. Dr. Bucca reported the histamine PC_{20} values of their study as figures in two separate reports [25,26]. In the current study, the individual-level values were measured from one of the figures [26]; see Additional file 2 for the data extraction. The reconstructed data set has the same means and gives the same F-statistics as Bucca et al. reported; see Additional files 2 and 3.

Statistical analysis
In 1980, Anah et al. reported the cumulative incidence of asthma attacks during the trial [27], which gives a rate ratio (RR) = 0.22 (95% confidence interval [CI]: 0.09-0.47) using the "poisson.test" program of the R-package [28]. However, Anah and colleagues did not publish the individual level data or standard deviations (SD) for the distribution of asthma attacks and therefore the variance per mean ratio could not be calculated (it is 1.0 for the Poisson distribution). Nevertheless, they published partial descriptions of the asthma attack distributions that were used to generate more realistic over-dispersed Poisson-type distributions for the treatment groups. The exact distribution of the severe and moderate asthma attacks in the vitamin C group could be inferred and thus the RR for severe and moderate attacks involves fewer imputations than the RR for all asthma attacks. The RRs and their 95% CIs were then calculated by using the "glm.nb" program of the R package, which fits the negative binomial regression model

Table 1 Characteristics of the included trials

Study	Item	Description
Anah et al. 1980 [27]	Participants	41 asthmatic subjects attending an asthma clinic in Nigeria. All had had asthma for at least 4 yrs. The participants had histories of increased asthma attacks during the rainy season. In all cases their attacks were precipitated by respiratory infections, which started with a sore throat and a dry cough. The trial was conducted during the rainy season. Patients with bronchitis were excluded. 22 M, 19 F; age 15 to 46 y (mean 27 y); 22 vit C 19 placebo.
	Duration	14 wk
	Intervention	1 g/d vit C or a placebo for 14 wk.
	Outcome	Frequency of asthma attacks. "Severe attacks" indicate those that needed emergency attendance at the hospital; "moderate attacks" those that necessitated the use of inhalers more frequently, and "mild attacks" those that caused some increase in wheezing and breathlessness.
	Notes	See calculations in Additional files 2 and 3.
Schertling et al. 1990 [30,31]	Participants	29 Participants with a diagnosis of infection-related asthma in former East-Germany. Patients with acute and serious purulent infections were excluded. 18 M, 11 F; age 18 to 60 y.
	Duration	Total duration 5 wk, composed of 2 periods of 2 wk intervention and a 1 wk washout between them.
	Intervention	5 g/d vit C or placebo for 1 wk before the histamine sensitivity test in the middle of the 2 wk intervention. Washout 1 wk between the 2-wk intervention phases.
	Outcomes	1) Sensitivity to histamine: positive result indicates that exposure to <1 µmol histamine increased respiratory tract resistance by 50%. 2) Asthma symptom score, 3) PEF
	Notes	See calculations in Additional file 2. The histamine sensitivity data are reported for 23 participants. There is no description for the missing data.
Bucca et al. 1989 [25,26]	Participants	9 members of hospital staff in Italy with a negative history of asthma and atopy. All suffered from the common cold with cough on the first vit C test day, and all had recovered on the second vit C test day 6 wk later. 5 M, 4 F; age 18 to 48 y (mean 29 y).
	Duration	Two study days separated by 6 wk.
	Intervention	Single dose 2 g of vit C.
	Outcome	PC_{20} was measured at baseline and 1 h after vit C administration on both study days.
	Notes	See calculations in Additional files 2 and 3.

Abbreviations:
PC_{20}: Concentration of histamine needed for a 20% FEV_1 decrease.
PEF: Peak Expiratory Flow.

[28,29]. These conservative RR estimates are shown as the findings of the Anah study (Table 3) see Additional files 2 and 3 for the calculations.

In 1990, Schertling et al. reported the numbers of participants who were sensitive to histamine on the vitamin C and the placebo phases of a cross-over study [30,31]. Bronchial hypersensitivity was defined as a cumulative dose of <1 µmol histamine that caused a 50% increase in respiratory tract resistance. In the current study, the *P*-value for the difference in the proportions of participants with bronchial hypersensitivity to histamine between the vitamin C and the placebo phases was calculated from the discordant observations using the binomial distribution. The 95% CI for the difference in the proportions was calculated using the Agresti-Caffo method [32]. See Additional file 2 for the calculations. Schertling and colleagues did not report the distribution for asthma symptom scores or PEF values, but they reported the

Wilcoxon-test *P*-values for the vitamin C and the placebo phase differences [30,31], which are shown in Table 3.

In 1989, Bucca et al. reported the histamine provocation concentrations that caused a 20% decline in FEV_1 level (PC_{20}) at baseline and at 1 hour after vitamin C administration for two study days that were separated by a 6 week interval [25,26]. On the first vitamin C test day, the participants suffered from the common cold, and 6 weeks later, on the second vitamin C test day, they had all recovered. In the current study, the effect of vitamin C was calculated as the difference in the $\log(PC_{20})$ levels between the baseline and 1 hour after vitamin C administration. A paired t-test was used to calculate the *P*-value and the 95% CI in the log-scale was also obtained. Thereafter the 95% CI was converted into the ratio scale. The paired t-test of the $\log(PC_{20})$ values was also used to calculate the interaction *P*-value between the vitamin C effect and the presence of the

Table 2 Methodological characteristics of the included trials

Study	Domain of interest	Description
Anah et al. 1980 [27]	Design	Parallel-group trial.
	Randomization	Reported as a randomized trial, but the method of randomization was not described.
	Allocation concealment	Not described, but double-blinding implies that allocation must have been concealed.
	Blinding of participants and personnel	Reported as double-blind, which implies that participants and personnel were blind; however, the persons who were blind are not explicitly described.
	Blinding of outcome assessment	Reported as double-blind, which implies that outcome assessment was blind; however, the persons who were blind are not explicitly described.
	Drop-outs	No description of drop-outs.
Schertling et al. 1990 [30,31]	Design	Cross-over trial.
	Randomization	Reported as a randomized trial, but the method of randomization was not described.
	Allocation concealment	Not described, but double-blinding implies that allocation must have been concealed.
	Blinding of participants and personnel	Reported as double-blind, which implies that participants and personnel were blind; however, the persons who were blind are not explicitly described.
	Blinding of outcome assessment	Reported as double-blind, which implies that outcome assessment was blind; however, the persons who were blind are not explicitly described.
	Drop-outs	Total number of participants was 29, but histamine sensitivity is reported for 23 participants. The reasons for the 6 missing participants are not given.
Bucca et al. 1989 [25,26]	Design	Self-controlled trial. Two series of histamine challenge tests were done before and after vit C. The first series was carried out when the participants suffered from the common cold, and the second series was carried out 6 wk later after the participants had recovered. On both study days, vit C was administered after the baseline histamine challenge test and the second histamine challenge test was carried out 1 h later. No placebo.
	Randomization	Not a randomized trial.
	Allocation concealment	Not applicable.
	Blinding of participants and personnel	Not blinded.
	Blinding of outcome assessment	Not blinded.
	Drop-outs	One participant out of 10 was excluded from the statistical analysis because she had whooping cough and not the common cold.

common cold. See Additional files 2 and 3 for the calculations.

In the analysis of the Bucca et al. data, linear modeling (lm program of the R package [28]) was used to determine whether the effect of vitamin C on the common-cold-day could be explained by the baseline $\log(PC_{20})$ level values a) on the common-cold-day or b) on the day the participant had recovered, or c) by the vitamin C effect on the day the participant had recovered. The improvement of model fit was assessed by the likelihood ratio test. The vitamin C effect on the common-cold-day was significantly explained by the baseline $\log(PC_{20})$ level on the common-cold-day and by the vitamin C effect on the day the participant had recovered. Compared with

the null model without the explanatory variables, the addition of these two variables improved the model fit by $\chi^2(2\ df) = 9.1$, $P = .011$. Since the vitamin C effect on the common-cold-day was explained by the vitamin C effect on the day the participant had recovered, the latter was subtracted from the former, which gave an adjusted vitamin C effect. In a linear model, the adjusted vitamin C effect was significantly explained by the baseline $\log(PC_{20})$ level: $\chi^2(1\ df) = 6.2$, $P = .013$ (Figure 1). See Additional file 3 for the calculations.

In the Bucca et al. data, the association between the histamine PC_{20} levels on the two study days separated by a 6 week period was analyzed using the "cor.test" and "lm" programs of the R package [28]. The influence of

Table 3 Findings of the included trials

Study	Outcome	P (2-tail) for the difference	Estimate of vitamin C effect (95% CI)	Notes
Anah et al. 1980 [27]	Incidence of all asthma attacks:	0.019	RR = 0.22 (0.06 to 0.81)	All asthma attacks: 9/22 and 35/19 (attacks/persons) in vit C and placebo groups, respectively. See Additional files 2 and 3 for the calculations.
	Incidence of severe and moderate asthma attacks:	0.003	RR = 0.11 (0.02 to 0.48)	Severe and moderate asthma attacks: 3/22 and 23/19 (attacks/persons) in vit C and placebo groups, respectively. See Additional files 2 and 3 for the calculations.
Schertling et al. 1990 [30,31]	Proportion of participants who were sensitive to histamine:	0.0005	52 percentage points decrease (25 to 71)	The P-value was calculated from the discordant observations: 12 were sensitive to histamine in the placebo phase but not in the vit C phase; 0 were sensitive to histamine in the vit C phase but not in the placebo phase. See Additional file 2 for the calculations.
	Asthma symptom score:	0.12	Placebo: 0.72, Vit C: 0.65	Scale 0 to 3; 0 indicates no symptoms. The P-value was calculated by Schertling et al. [30,31].
	PEF:	0.12	Placebo: 400 L/min, Vit C: 409 L/min	The P-value was calculated by Schertling et al. [30,31].
Bucca et al. 1989 [25,26]	Histamine PC_{20}:	0.0003	3.2 fold increase in PC_{20}, (2.0 to 5.1 fold)	Vit C increased histamine PC_{20} geometric mean from 7.8 to 25.1 mg/ml. See Additional files 2 and 3 for the calculations.
	Interaction between the vitamin C effect and the common cold:	0.003		Interaction test for the vit C effect on PC_{20} (before/after vit C) and the presence of the common cold (yes/no). See Additional file 2 for the calculations.

Abbreviations:
CI: Confidence Interval.
PC_{20}: Concentration of histamine needed for a 20% FEV_1 decrease.
PEF: Peak Expiratory Flow.
RR: Rate Ratio.

vitamin C administration on the association between the $\log(PC_{20})$ levels on the two study days was analyzed with linear modeling as follows. First, the baseline histamine $\log(PC_{20})$ determined when the participant was suffering from the common cold was modeled using the baseline $\log(PC_{20})$ determined after the participant had recovered as the explanatory variable. Second, the difference in the vitamin C effects on the two study days was added to the linear model. The comparison of these two models tested whether vitamin C administration significantly improved the association between the PC_{20} levels on the two study days separated by 6 weeks and gave $\chi^2(1 \ df) = 9.2$, $P = .0024$. See Additional file 3 for the calculations.

The Bucca et al. study did not use a placebo and the second histamine challenge test was carried out at 1 hour after the baseline test. Therefore, studies that give information on the role of placebo on the histamine challenge test [7-9,33-35] and about tachyphylaxis [35-40] were searched; see Additional file 2 for the data of two reports [33,36]. Furthermore, one day before the first vitamin C test day, Bucca et al. ascertained the reproducibility of the histamine challenge test. The baseline test and the test 1 hour later had a very close correlation (r = .96).

The coefficient of variation was on average 6% for three measurements comprising the two reproducibility day measurements and the baseline histamine test on the first vitamin C day [25].

The 2-tailed *P*-values are presented in this text.

The statistical analyses in this systematic review were not planned in a protocol prior to the review. Instead the statistical approaches were formulated after the data of the selected studies became available.

Results

Three intervention studies that give information on the effect of vitamin C on common cold-induced asthma were identified. A total of 79 people participated in the three trials (Table 1). The three studies are clinically heterogeneous and the outcomes are different. Therefore no pooled effect can be calculated. Instead the studies are analyzed separately. The methodological characteristics of the three studies are described in Table 2.

The study by Anah et al. was a randomized double-blind placebo-controlled trial with parallel groups (N = 41) [27]. The effect of 1 g/day of vitamin C on participants who had histories of increased asthma attacks during the rainy

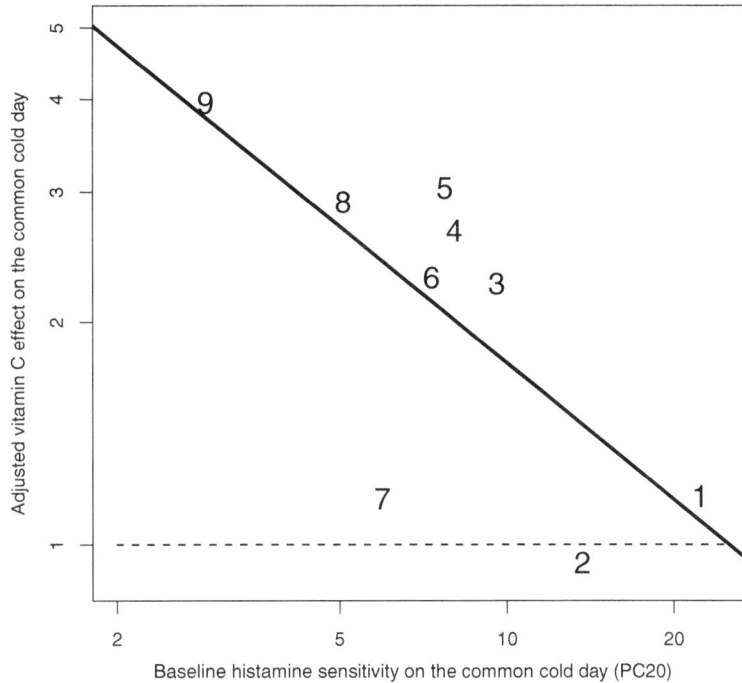

Figure 1 The association between vitamin C effect and baseline histamine PC$_{20}$ level on the common-cold-day. Baseline PC$_{20}$ level indicates the histamine PC$_{20}$ level before vitamin C administration on the common-cold day in the Bucca et al. study [25,26]. Adjusted vitamin C effect indicates that the vitamin C effect of the second day (after recovery at 6 wk) is subtracted from the vitamin C effect on the common-cold-day. For example, participant #9 had a 7.45-fold increase in PC$_{20}$ level on the common-cold-day and a 1.88-fold increase in PC$_{20}$ level on the second day. This gives an adjusted vitamin C effect of 3.96 (7.45/1.88). Adding the baseline histamine PC$_{20}$ level to the null model increased the model fit by χ^2(1 df) = 6.2, P = .013. The horizontal dash (−) line indicates the level of vitamin C effect after recovery. The numbers indicate the identification numbers used in Additional file 2. See the Additional file 3 for the calculations of the linear model.

season in Nigeria was investigated. In all previous cases their attacks were precipitated by respiratory infections, which started with a sore throat and a dry cough. The 14-week trial was carried out during the Nigerian rainy season. The study recorded 35 asthma attacks in the placebo group (n = 19), but only 9 attacks in the vitamin C group (n = 22). Thus, vitamin C decreased the incidence of all asthma exacerbations by 78% (Table 3). The effect appeared even greater on those asthma exacerbations that were classified as severe or moderate, which decreased by 89% (Table 3). Furthermore, Anah et al. reported that there was a recurrence of asthma attacks in the vitamin C group within 8 weeks after vitamin administration was discontinued, though no quantitative data were published.

The study by Schertling et al. was a randomized double-blind placebo-controlled cross-over trial conducted in the former East Germany (N = 29) [30,31]. The effect of 5 g/day of vitamin C was studied on participants who had a diagnosis of infection-related asthma. Schertling et al. tested bronchial responsiveness to histamine so that hypersensitivity was defined as increase in respiratory tract resistance of 50% for a cumulative exposure to <1 μmol histamine. Vitamin C decreased the proportion of participants who were sensitive to histamine by 52 percentage

points (Table 3). The decrease in prevalence was from 91% (21/23) during the placebo phase to 39% (9/23) during the vitamin C phase. The mean symptom scores and PEF values were also reported and, though non-significant, their differences were in favor of vitamin C (Table 3).

Bucca et al. investigated the effect of a single dose 1 g vitamin C on histamine challenge test of common cold patients in a self-controlled study (n = 9) [25,26]. A second pair of histamine challenge tests was carried out 6 weeks later after the participants had recovered. When the participants suffered from the common cold, the baseline PC$_{20}$ level was 50% lower than after they had recovered (P = .005), which indicates that the common cold increased bronchial sensitivity to histamine. When the participants suffered from the common cold, vitamin C administration caused a 3.2-fold increase in the geometric mean histamine PC$_{20}$ level in the baseline values of 7.8 to 25.1 mg/ml (Table 3). After the participants had recovered from the common cold 6 weeks later, vitamin C increased the PC$_{20}$ level by just 1.6 fold.

A comparison between the two study days found that there was a significant interaction between the vitamin C effect and the presence of the common cold (P = .003), which indicates that the effect of vitamin C on bronchial hypersensitivity was different between the two test days separated by 6 weeks. Furthermore, a linear regression analysis revealed that the difference in the vitamin C effect between the two study days depended significantly on the baseline histamine PC_{20} level determined on the common-cold-day (Figure 1). If there are factors causing bias in the self-controlled comparison and if the factors are constant on both study days, they would be removed from the calculation of the adjusted vitamin C effect, i.e., the difference in effect between the two study days. Such potential factors include the placebo effect and tachyphylaxis. The linear regression model indicated there were no differences in the vitamin C effects between the two study days when the baseline histamine PC_{20} level was 25 mg/ml on the common-cold-day (Figure 1). However, when the baseline PC_{20} level was 2 mg/ml on the common-cold-day, the model predicted that vitamin C administration would increase the histamine PC_{20} level 4.7-fold over the corresponding effect after recovery from the cold.

In the study by Bucca et al., there was a significant correlation between the histamine PC_{20} levels on the two study days after vitamin C administration (r = 0.81, P = .008). After vitamin C administration the geometric means of the PC_{20} levels on the two days were essentially identical: 25.1 vs. 25.7 mg/ml [25]. Before vitamin C administration the correlation between the PC_{20} levels for the two days was weak (r = 0.66, P = .054). Linear modeling was used to determine whether the increase in correlation caused by vitamin C administration was statistically significant. Adding the difference between the vitamin C effects for the two study days as a factor to the linear model explaining the baseline PC_{20} levels on the common-cold-day by the baseline PC_{20} levels after recovery improved the fit of the linear model significantly (P = .003). Consequently, the closer association between the PC_{20} values after vitamin C administration cannot be explained by random variation alone.

Bucca et al. did not use a placebo [25], and therefore data on the possible role of placebo on the histamine challenge test was assessed from other studies. One study reported that the histamine sensitivity on the placebo day did not differ from the levels on the no-treatment day (95% CI: -22% to +21%) [33]. Other studies also found no effect of placebo on histamine sensitivity [7-9,34,35]. Another potential problem in the Bucca group's study design was tachyphylaxis, which indicates that a second histamine challenge test carried out too soon after the first test might lead to increased PC_{20} values. Although this phenomenon has been reported, in one study the increase in histamine PC_{20} value was less than 1.5-fold for the second challenge test carried out at 1 hour after the first test [36]. Other studies have found small or no

tachyphylaxis effects [35,37-40]. Furthermore, the close reproducibility of the histamine challenge test in the Bucca et al. study is also inconsistent with a substantial tachyphylaxis effect [25]. Finally, if there is a constant placebo effect or tachyphylaxis that would cause bias, such effects would be eliminated from the calculation of the adjusted vitamin C effect, i.e., the difference in effects between the two study days. Therefore, the strong association between the adjusted vitamin C effect and the baseline histamine PC_{20} level is a further argument against the placebo effect and the tachyphylaxis effect (Figure 1). In conclusion, the placebo effect is not an issue and tachyphylaxis does not explain the 3.2-fold increase in the histamine PC_{20} level of common cold patients who were administered vitamin C.

Discussion

The three identified studies give relevant information for assessing the potential role of vitamin C on alleviating asthma exacerbations caused by the common cold. The studies differ substantially in their methods, participants, settings and outcomes, yet each of them found a benefit from vitamin C administration.

Anah et al. [27] recorded the occurrence of asthma exacerbations, whereas Schertling et al. [30] and Bucca et al. [25] studied bronchial sensitivity to histamine. The common cold can lead to a transient bronchial hypersensitivity, which is a characteristic feature of asthma [7-12,25]. Challenge tests with histamine and methacholine have been widely used for the examinations of asthma patients [41]. Furthermore, reducing the airway hypersensitivity of asthmatics led to a significant reduction in asthma exacerbations, which implies that bronchial hypersensitivity is a clinically important measure of the asthma severity [42].

Two of the identified studies [27,30] were randomized double-blind placebo-controlled trials. Both studies used patients who suffered from infection-related asthma. Anah et al. found that vitamin C decreased the occurrence of respiratory infection-induced asthma attacks by 78% [27]. Schertling et al. found that vitamin C decreased the proportion of asthma patients who suffered from bronchial hypersensitivity to histamine by 58 percentage points [30]. In the Schertling group's study, vitamin C did not influence asthma symptoms or PEF values. However, the number of participants in that study was small and therefore the study had insufficient statistical power to test the effect on these outcomes. The Anah et al. study was carried out in Nigeria in the 1970s, and Schertling et al. study was carried out in former East Germany in the 1980s. Thus, those findings cannot be directly extrapolated to Western countries in the 2010s. Nevertheless, these two trials were methodologically strong. The highly significant effects caused by vitamin C administration indicate a genuine biological effect on the lungs of some people who suffer from common cold-induced asthma exacerbations.

Bucca et al. found that vitamin C administration caused a 3.2-fold increase in histamine PC_{20} levels of common cold patients, which indicates that vitamin C decreased bronchial hypersensitivity caused by the common cold [25]. The effect of vitamin C was significantly smaller after the participants had recovered from the colds. Furthermore, on the two vitamin C test days, which were separated by 6 weeks, histamine PC_{20} levels correlated significantly after vitamin C was administered, but did not do so before its administration. This indicates that vitamin C administration was associated with a kind of normalization of bronchial sensitivity. The study by Bucca and colleagues is methodologically weaker than the two other studies, but analyzing the two study days gives much strength compared with measuring participants only on the common-cold-day. In any case, placebo effect and tachyphylaxis do not readily explain the effect of vitamin C found in the participants when they were suffering from the common cold.

Publication bias might be a problem in the case where a few studies have been published. However, publication bias cannot reasonably explain the remarkably small P-values found in each of the three studies reviewed here. Furthermore, publication bias cannot explain findings that are not published in the original study reports. Therefore, publication bias cannot explain the association between the PC_{20} level on the common-cold day and the adjusted vitamin C effect (Figure 1). This systematic review was done by one person and one person might have a higher error rate in the extraction of data than a group. However, only three studies are included and the extracted data were several times compared against the original study reports. It is unlikely that errors would have remained. Furthermore, to increase transparency in this systematic review, the extracted data and the calculations are described in Additional files 2 and 3.

Asthma is a heterogeneous syndrome, an "umbrella concept," that comprises a collection of different phenotypes with different underlying pathophysiologies, rather than a single disease [43,44]. A previous meta-analysis found that vitamin C may alleviate exercise-induced bronchoconstriction [24] and the current study revealed that vitamin C may alleviate common cold-induced asthma exacerbations. It is noteworthy that both of these conditions involve short-term stress, caused either by physical exertion or by an infectious disease. Given the diverse asthma phenotypes that exist, it is relevant to consider whether vitamin C might influence other asthma phenotypes.

In a four-month study of British asthmatics who regularly used inhaled corticosteroids, Fogarty et al. found no effect of 1 g/day vitamin C on the FEV_1 level, on bronchial

sensitivity to methacholine, or on asthma symptoms [45]. However, those authors found that the need for inhaled corticosteroids was slightly lower in the vitamin C group [46]. The Fogarty et al. study indicates that regular vitamin C administration is not substantially beneficial for patients with persistent asthma without acute problems. However, their study does not conflict with the possibility that vitamin C may be beneficial for pulmonary functions of some asthmatics under certain forms of acute stress, such as people who endure heavy physical activity or suffer from a viral respiratory tract infection.

Evidently, more research on the role of vitamin C on common cold-induced asthma is needed. On the other hand, vitamin C costs only a few pennies per gram and it is safe in gram doses [16,17,47]. Given the strong evidence that shows that vitamin C alleviates common cold symptoms [14-17], and the findings of this systematic review, it may be reasonable for asthmatic patients to test vitamin C on an individual basis when they have exacerbations of asthma caused by respiratory infections.

Abbreviations

CI: Confidence interval; FEV_1: Forced expiratory volume in 1 second; PC_{20}: Concentration of histamine needed for a 20% FEV_1 decrease; PEF: Peak expiratory flow; RR: Rate ratio.

Competing interests

The author declares that he has no competing interests.

Acknowledgements

The author is grateful to Silvia Maggini (Roche, Switzerland) for arranging the translation of the Schertling et al. report [30] into English.

This research has received no grant from any funding agency in the public, commercial or not-for-profit sectors.

References

1. Rosenthal LA, Avila PC, Heymann PW, Martin RJ, Miller EK, Papadopoulos NG, Peebles RS, Gern JE: Viral respiratory tract infections and asthma: the course ahead. *J Allergy Clin Immunol* 2010, **125**:1212–1217. http://dx.doi.org/10.1016/j.jaci.2010.04.002.
2. Minor TE, Dick EC, DeMeo AN, Ouellette JJ, Cohen M, Reed CE: Viruses as precipitants of asthmatic attacks in children. *JAMA* 1974, **227**:292–298. http://dx.doi.org/10.1001/jama.1974.03230160020004.
3. Nicholson KG, Kent J, Ireland DC: Respiratory viruses and exacerbations of asthma in adults. *BMJ* 1993, **307**:982–986. http://www.ncbi.nlm.nih.gov/pmc/articles/PMC1679193.
4. Johnston SL, Pattemore PK, Sanderson G, Smith S, Lampe F, Symington P, O'Toole S, Myint SH, Tyrrell DA: Community study of role of viral infections in exacerbations of asthma in 9–11 year old children. *BMJ* 1995, **310**:1225–1229. http://www.ncbi.nlm.nih.gov/pmc/articles/PMC2549614.

5. Gern JE: **The ABCs of rhinoviruses, wheezing, and asthma.** *J Virol* 2010,
    84:7418–7426. http://dx.doi.org/10.1128/JVI.02290-09, http://www.ncbi.nlm.
    nih.gov/pubmed/20375160.
6. Walter MJ, Castro M, Kunselman SJ, Chinchilli VM, Reno M, Ramkumar TP,
    Avila PC, Boushey HA, Ameredes BT, Bleecker ER, Calhoun WJ, Cherniack
    RM, Craig TJ, Denlinger LC, Israel E, Fahy JV, Jarjour NN, Kraft M, Lazarus SC,
    Lemanske RF Jr, Martin RJ, Peters SP, Ramsdell JW, Sorkness CA, Sutherland
    ER, Szefler SJ, Wasserman SI, Wechsler ME: **National Heart, Lung and Blood
    Institute's Asthma Clinical Research Network: Predicting worsening
    asthma control following the common cold.** *Eur Respir J* 2008,
    32:1548–1554. http://dx.doi.org/10.1183/09031936.00026808.
7. Empey DW, Laitinen LA, Jacobs L, Gold WM, Nadel JA: **Mechanisms of
    bronchial hyperreactivity in normal subjects after upper respiratory tract
    infection.** *Am Rev Respir Dis* 1976, **113**:131–139. http://www.ncbi.nlm.nih.
    gov/pubmed/1247226.
8. Grünberg K, Timmers MC, Smits HH, de Klerk EP, Dick EC, Spaan WJ,
    Hiemstra PS, Sterk PJ: **Effect of experimental rhinovirus 16 colds on
    airway hyperresponsiveness to histamine and interleukin-8 in nasal
    lavage in asthmatic subjects in vivo.** *Clin Exp Allergy* 1997, **27**:36–45.
    http://www.ncbi.nlm.nih.gov/pubmed/9117878.
9. Grünberg K, Timmers MC, de Klerk EP, Dick EC, Sterk PJ: **Experimental
    rhinovirus 16 infection causes variable airway obstruction in subjects
    with atopic asthma.** *Am J Respir Crit Care Med* 1999, **160**:1375–1380.
    http://www.ncbi.nlm.nih.gov/pubmed/10508832.
10. Lemanske RF, Dick EC, Swenson CA, Vrtis RF, Busse WW: **Rhinovirus upper
    respiratory infection increases airway hyperreactivity and late
    asthmatic reactions.** *J Clin Invest* 1989, **83**:1–10. http://www.ncbi.nlm.nih.
    gov/pubmed/2536042.
11. Cheung D, Dick EC, Timmers MC, de Klerk EP, Spaan WJ, Sterk PJ:
    **Rhinovirus inhalation causes long-lasting excessive airway narrowing
    in response to methacholine in asthmatic subjects in vivo.** *Am J
    Respir Crit Care Med* 1995, **152**:1490–1496. http://www.ncbi.nlm.nih.gov/
    pubmed/7582282.
12. Fraenkel DJ, Bardin PG, Sanderson G, Lampe F, Johnston SL, Holgate ST:
    **Lower airways inflammation during rhinovirus colds in normal and in
    asthmatic subjects.** *Am J Respir Crit Care Med* 1995, **151**:879–886.
    http://www.ncbi.nlm.nih.gov/pubmed/7881686.
13. Carpenter KJ: *The History of Scurvy and Vitamin C.* New York, NY: Cambridge
    University Press; 1986.
14. Hemilä H: **Vitamin C supplementation and common cold symptoms:
    problems with inaccurate reviews.** *Nutrition* 1996, **12**:804–809. http://hdl.
    handle.net/10250/7979, http://dx.doi.org/10.1016/S0899-9007(96)00223-7.
15. Hemilä H: **Vitamin C supplementation and common cold symptoms:
    factors affecting the magnitude of the benefit.** *Med Hypotheses* 1999,
    52:171–178. http://hdl.handle.net/10250/8375, http://dx.doi.org/10.1054/
    mehy.1997.0639.
16. Hemilä H, Chalker EB: **Vitamin C for preventing and treating the common
    cold.** *Cochrane Database Syst Rev* 2013, **1**:CD000980. http://dx.doi.org/
    10.1002/14651858.CD000980.pub4.
17. Hemilä H: *Do vitamins C and E affect respiratory infections*, PhD Thesis.
    Helsinki, Finland: University of Helsinki; 2006:11–16. 46–51, 62–63.
    http://hdl.handle.net/10138/20335.
18. Hemilä H: **Vitamin C intake and susceptibility to the common cold.**
    [discussion in: 1997, 78:857–866]. *Br J Nutr* 1997, **77**:59–72.
    http://dx.doi.org/10.1017/S0007114500002889.
19. Elwood PC, Lee HP, St Leger AS, Baird M, Howard AN: **A randomized
    controlled trial of vitamin C in the prevention and amelioration of the
    common cold.** *Br J Prev Soc Med* 1976, **30**:193–196. http://www.ncbi.nlm.
    nih.gov/pmc/articles/PMC478963.
20. Anderson TW, Reid DBW, Beaton GH: **Vitamin C and the common cold**
    [correction of: 1972, 107:503–508]. *Can Med Assoc J* 1973, **108**:133.
    http://www.ncbi.nlm.nih.gov/pmc/articles/PMC1941144.
21. Hemilä H, Louhiala P: **Vitamin C may affect lung infections.** *J R Soc Med*
    2007, **100**:495–498. http://www.ncbi.nlm.nih.gov/pmc/articles/PMC2099400.
22. Goldsmith GA, Ogaard AT, Gowe DF: **Vitamin C (ascorbic acid) nutrition in
    bronchial asthma: an estimation of the daily requirement of ascorbic
    acid.** *Arch Intern Med* 1941, **67**:597–608.
23. Silbert NE: **Vitamin C: a critical review of the use of vitamin C in allergic
    disorders and a preliminary report comparing it therapeutically with
    antihistamines, antiasthmatics and sedatives.** *Med Times* 1951, **79**:370–376.
    http://www.ncbi.nlm.nih.gov/pubmed/14852293.
24. Hemilä H: **Vitamin C may alleviate exercise-induced bronchoconstriction:
    a meta-analysis.** *BMJ Open* 2013, **3**:e002416. http://dx.doi.org/10.1136/
    bmjopen-2012-002416.
25. Bucca C, Rolla G, Arossa W, Caria E, Elia C, Nebiolo F, Baldi S: **Effect of
    ascorbic acid on increased bronchial responsiveness during upper
    airway infection.** *Respiration* 1989, **55**:214–219. http://www.ncbi.nlm.nih.
    gov/pubmed/2595105, http://dx.doi.org/10.1159/000195737.
26. Bucca C, Rolla G, Farina JC: **Effect of vitamin C on transient increase of
    bronchial responsiveness in conditions affecting the airways.** *Ann NY
    Acad Sci* 1992, **669**:175–187. http://www.ncbi.nlm.nih.gov/pubmed/1444023,
    http://dx.doi.org/10.1111/j.1749-6632.1992.tb17098.x.
27. Anah CO, Jarike LN, Baig HA: **High dose ascorbic acid in Nigerian
    asthmatics.** *Trop Geogr Med* 1980, **32**:132–137. http://www.ncbi.nlm.nih.gov/
    pubmed/7423602.
28. **The R Project for Statistical Computing** http://www.r-project.org.
29. Glynn RJ, Buring JE: **Ways of measuring rates of recurrent events.** *BMJ*
    1996, **312**:364–367. http://www.ncbi.nlm.nih.gov/pmc/articles/PMC2350293.
30. Schertling M, Winsel K, Müller S, Henning R, Meiske W, Slapke J: **Action of
    ascorbic acid on clinical course of infection related bronchial asthma
    and on reactive oxygen metabolites by BAL cells [in German].** *Z Klin Med*
    1990, **45**:1770–1774. English translation available at: http://www.mv.helsinki.
    fi/home/hemila/T9.pdf.
31. Schertling M: *Einfluss von Ascorbinsäure auf den klinischen Verlauf des
    infektbedingten Asthma bronchiale und die Bildung von reaktiven
    Sauerstoffmetaboliten durch BAL-Zellen.* Berlin, East Germany: PhD thesis;
    1989. Excerpts available at: http://www.mv.helsinki.fi/home/hemila/A/
    Schertling.htm.
32. Fagerland MW, Lydersen S, Laake P: **Recommended confidence intervals
    for two independent binomial proportions.** *Stat Methods Med Res* 2011.
    (in press). http://dx.doi.org/10.1177/0962280211415469.
33. Nathan RA, Segall N, Glover GC, Schocket AL: **The effects of H1 and H2
    antihistamines on histamine inhalation challenges in asthmatic patients.**
    Am Rev Respir Dis 1979, **120**:1251–1258. http://www.ncbi.nlm.nih.gov/
    pubmed/42333.
34. Malo JL, Fu CL, L'Archevêque J, Ghezzo H, Cartier A: **Duration of the effect
    of astemizole on histamine-inhalation tests.** *J Allergy Clin Immunol* 1990,
    85:729–736. http://www.ncbi.nlm.nih.gov/pubmed/1969870.
35. Lemire I, Cartier A, Malo JL, Pineau L, Ghezzo H, Martin RR: **Effect of sodium
    cromoglycate on histamine inhalation tests.** *J Allergy Clin Immunol* 1984,
    73:234–239. http://www.ncbi.nlm.nih.gov/pubmed/6421918.
36. Strban M, Manning PJ, Watson RM, O'Byrne PM: **Effect of magnitude of
    airway responsiveness and therapy with inhaled corticosteroid on
    histamine tachyphylaxis in asthma.** *Chest* 1994, **105**:1434–1438.
    http://www.ncbi.nlm.nih.gov/pubmed/8181332.
37. Schoeffel RE, Anderson SD, Gillam I, Lindsay DA: **Multiple exercise and
    histamine challenge in asthmatic patients.** *Thorax* 1980, **35**:164–170.
    http://dx.doi.org/10.1136/thx.35.3.164.
38. Ruffin RE, Alpers JH, Crockett AJ, Hamilton R: **Repeated histamine
    inhalation tests in asthmatic patients.** *J Allergy Clin Immunol* 1981,
    67:285–289. http://www.ncbi.nlm.nih.gov/pubmed/7204784.
39. Polosa R, Finnerty JP, Holgate ST: **Tachyphylaxis to inhaled histamine in
    asthma: its significance and relationship to basal airway responsiveness.**
    J Allergy Clin Immunol 1990, **86**:265–271. http://www.ncbi.nlm.nih.gov/
    pubmed/2384654.
40. Roorda RJ, Gerritsen J, van Aalderen WM, Schouten JP, Knol K: **Repeated
    provocation tests in asthmatic children for testing tachyphylaxis to
    histamine.** *Pediatr Pulmonol* 1991, **10**:106–111. http://dx.doi.org/10.1002/
    ppul.1950100212.
41. Crapo RO, Casaburi R, Coates AL, Enright PL, Hankinson JL, Irvin CG,
    MacIntyre NR, McKay RT, Wanger JS, Anderson SD, Cockcroft DW, Fish JE,
    Sterk PJ: **Guidelines for methacholine and exercise challenge testing-
    1999.** *Am J Respir Crit Care Med* 2000, **161**:309–329. http://www.ncbi.nlm.
    nih.gov/pubmed/10619836.
42. Sont JK, Willems LN, Bel EH, van Krieken JH, Vandenbroucke JP, Sterk PJ:
    **Clinical control and histopathologic outcome of asthma when using
    airway hyperresponsiveness as an additional guide to long-term treat-
    ment.** *Am J Respir Crit Care Med* 1999, **159**:1043–1051. http://www.ncbi.nlm.
    nih.gov/pubmed/10194144.
43. Fajt ML, Wenzel SE: **Asthma phenotypes in adults and clinical
    implications.** *Expert Rev Respir Med* 2009, **3**:607–625. http://www.ncbi.nlm.
    nih.gov/pubmed/20477351, http://dx.doi.org/10.1586/ers.09.57.

44. Lötvall J, Akdis CA, Bacharier LB, Bjermer L, Casale TB, Custovic A, Lemanske RF Jr, Wardlaw AJ, Wenzel SE, Greenberger PA: **Asthma endotypes: a new approach to classification of disease entities within the asthma syndrome.** *J Allergy Clin Immunol* 2011, **127**:355–360.

45. Fogarty A, Lewis SA, Scrivener SL, Antoniak M, Pacey S, Pringle M, Britton J: **Oral magnesium and vitamin C supplements in asthma: a parallel group randomized placebo-controlled trial.** *Clin Exp Allergy* 2003, **33**:1355–1359. http://dx.doi.org/10.1046/j.1365-2222.2003.01777.x.

46. Fogarty A, Lewis SA, Scrivener SL, Antoniak M, Pacey S, Pringle M, Britton J: **Corticosteroid sparing effects of vitamin C and magnesium in asthma: a randomised trial.** *Respir Med* 2006, **100**:174–179. http://dx.doi.org/10.1016/j.rmed.2005.03.038.

47. Padayatty SJ, Sun AY, Chen Q, Espey MG, Drisko J, Levine M: **Vitamin C: intravenous use by complementary and alternative medicine practitioners and adverse effects.** *PLoS One* 2010, **5**:e11414. http://dx.doi.org/10.1371/journal.pone.0011414.

9

Influence of the programmed cell death of lymphocytes on the immunity of patients with atopic bronchial asthma

Cyrille Alode Vodounon[1,2,4*], Christophe Boni Chabi[4], Ylia Valerevna Skibo[1], Vincent Ezin[2], Nicolas Aikou[2], Simeon Oloni Kotchoni[3], Simon Ayeleroun Akpona[4], Lamine Baba-Moussa[2] and Zinaida Ivanovna Abramova[1]

Abstract

Background: Fairly recent data highlight the role of programmed cell death and autoimmunity, as potentially important factors in the pathogenesis of chronic obstructive airway diseases. The purpose of our research was to determine the influence of apoptotic factors on the immunity of patients with atopic bronchial asthma according to the degree of severity.

Method: The study was performed on the peripheral blood of patients with atopic bronchial asthma with different severity. The Immunological aspects were determined with ELISA, the fluorimetric method and the method of precipitation with polyethylene glycol. And the quantification of the parameters of the programmed cell death was performed by the method of flow cytometry and electron microscopy method.

Results: The data obtained from morphological and biochemical parameters show the deregulation of Programmed Death of lymphocytes of patients with atopic bronchial asthma but individual for each group of patients. This dysfunction might induce the secretion of autoantibodies against DNA. This could explain the accumulation of circulating immune complex with average size considered as the most pathogenic in patients with bronchial asthma especially in the patients of serious severity. It should be noted that Patients with bronchial asthma of mild and severe severity had different way and did not have the same degree of deficiency of the immune system.

Conclusion: These data suggested that apoptotic factor of lymphocytes may play an important role in controlling immunity of patients with atopic bronchial asthma.

Keywords: Programmed cell death, Immunity, Atopic Bronchial Asthma

Introduction

Each pathological process resembles a stereotypical reaction of the organism due to the action of various pathogens. Although there is a genetic and immunological specificity, all species highly organized (including humans) show practically the same stereotyped responses. Programmed cell death (PCD), which is similar to a natural physiological process [1-3] is a very illustrative example of the stereotypical reactions. An important progress in the study of the PCD concern the morphobiochemical changes observed during apoptosis [4-6]. In this respect, with the current classification of programmed cell death we can note: PCD of type I- apoptosis, PCD of type II - autophagy and necrosis as PCD of type III [7]. If before, the decisive role of PCD was attributed to induce this process (physiological: during apoptosis, supra-physiological during necrosis), now the differences from apoptosis and necrosis of the surrounding cells and the organism are in the foreground. On the other hand, the process of autophagy in normal cells is a possibility of renewal of organelles [8-10]. It was established that autophagy plays a vital role during

* Correspondence: sweetiebj@yahoo.fr
[1]Laboratory Acid Nucleic, Institute of Fundamental Medicine and Biology, Kazan Federal University (KFU-Russian), Kremlyovskaya str. 18, Kazan 480008, Republic of Tatarstan, Russian Fédération
[2]Laboratoire de Biologie et de Typage Moléculaire en Microbiologie, Département de biochimie et biologie cellulaire, Faculté des sciences et Techniques (FAST), Université d'Abomey-Calavi (UAC-Benin), 05PB1604 Cotonou, Benin
Full list of author information is available at the end of the article

embryogenesis and in the post-embryonic metamorphosis [11]. The deregulation of this process plays an important role in many diseases such as: neurodegenerative diseases (Alzheimer's and Parkinson's) [7,10,12], myodystrophy and cardiomyopathy diseases [13,14], the aging and infections [12] and malignant tumors [7]. The intensification of the study on the process of cell death is due to the fact that there are several methods existing nowadays available to record the various manifestations of PCD and to analyze molecular mechanisms [15] which are tightly related to mechanisms of other important events (eg cell activation and associated biological signaling). The study of PCD proved to be productive and fruitful for the understanding of a certain number of important processes, including immune homeostasis and oncogenesis. In connection with the phenomenon of PCD, it was necessary to review a certain number of conceptual data of pathophysiology. In eukaryotes, PCD was previously considered as a negative process in view of the importance of identifying the phenomenon of necrosis. Nowadays, we have a better understanding of PCD: on the one hand, the death of cells in the body is seen as a natural process, and the existence of a multicellular organism requires a balanced relationship between life and death. Nevertheless, the role of apoptosis in the development of the pathological process is less obvious. It seems that this form of cell death (as opposed to necrosis) is not an indispensable component of the typical pathological process, but rather the malfunction of apoptosis is the cause of a certain number of diseases [6,16,17]. Thus, the relevance of this problem is defined by a correlation of the malfunction of PCD process with most diseases, including autoimmune diseases. The identification of the mechanisms of deregulation of the PCD associated with some specific diseases allows understanding the etiopathology of these diseases. The goal of our research was to determine the immunological characteristics and the biochemical and morphological parameters of PCD of lymphocytes of patients with atopic bronchial asthma (ABA) according to their degree of severity.

Materials and methods
Patients and blood sampling
The study was carried on the peripheral blood from relatively healthy individuals (n = 21) and asthmatic patients (n = 92). The group of patients was composed of individuals with different severity of asthma: 38 patients of mild severity with an average of 39 +/- 5 years, 20 patients of moderate severity (42+/- 5) and 34 patients of severe severity (42 +/- 5). At the time of blood collection, patients were hospitalized in the detachment of Pneumology and were not treated with glucocorticoid. All the donors were non smokers and were selected after consent. The collection of venous blood from donors was done in the morning before taking breakfast. The diagnosis of atopic bronchial asthma was

established by medical doctors on the basis of data from the allergic anamnesis, the results of allegen skin prick test, epidemiology, and the experiments of nasal provokers and inhalers. The work was conducted under the rules of the Committee of Ethics in the Laboratory of Clinical Immunology and Allergy of RKB.

Detection of antibody - antiDNA by enzyme immunoassay
The determination of the rate of antibody anti-double stranded DNA was performed by enzyme-linked immunosorbent assay (ELISA) [18], previously optimized in the laboratory of the State University of Kazan. The lyophilized DNA of erythrocyte of chicken was used as antigen. The blood serum samples were incubated for 40 minutes at 56 degrees of Celsius to inactivate the proteins of the complement system and to dissociate the immune complex. For the detection of the antibodies associated with DNA in the wells of the ELISA plate, peroxidase-conjugated to antibody against human anti-IgG was used. The response of the coloring of ELISA reaction was detected by spectrophotometer "Multiskan" in units of optical density at a wavelength of 492 nm.

Determination of extracellular DNA concentration
The determination of the concentration of extracellular DNA was performed by the fluorimetric method with the aid of the colouring Hoechst 33342 (bisbenzimide) as fluorochrome. The level of fluorescence in solutions was measured in quartz cuvettes with 0.6 ml of volume using a fluorescence spectrophotometer "Hitachi MPF-4" (Japan) at an excitation wavelength of 358 nm and an emission wavelength of 458 nm. To determine the rate of fluorescence of DNA in solution, we took into account the fluorescence of Hoechst solution (0.24 µg) contained in a TNE buffer.

Determination of circulating immune complexes (CIC) by the method of precipitation with polyethylene glycol (PEG)
The rate of CIC in the serum was determined by the method based on the selective precipitation of antigen-antibody complexes in 4.17% PEG having a molecular weight of 6000, followed by a photometric determination of the density of the precipitate.

Separation of CIC by the precipitation method with PEG
to obtain CIC from the blood serum of patients with atopic bronchial asthma, 0.5 ml of serum was incubated with 0.5 ml of 7.5% PEG in 0.1 M borate buffer for 1 hour at 4°C. The precipitate was washed twice with 3.5% PEG in 0.1 M buffer, and centrifuged at 2500 rpm/min for 20 min at 4°C. And then the sediment suspended in 0.5 ml of phosphate buffered saline (PBS) was added.

Isolation of T-lymphocytes

Lymphocytes were isolated by the standard method of zonal centrifugation proposed by Patel et al. [19] with a mixture of Ficoll-verograffin ($\rho = 1077$ g cm-1) [20,21]. This method consists of isolating 95% of T- lymphocytes and their viability was determined by the trypan blue exclusion method [22].

Culture of lymphocytes

The cells obtained (2×10^6) were diluted in 1 ml of the RPMI-1640 medium in plank made of plastic with flat bottom (Nung), then supplemented with 10% serum of foetal calf and 10 µl of L-glutamine (200 µg/ml) (Flow) [23]. The cells were cultured with or without dexamethasone (final concentration of 10^{-4}M) and then samples were incubated in CO_2-incubator (5% CO_2) for 1 - 6 days [24,25].

Ultrastructural study

To study the morphology of the cells, cells obtained after zonal centrifugation were precipitated successively in 2.5% glutaraldehyde and 1% OsO4 for 1 hour [26]. The sample was then immersed in Epon 810 after being dehydrated with ethanol (30-96 degrees of Celsius), in acetone and propylene oxide. Then the cutting was realized with the aid of ultra-microtome LKB-3 followed by the observation with an electronic microscope (Hitachi 125, Japan) [27] after placing the material in the uranyl acetate and lead citrate for the contraction.

Determination of apoptosis

the quantification of apoptosis of lymphocytes was performed by the method of flow cytometry on FACSCalibur device ("Becton Dickinson") with the use of some parameters, such as the determination of the fragmentation of DNA by the iodide propidium (IP) ("Sigma") [28], the translocation of membrane phosphatidylserines to the surface of lymphocytes using merocyanine (MC540), the measuring of the variation in mitochondrial membrane potential of lymphocytes according to the fluorescence intensity CMX-Ros ("Molecular Probes") [29]. More than 10, 000 cells were counted on each variant of the experiment.

Statistical analysis

the analysis was performed using Excel program and Statistics 5.0. Comparison of ranges of variation was done with non-parametric criteria of Kryckaya Yollica and T- criteria of Manna Yitni. The authenticity of the frequency difference of the indices encountered was determined using the method of Fischer and t-test and partly with correction of Bonfferoni. The correctional analysis was performed by the method of Rank and Cpirmena-rs.

Results

Immunological aspects

The content of antibodies against double-stranded DNA and the content of CIC in the blood of patients with ABA

The rate of antibodies against double-stranded DNA in the serum of patients with ABA and relatively healthy donors was examined using enzyme immunoassay (Figure 1). A minimum level of antibodies in all patient groups was observed (Figure 1b). With the method of correlational analysis we established a direct relationship of dependence between the high level of IgG antibodies – anti DNA and the severity of asthma ($p = 0.0005$). A significant and direct relationship of dependence between the level of extracellular DNA levels and that of antibodies (IgG anti-nDNA) was also established (Figure 2). The attention was on the value of p (0.00006), reflecting the strong correlation between its significant data. The results of Figure 3 show a significant increase ($p < 0.05$) of the concentration of circulating immune complexes (CIC) in the blood of asthmatic patients compared with controls. And the concentration was significant in asthmatic patients with serious severity. In determining the size of the CIC, we observed that 85.6% of patients with bronchial asthma had CIC of small and medium size in the blood. On the other hand, in relatively healthy individuals, CIC of large size were recorded in 86% of donors and while 14% had CIC of medium size. Thus, the results of this study showed an increase in the concentration of CIC in asthmatic patients with a change in the size of the CIC towards the dominant formation of CIC of small and medium size and this rate of distribution was related to the severity of asthma. Using the method of correlational analysis, we have established with certainty a direct dependency relationship between the formation of CIC and antibodies to native DNA (Figure 4a) and on the other hand, the concentration of CIC was inversely proportional to the concentration extracellular DNA.

Programmed cell death of lymphocytes of patients with ABA

Given that changes were observed rapidly at cellular level, we found interesting the study of biochemical and morphological parameters of lymphocytes of patients with asthma in vitro after reviewing the immunological aspects. Therefore, we conducted a comparative analysis of morphological characteristics of lymphocytes of relatively healthy donors and patients with asthma of mild and serious severity. Thus, with the aid of transmission electron microscopy morphological differences were identified between the lymphocytes of control group and the lymphocytes of patients with asthma. The electron microscope revealed morphological and structural changes in lymphocytes especially in the nucleus, the chromatin and plasma membrane of patients with

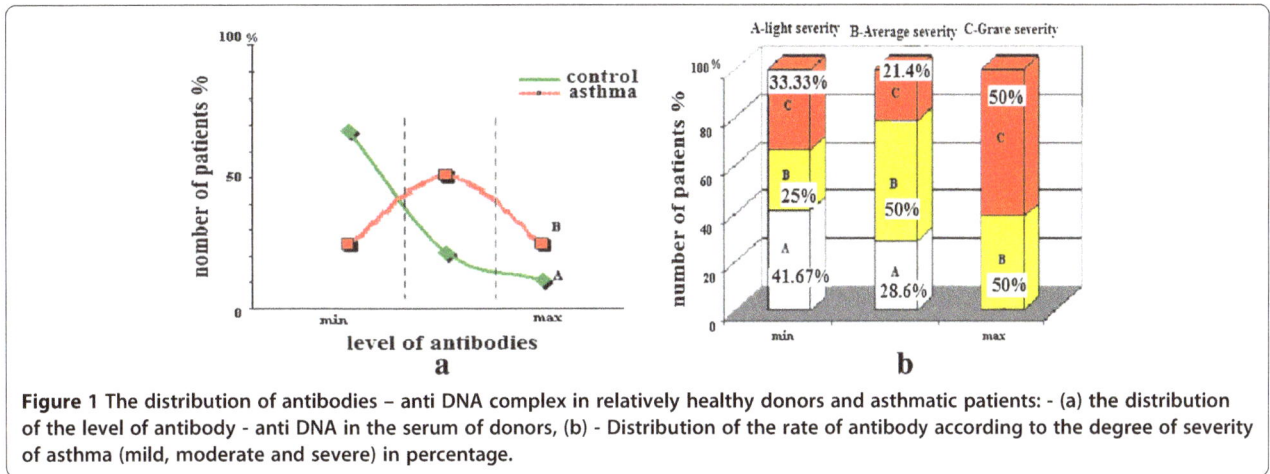

Figure 1 The distribution of antibodies – anti DNA complex in relatively healthy donors and asthmatic patients: - (a) the distribution of the level of antibody - anti DNA in the serum of donors, (b) - Distribution of the rate of antibody according to the degree of severity of asthma (mild, moderate and severe) in percentage.

asthma and this according to the severity degree of the disease. Cells with a modified structure were observed: on the cell surface outgrowths appeared on the cell membrane, deep invaginations and chromatin condensation and orientation of the nucleus towards the periphery with intussusceptions. The structure of the lymphocytes of the peripheral blood from asthmatic patients with serious severity differs from the structure of the cells of clinically healthy donors and that of asthmatics with mild severity (Figure 5). The buddings known as the blebbing were observed on the cell membrane [30]. Besides, some cells contain phagosomes with cellular debris inside which are generally characteristics of autophagic cells (Figure 5a,b). The study of apoptosis in vitro now provides a better understanding of malfunction of the molecular processes during asthma. In the culture media most of the cells die by apoptosis. But our present study showed that this statement is not always

true in asthmatics. To study the biochemical parameters in vitro, we compared the level of lymphocytes for 3 and 6 days of growth in the presence or in the absence of dexamethasone which is an inductor of apoptosis. As shown in Figure 6, the rate of lymphocytes increased after 3 days of growth at all the groups studied, particularly in clinically healthy donors and asthmatic patients with mild severity. On the other hand, after 6 days of growth there was a decrease in the rate of lymphocytes at all groups studied compared to those observed after 3 days of culture (Figure 6). The use of dexamethasone as inductor of apoptosis resulted in an increase of 5% (Figure 7) of the level of lymphocytes in clinically healthy donors after 3 days of culture and a decrease of 70% (compared to 3rd day) after 6 days of culture (Figure 8). The structure of these lymphocytes underwent significant changes, which may indicate an inhibition of mitotic activity of the cells of clinically healthy donors in the presence of dexamethasone. The lymphocytes of asthmatic patients with mild severity in the presence of dexamethasone continue to proliferate with a slight

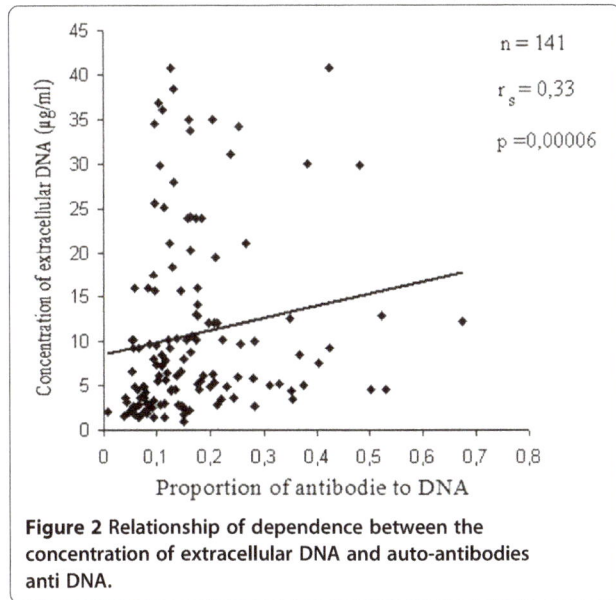

Figure 2 Relationship of dependence between the concentration of extracellular DNA and auto-antibodies anti DNA.

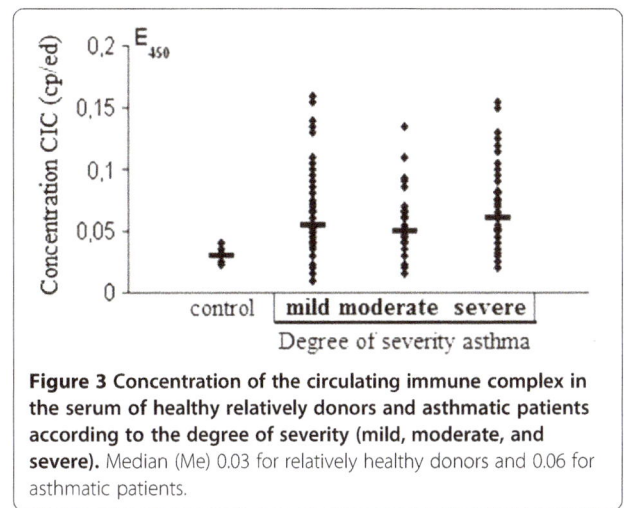

Figure 3 Concentration of the circulating immune complex in the serum of healthy relatively donors and asthmatic patients according to the degree of severity (mild, moderate, and severe). Median (Me) 0.03 for relatively healthy donors and 0.06 for asthmatic patients.

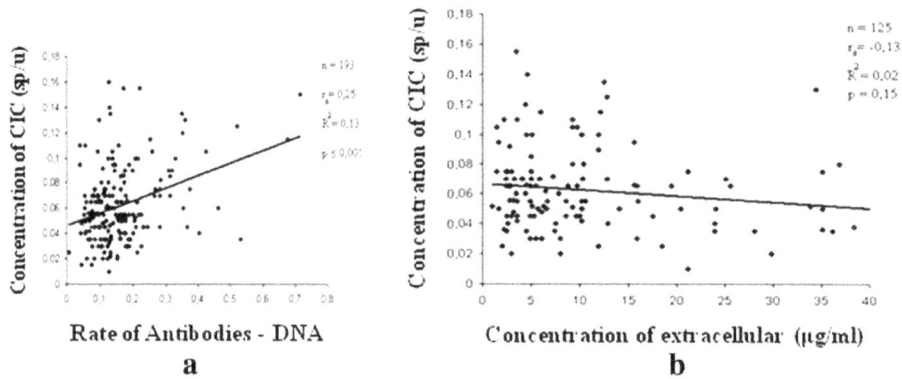

Figure 4 Determination of dependency relationships between immunological markers of patients with asthma: a- The dependency relationship between the concentration of CIC and the rate of antibodies anti-DNA, b- Dependency relationship between the concentration of CIC and the concentration of extracellular DNA in the blood serum of patients with atopic bronchial asthma.

decrease in the proliferative activity of its lymphocytes, which could explain the death of its cells following apoptotic induction. After 6 days of culture, there was a decrease in lymphocytes of patients with mild severity (Figure 8). More attention should be paid to the lymphocytes of asthmatic patients with serious severity: if in the absence of dexamethasone, the level of lymphocytes increased by 15% while in the presence of the apoptotic inductor this level declining by 10% after 3 days of culture as compared to the level before the cell culture. With cytometry method the quantification of apoptosis of lymphocytes with the use of some biochemical parameters was performed. During the study of the mechanism of PCD, great importance was given to mitochondria as it releases a large amount of biologically active substance necessary for the transition from apoptosis to the final and irreversible phase [30]. From the analysis of Figure 9, a correlation between the number of cells with a decrease of mitochondrial membrane potential and the expression of phosphatidilserine on the membrane wall of lymphocyte of clinically healthy donors and asthmatic was

observed. After 3 days of culture, no significant difference was found between the numbers of lymphocytes with a decrease in membrane potential which underwent a translocation of phosphatidylcholine on the cell membrane (Figure 9). The level of lymphocytes with a decrease in membrane potential in clinically healthy donors has increased by 70% and 110% in asthmatics with mild severity. On the other hand, this level is not as expressive in asthmatic of serious severity after 6 days of culture. The incubation of lymphocytes in the presence of dexamethasone leads to a decrease in the size of mitochondrial membrane potential in some lymphocytes but the dynamics vary considerably from one group to another. In the presence of dexamethasone, a slight resistance of lymphocytes of clinically healthy donors compared to a spontaneous apoptosis was observed (Figure 10). After 3 days of incubation with dexamethasone, that the number of lymphocytes with decreased mitochondrial membrane potential was higher in asthmatics compared to clinically healthy donors was recorded. The lymphocytes of patients with ABA showed

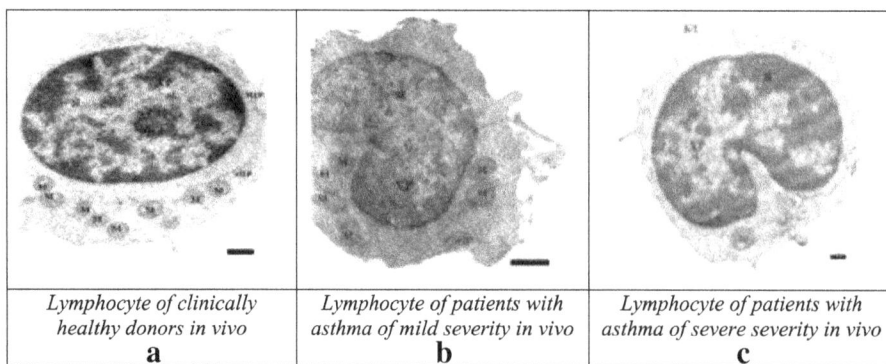

Lymphocyte of clinically healthy donors in vivo	Lymphocyte of patients with asthma of mild severity in vivo	Lymphocyte of patients with asthma of severe severity in vivo
a	b	c

Figure 5 Comparative study of Ultrastructure of lymphocytes of clinically healthy donors (a) and of patients with asthma according to the degree of severity: (b)-mild severity (c) severe severity in vivo.

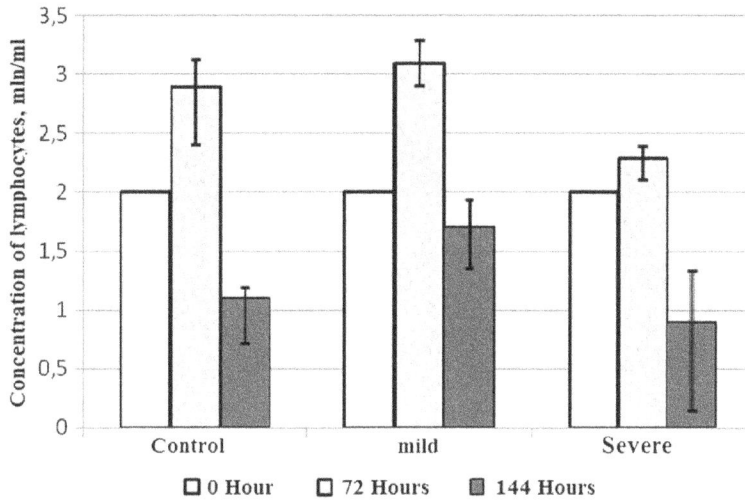

Figure 6 Evolution of the concentration of lymphocytes of clinically healthy donors and asthmatics with mild and severe severity after 0, 3 and 6 days cultures in vitro.

resistance to the development of apoptosis while clinically healthy donor lymphocytes were characterized by a progressive increase in PCD after 6 days of culture. A small demonstration of early signs of spontaneous apoptosis and induced lymphocytes of patients with asthma of mild and serious severity after 6 days of culture in vitro might lead us to think of a disruption of this process of PCD of type 1. The use of iodide propidium revealed cells with fragmented DNA (Figure 11). According to some authors, the morphological characteristics of DNA fragmentation were characterized by an invagination of the nuclear membrane and condensation of chromatin at the nuclear periphery level. In vitro studies showed no significant difference in DNA fragmentation of lymphocytes (Figure 12). Even after 6 days of incubation, the DNA fragmentation of lymphocytes of asthmatics was less pronounced compared to controls. The results showed that there were cells with fragmented DNA both in asthmatics and in clinically healthy donors. Culture of cells without dexamethasone (spontaneous apoptosis) for 3-6 days resulted in a fragmentation of the DNA of lymphocytes (Figure 12). The number of cells with fragmented DNA almost doubled in the culture medium of relatively healthy donors (9% -18%) and in asthmatics with mild severity this variation was 8% to 15% while it was 14% to 21% in asthmatics patients with serious severity. When comparing among themselves, the development of the process in some cultures (for 3 and 6 days) in the presence of dexamethasone, there was a 3-fold increase in the number of cells with characteristic traits of the

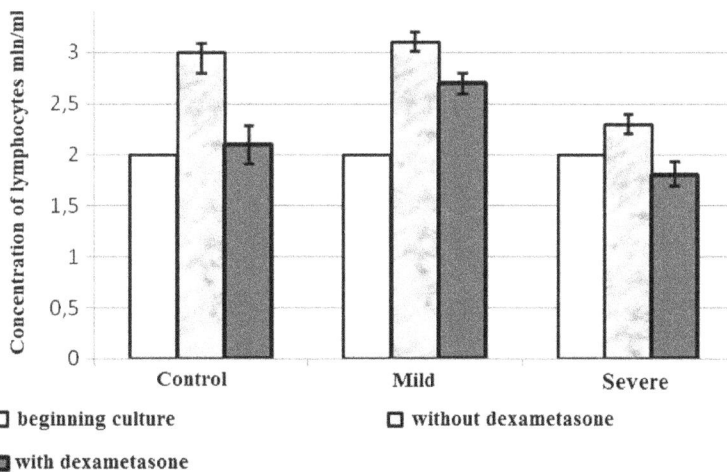

Figure 7 Variation of the number of lymphocytes (mln/ml) of clinically healthy donors (control) and of patients with asthma (mild and severe severity) during 3 and 6 days of culture with or without dexamethasone in vitro.

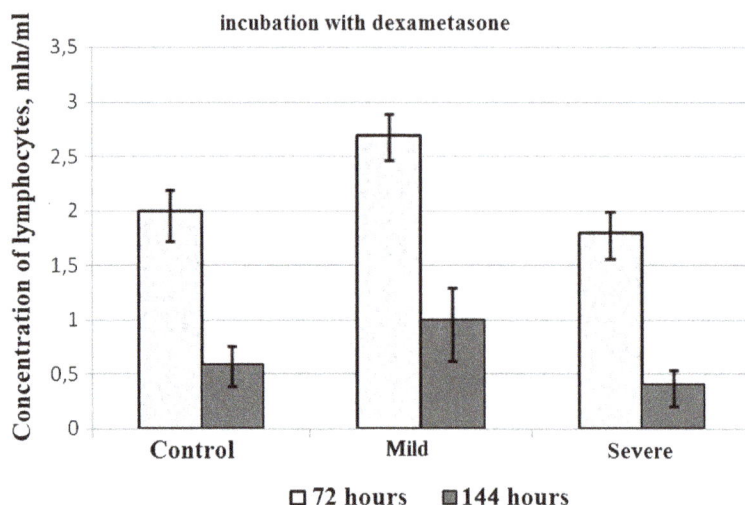

Figure 8 Comparative study of evolution of lymphocytes of clinically healthy donors and patients with asthma of mild and severe severity after 3 and 6 days of culture in the presence of dexamethasone.

final phase of apoptosis (ie 187%) in relatively healthy donors (Figure 12) and 25% (from 8% to 10%) in asthmatics with mild severity and 14% (ie from 14 to 16%) in asthmatics with serious severity. We followed the dynamics of the induction of spontaneous apoptosis and apoptosis induced by dexamethasone of lymphocytes in vitro in different groups studied and it was found that the lymphocytes of relatively normal donors responded to the induction of spontaneous apoptosis and induced by dexamethasone with a significant increase in the number of apoptotic cells in the final

phase of 67% after 3 days of culture and 190% after 6 days of culture (Figure 12). As the results show, the asthmatic cells demonstrate a resistance to apoptosis induced by dexamethasone.

Discussion

In a physiopathological context, asthma is a chronic inflammatory disease of the respiratory airways [31] and the choice of the study of programmed cell death is particularly due to the fact that these lymphocytes play an irrecusable role in the pathogenesis of asthma [17,32,33].

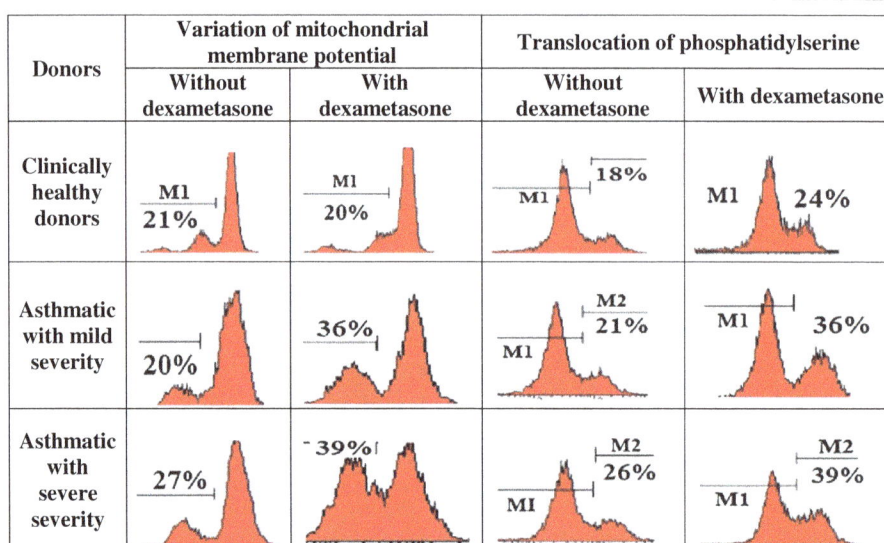

Figure 9 Cytofluorogramme showing the quantification of the apoptosis of lymphocytes of relatively healthy donors and of asthmatic with mild and severe severity by using some parameters such as the translocation of phosphatidylserine at the surface of lymphocytes with MC540 and the variation of mitochondrial membrane potential according to the fluorescence intensity of CMX -Ros during 3 days of culture with dexamethasone.

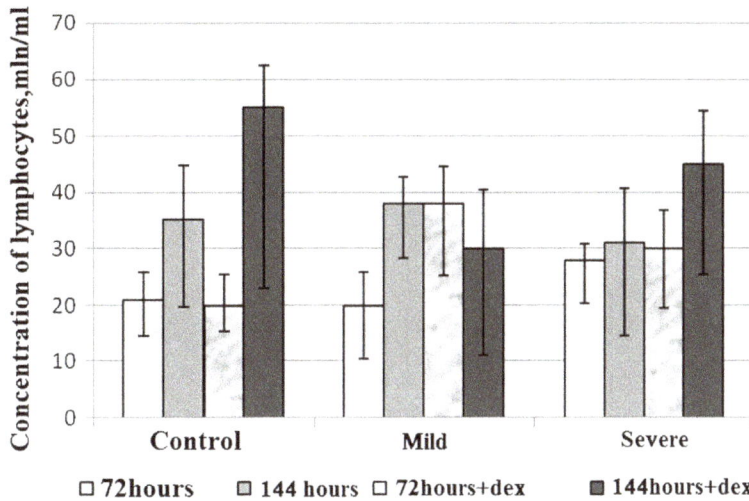

Figure 10 Variation of mitochondrial membrane potential of lymphocytes of relatively healthy donors and patients with atopic bronchial asthma (mild and severe severity) after 3 and 6 days of culture with or without dexamethasone in vitro.

Despite the plentiful data on asthma, the concept of PCD in the pathogenesis of asthma is and remains misunderstood and controversial [34,35]. Increasing interest in this process of PCD [36] in recent years was fundamental to conduct this present study. During the development of asthma a multitude of Immunogenetic mechanism and cells of immune systems might be involved [37]. The results of immunological studies suggest a number of changes in the functional state of lymphocytes in patients with asthma. In 1995 Szczeklik et al. [38] while studying the autoimmune status of patients suffering from Bronchial asthma, found in the blood some antinuclear antibodies, in any case, none of the patients got some antibodies with $_{N}$DNA, however, the quantity of autoimmunity of the patients suffering from bronchial pulmonary system reveal the advantage of the synthesis of specific organ antibody, for example $_{N}$DNA and/or

$_{DN}$DNA autoantibodies [39]. Therefore, the level of IgG anti -$_{N}$DNA increased significantly according to the degree of severity of asthma (Figure 2) and given that IgG have the ability to be locked up in the tissues, one could think of a lesion of target tissues in progressive course with the severity degree of the disease. It was revealed in patients with asthma the significant presence of CIC of average size and considered as the most pathogenic of CIC which was formed during a slight plethora of antigens. In relatively healthy donors, a process of enlargement of chronic CIC was observed and this in accordance with a proportional relationship of the level of antigen and antibody corresponding to their elimination. It should be noted that we recorded a direct relationship of dependence between the concentration of CIC and the level of antibodies against DNA and inverse dependence between the concentration of CIC and the concentration of

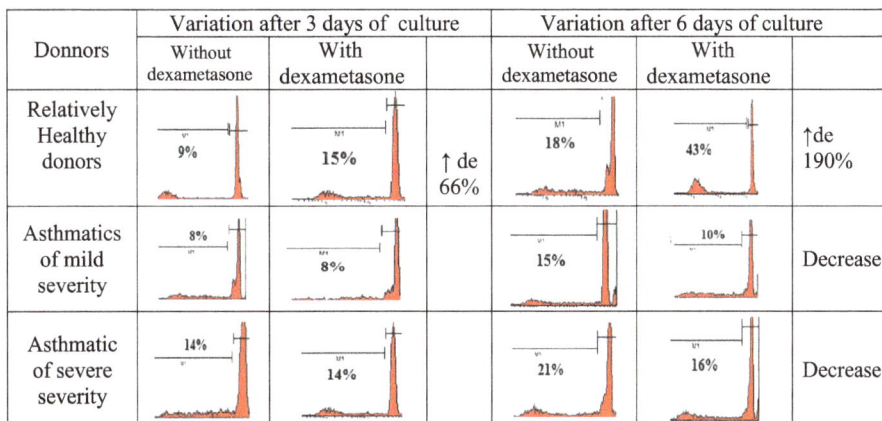

Donnors	Variation after 3 days of culture			Variation after 6 days of culture		
	Without dexametasone	With dexametasone		Without dexametasone	With dexametasone	
Relatively Healthy donors	9%	15%	↑ de 66%	18%	43%	↑de 190%
Asthmatics of mild severity	8%	8%		15%	10%	Decrease
Asthmatic of severe severity	14%	14%		21%	16%	Decrease

Figure 11 Cytofluorogramme showing the quantification of the apoptosis of lymphocytes of relatively healthy donors and of asthmatic with mild and severe forms by using some parameter such as the determination of DNA fragmentation with propidium iodide after 3 days and 6 days of culture without or with dexametasone.

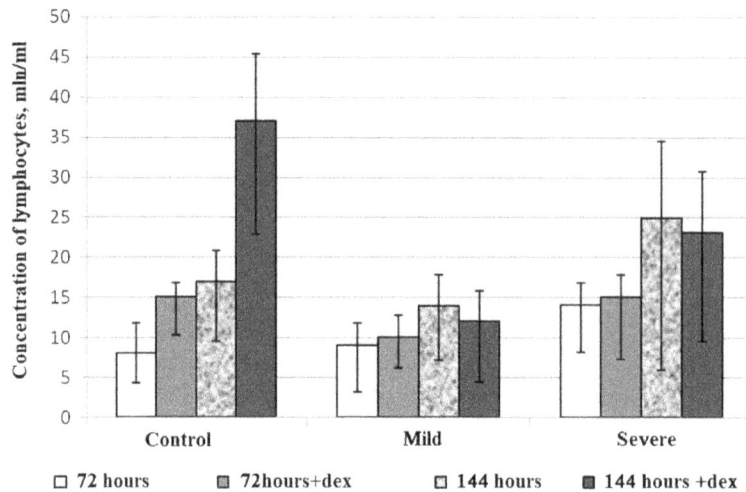

Figure 12 Variation of the concentration of lymphocytes during the advance phase of apoptosis in clinically healthy donors and asthmatics with mild and severe severity after 3 and 6 days of culture with or without dexamethasone.

extracellular DNA in the blood (Figure 6). This leads us to suggest the absence of a relation of equivalence between the antibody and the antigen during the progression of the severity degree of asthma. The existence of CIC in the blood is a normal and natural phenomenon of immune reactions. But their high level constitutes a means of diagnosing the pathology. Circulating immune complexes of large size are less soluble and can be easily removed by macrophages unlike CIC of medium and small size. They dissolve easily, making their removal difficult, which explains the CIC concentrations of medium and small size in asthmatics with serious severity. Therefore, the conception of the role played by the immune process in the pathogenesis of asthma is widely acknowledged, however, the importance of indicators of diagnosis and individual prognosis of the immune system remains poorly studied and in particular the accumulation in biological fluids IG antibodies - anti DNA, abzymes with DNAse activities, extracellular DNA, and CIC according to the degree of severity of the disease. The results obtained in this study allow us to suggest that these markers play a vital role in the pathogenesis of autoimmune process during asthma. And it is not excluded that these immunological characteristics stemmed from other natural physiological process. Thus, the observed difference underlined in the mitotic activity and the variation of the level of lymphocytes in culture of clinically healthy donors and asthmatic shows varying degrees of cell survival according to the severity of the disease. From the results of our work we could note that, based on a slowing of cell growth of lymphocytes from asthmatics with severe severity, the lymphocytes of asthmatics with mild severity are characteristic of lymphoproliferous activity in vitro. For the researches on asthma we do not often take into account the severity of asthma. Patients with asthma of mild and severe severity have different backgrounds and do not have the same degree of deficiency of

the immune system. Failure to take into account the degree of severity could lead to false reasoning of statistical analysis. We found after our study that PCD of lymphocytes of patients manifested differently based on their degree of severity. Further to the adoption of the concept of PCD of type 1, the death of lymphocytes under the influence of certain doses of glucocorticoids was considered a classic model of apoptosis [40,41]. Recently data were published on the sensitivity of subpopulations of lymphocytes of peripheral blood particularly cytotoxic and NK lymphocytes at a high dose of dexamethasone [42,43]. The use of systemic glucocorticoids increases systematically the number of lymphocytes in the dipodiploide area. This confirms the hypothesis that the use of corticosteroids inhibit cytokine production (Ile 3, 4, 5) which keeps the high level of Bcl-2 anti apoptotic protein) and consequently leads to an acceleration of apoptosis lymphocytes [24,44]. On the other hand, studies showed that the use of dexamethasone leads to a decrease in the number of migrating cells in the lungs after inhalation of specific allergens [45]. The dexamethasone as inductor of apoptosis is expected to influence the number of proliferating cells especially their reduction [46,47]. But according to our data, the lymphocytes of asthmatic patients with mild severity showed resistance to glucocorticoids followed by active proliferation of its cells. There was also a decrease in the number of cells in the late phase of apoptosis. This may be due to a malfunction of the expression of DNase responsible for DNA degradation. It is conceivable in view of these results that there are indeed particularities in the course of apoptosis, in asthmatics and this according to the degree of severity of the disease. However, even if the conditions of the body seem to be met to artificially induce apoptosis, the results obtained could not totally be those of internal conditions. Several parameters can influence the results. Researches on apoptosis still continue nowadays, it may be other unknown physiological parameters which determine the course of this process, of which the absence would influence the results. Asthma can also be linked to a genetic predisposition, and even from a race to another, differences can be observed. Thus, results on the morphology of lymphocytes of asthmatics were obtained. And most of lymphocytes had specific morphological characteristics. Sometimes, cells with characteristics of autophagosomes autophagy were found [29,48]. The presence of autophagy could explain the decrease of apoptotic cells in asthmatics with mild severity. And the PCD is universally prevalent in the world of multicellular organisms, and affects all types of tissues. It operates according to the biochemical and morphological parameters strictly defined and do not depend on the causes leading to the initiation of this process. In addition, the study of PCD is very productive to understand a certain number of important processes including immune homeostasis. Finally, according to new data, it has become essential and indispensable to review a certain number of conceptual bases of physiopathology and immunopathology.

Conclusion

Autoimmunity and Programmed Cell Death are a highly conserved and integrated response in normal physiological processes playing a vital role in the pathogenesis of various diseases, especially in the development of asthma.

Competing interests
We have no competing interests.

Authors' contributions
ZIA, CAV, LBM, SAA designed the study. CAV, YVS, VE, CBC participated in the technical work and the acquisition and interpretation of data. CBC, AN, SOK, SOK, CAV evaluated the literature. CAV, LBM, ZIA, YVS, YVS carried out the experiments of this study. SOK, LBM, VE, SAA, SOK, CAV and ZIA have given final approval of the version to be published. All authors have read and approved the final manuscript.

Acknowledgement
The authors thank Federation of Russia and University of Parakou.

Author details
[1]Laboratory Acid Nucleic, Institute of Fundamental Medicine and Biology, Kazan Federal University (KFU-Russian), Kremlyovskaya str. 18, Kazan 480008, Republic of Tatarstan, Russian Fédération. [2]Laboratoire de Biologie et de Typage Moléculaire en Microbiologie, Département de biochimie et biologie cellulaire, Faculté des sciences et Techniques (FAST), Université d'Abomey-Calavi (UAC-Benin), 05PB1604 Cotonou, Benin. [3]Department of Biology and Center for Computational & Integrative Biology, Rutgers University, Camden, NJ 08102, USA. [4]Laboratoire de Biochimie et Biologie Moléculaire, Faculté de Médecine, Université de Parakou, BP: 123 Parakou, Parakou, Benin.

References
1. Nagata S: Apoptosis by death factor. *Cell* 1997, **88**:355–365.
2. Jacobson MD, Weil M, Raff MC: Programmed cell death in animal development. *Cell* 1997, **88**:347–354.
3. Barber GN: Host defense, viruses and apoptosis. *Cell Death Differ* 2001, **8**:113–126.
4. Okada H, Mak TW: Pathways of apoptotic and non-apoptotic death in tumor cells. *Nat Rev Cancer* 2004, **4**:592–603.
5. Vodounon ACJ, Baba-Moussa L, Skibo YV, Sezan A, Abramova ZI: The Implication of Morphological Characteristics in the Etiology of Allergic asthma Disease and in Determining the Degree of Severity of Atopic and Bronchial Asthma. *Asian J Cell Biol* 2011, **6**:65–80.
6. Moskaleva E, Severin SE: Possible mechanisms of adaptation of cells damage, inducing programmed death, the relationship with the pathology. *Pathol Physiol Exp Ther* 2006, **2**:2–16.
7. Mansky BH: Ways to cell death and their biological significance. *Cytology* 2007, **49**(11):909–914.
8. Edinger AZ, Thompson C: Death by design: apoptosis, necrosis and autophagy. *Curr Opin Cell Biol* 2004, **16**:663–669.
9. Lockshin RA, Zakeri Z: Apoptosis, autophagy, and more. *JBCB* 2004, **36**:2405–2419.
10. Kando Y, Kanzawa T, Sawaya R, Kondo S: The role of autophagy in cancer development and response to therapy. *Nat Rev Canc* 2005, **5**:726–734.
11. Levine B, Klionsky DJ: Development by self-digestion: molecular machanisms and biological functions of autophagy. *Dev Cell* 2004, **6**:463–477.
12. Levine B, Yuan J: Autophagy in cell death: an innocent convict? *J Clin Investig* 2005, **115**:2679–2688.
13. Nishino I: Autophagic vacuolar myopathies. *Curr Neurol Neurosci Rep* 2003, **3**:64–69.
14. Meijer AJ, Codogno JP: Regulation and role of autophagy in mammalian cells. *IJBCB* 2004, **36**:2445–2462.
15. Urbonien D, Skalauskas R, Sitkauskiene B: Autoimmunity in pathogenesis of chronic obstructive pulmonary disease. *Medicina (Kaunas)* 2005, **41**(3):190–195.
16. Yarilin AA: *Fundamentals of Immunology.* Moscow: Meditsina Publishers; 1999.
17. Barnes PJ, Adcock IM: How do corticosteroids work in asthma? *Ann Intern Med* 2003, **139**:359–370.
18. Goldsby RA, Kindt TJ, Osborn BA: Enzyme-linked Immunosorbent Assay. *Immunology* 2003, **5**:148–150.
19. Patel D, Rubbi CP, Rickwood D: Separation of T and B lymphocytes from human peripheral blood mononuclear cells using density perturbation methods. *Clin Chim Acta* 1995, **240**:187–193.
20. Heyfits LB, Abalkin VA: Separation of human blood cells in a density gradient Ficoll-verografin. *Lab Work* 1973, **10**:579–581.
21. Antoneeva II: Differentiation and activation-associated markers of peripheral blood lymphocytes in the patients with ovarian in the course of tumor progression. *Med Immunol* 2007, **6**:649–652.
22. Khorshid FA, Moshref SS: In vitro anticancer agent, I-tissue culture study of human lung cancer cells A549 II-tissue culture study of mice leukemia cells L1210. *Int J Canc Res* 2006, **2**:330–344.
23. Soroka NF, Svirnovski AI, Rekun AL: Effect of immunosuppressive drugs on apoptosis of lymphocytes of patients with systemic lupus erythematosus in vitro. *Sci Pratic Rheumatol* 2007, **1**:15–21.
24. Boychuk SV, Mustafin IG, Fassahov RS: Mechanisms of dexamethasone-induced apoptosis of lymphocytes in atopic asthma. *Pulmonology* 2003, **2**:10–16.
25. Doering J, Begue B, Lentze MJ, Rieux-Laucat F, Goulet O: Induction of T-lymphocytes apoptosis by sulphasalazine in patients with Crohn's disease. *Gut* 2004, **53**:1632–1638.
26. Abdelmeguid NE, Mostafa MH, Abdel-Moneim AM, Badawi AF, Abou Zeinab NS: Tamoxifen and melatonin differentially influence apoptosis of normal mammary gland cells: Ultrastructural evidence and p53 expression. *Int J Canc Res* 2008, **4**:81–91.
27. Sanders EJ, Wride MA: Ultrastructural identification of apoptotic nuclei using the TUNEL technique. *Histochem J* 1996, **28**:275–281.
28. Nicoletti I, Migliorati G, Pagliacci MC, Grignani F, Riccardi C: A rapid and simple method for measuring thymocyte apoptosis by propidium iodide staining and flow cytometry. *J Immunol Meth* 1991, **139**:271–279.
29. Melis M, Siena L: Fluticasone induces apoptosis in peripheral T-lymphocytes: a comparison between asthmatic and normal subjects. *Eur Respir J* 2002, **19**:257–266.
30. Reichlin NT, Reichlin AN: Apoptosis regulation and manifestation in physiological conditions and tumors. *Probl Oncol* 2002, **48**:159–171.
31. Lee J-H, Yu H-H, Wang L-C, Yang Y-H, Lin Y-T, Chiang B-L: The levels of CD4[+]CD25[+] regulatory T cells in paediatric patients with allergic rhinitis and bronchial asthma. *Clin Exp Immunol* 2007, **148**(1):53–63.

32. Vignola AM: **Airway Inflammation in Mild Intermittent and in Persistent Asthma.** *Am J Respir Crit Care Med* 1998, **157**(2):403–409.

33. Mammoth TV, Kaidashev IP: **New aspects of the apoptosis of mononuclear cells in the pathogenesis of atopic asthma.** *Allergology* 2005, **4**:15–23.

34. Deponte M: **Programmed cell death in protists.** *Biochem Biophys Acta* 2008, **1783**:1396–1405.

35. Jiménez C, Capasso JM, Edelstein CL: **Different ways to die: cell death modes of the unicellular chlorophyte Dunaliella viridis exposed to various environmental stresses are mediated by the caspase-like activity DEVDase.** *J Exp Bot* 2009, **3**:815–828.

36. Bidle KD, Falkowski PG: **Cell death in planktonic, photosynthetic microorganisms.** *Nat Rev Microbiol* 2004, **2**:643–655.

37. Wiik AS, Gordon TP, Kavanaugh AF, Lahita RG, Reeves W, van Venrooij WJ, Wilson MR, Fritzler M: **Cutting edge diagnostics in rheumatology: the role of patients, clinicians, and laboratory scientists in optimizing the use of autoimmune serology.** *Arthritis Rheum* 2004, **51**:291–298.

38. Szczeklik A, Nizankowska E, Serafin A: **Autoimmune phenomena in bronchial asthma with special reference to aspirin intolerance.** *Am J Respir Crit Care Med* 1995, **6**:1753–1756.

39. Markin OA, Yastrebova HE, Vaneva HP: **Autoantibodies in children with chronic inflammatory lung diseases.** *Zh Mikrobiol Epidemiol Immunobiol* 2001, **6**:52–55.

40. Kaznatheev K, Kaznatheev KS, LF Kaznacheeva LF, Molokov AV: **Apoptosis cell in children with atopic dermatitis during the application of the cream "Skin-Cap".** *Allergy* 2006, **3**:7–11.

41. Majino G, Majino G, Joris I: **Apoptosis, oncosis and necrosis. An overview of cell death.** *J Pathol* 1995, **146**(1):3–15.

42. Leung D: **Pathogenesis of atopic dermatitis.** *J Allergy Clin Immunol* 1999, **104**:99–108.

43. Kungurov NV, Gerasimov NM, Kohan MM: *Atopic dermatitis. Types of course, the principles of therapy.* Ekaterinburg; 2000:272.

44. Mineev VN, Nesterovich II, Orange ES, Tafer AL: **Apoptosis and the activity of ribosomal cistrons in peripheral blood cells in bronchial asthma.** *Allergology* 2003, **3**:15–19.

45. O'Sullivan S, Cormican L, Burke CM: **Fluticasone induces T cell apoptosis in the bronchial wall of mild to moderate asthmatics.** *Asthma* 2004, **59**(8):657–661.

46. Tuckermann JP, Kleiman A, McPherson KG, Reichardt HM: **Molecular mechanisms of glucocorticoids in the control of inflammation and lymphocyte apoptosis.** *Crit Rev Clin Lab Sci* 2005, **42**:71–104.

47. Frankfurt O, Rosen ST: **Mechanisms of glucocorticoid-induced apoptosis in hematologic malignancies: updates.** *Curr Opin Oncol* 2004, **16**:553–563.

48. Degenhardt K, Mathew R, Beaudoin B, Chen G: **Autophagy promotes tumor cell survival and restricts necrosis, inflammation, and tumorigenesis.** *Cancer Cell* 2006, **10**:51–64.

10

A detailed phenotypic analysis of immune cell populations in the bronchoalveolar lavage fluid of atopic asthmatics after segmental allergen challenge

Jonathan S Boomer[1], Amit D Parulekar[1,2], Brenda M Patterson[1], Huiqing Yin-Declue[1], Christine M Deppong[1], Seth Crockford[1], Nizar N Jarjour[3], Mario Castro[1] and Jonathan M Green[1*]

Abstract

Background: Atopic asthma is characterized by intermittent exacerbations triggered by exposure to allergen. Exacerbations are characterized by an acute inflammatory reaction in the airways, with recruitment of both innate and adaptive immune cells. These cell populations as well as soluble factors are critical for initiating and controlling the inflammatory processes in allergic asthma. Detailed data on the numbers and types of cells recruited following allergen challenge is lacking. In this paper we present an extensive phenotypic analysis of the inflammatory cell infiltrate present in the bronchoalveolar lavage (BAL) fluid following bronchoscopically directed allergen challenge in mild atopic asthmatics.

Methods: A re-analysis of pooled data obtained prior to intervention in our randomized, placebo controlled, double blinded study (costimulation inhibition in asthma trial [CIA]) was performed. Twenty-four subjects underwent bronchoscopically directed segmental allergen challenge followed by BAL collection 48 hours later. The BAL fluid was analyzed by multi-color flow cytometry for immune cell populations and multi-plex ELISA for cytokine detection.

Results: Allergen instillation induced pro-inflammatory cytokines (IL-6) and immune modulating cytokines (IL-2, IFN-γ, and IL-10) along with an increase in lymphocytes and suppressor cells (Tregs and MDSC). Interestingly, membrane expression of CD30 was identified on lymphocytes, especially Tregs, but not eosinophils. Soluble CD30 was also detected in the BAL fluid after allergen challenge in adult atopic asthmatics.

Conclusions: After segmental allergen challenge of adult atopic asthmatics, cell types associated with a pro-inflammatory as well as an anti-inflammatory response are detected within the BAL fluid of the lung.

Keywords: T lymphocyte, CD30 expression, Segmental allergen challenge, Asthma

Background

Asthma is a complex immunological disease affecting approximately 8-10% of the population of the United States [1-3]. The pathology of asthma includes pulmonary inflammation, airway eosinophilia, mucus hypersecretion and airway hyperreactivity (AHR), induced by specific and nonspecific stimuli which lead to an inappropriate Th2 response [1-3]. T lymphocytes of a Th2 type secrete IL-3, IL-4, IL-5, IL-9, and IL-13 [1-3], cytokines which play important roles in Th2 lymphocyte survival, B cell isotype switching to IgE and mast cell, basophil and eosinophil differentiation and survival [1-4]. This complex inflammatory cascade is controlled by soluble factors as well as interactions between cell types involving surface receptors such as CD80/86 on dendritic cells (DC) and CD28/CTLA-4 on T cells [5-9], ultimately resulting in the asthma phenotype [1-3].

* Correspondence: jgreen@wustl.edu
[1]Department of Internal Medicine, Washington University School of Medicine, St Louis, MO 63110, USA
Full list of author information is available at the end of the article

Although inflammation is critical to the pathogenesis of asthma, the exact cell types present in the lung and their differentiation state remain not well defined. In this report, we characterized the immune cell populations and cytokines present within the lungs of mild atopic asthmatics that underwent bronchoscopy with broncho-alveolar lavage (BAL) after segmental allergen challenge (SAC). We detected an increase in pro-inflammatory cytokines (IL-6) and immune modulating cytokines (IL-2, IFN-γ and IL-10) along with an increase in lymphocytes and the suppressor cells, regulatory T (Treg) and myeloid derived suppressor cells (MDSC). Although we did not detect expression of CD30 on eosinophils, we did detect significant membrane expression of CD30 on Tregs and the presence of sCD30 in the BAL fluid of adult atopic asthmatics.

Methods

Data collected from the Costimulation Inhibition in Asthma (CIA) trial (ClinicalTrials.gov NCT00784459) [10] was pooled and re-analyzed for this manuscript. For detailed methods and a description of the participant population and inclusion/exclusion criteria, please refer to reference [10]. In brief, nonsmoking males and females between 18 and 50 years of age with previously diagnosed mild asthma by NAEPP guidelines were identified. At screening, participants underwent skin prick testing of cat allergen extract, short ragweed allergen extract (Ambrosia artemisiifolia), and standardized dust mite allergen extracts (Dermatophagoides farinae and/or Dermatophagoides pteronyssinus) (all from Greer Laboratories, Lenoir NC) to determine their reactivity using standard methods [10-13] (Table 1). Eligible participants underwent bronchoscopy with segmental allergen challenge (SAC) with instillation of 5 ml allergen solution at a concentration 1000X the minimum skin reactive test dose, with a maximum of 1:100 dilution of the stock allergen . Repeat bronchoscopy was performed 48 hours later with BAL performed in the same subsegment in which allergen had previously been instilled. The study was approved by the Washington University Institutional Review Board.

Table 1 Allergens used for titrated skin prick testing

	1:100000	1:1000000	1:10000000	Total
Cat	2	3	5	10
Ragweed	4	5	2	11
D farinae	1	0	1	2
D Pteronyssinus	1	0	0	1

The dilution of allergen that provoked a positive test during titrated skin prick testing is shown. Shown is the number of subjects that had a positive test at the indicated dilution of allergen. 24 subjects were recruited for the initial trial with pre-randomization data re-analyzed for this study. Adapted from Table E8 (reference [10]).

Measurement of BAL total cell counts and differentials

In the research laboratory, total cell counts were determined, cytospins prepared and manual differentials performed immediately following bronchoscopy [10]. The BAL fluid was centrifuged and the supernatant concentrated, using Ultracentrifugation Filter Units (Millipore, Billerica MA), to approximately $1/20^{th}$ of the original volume, aliquoted and frozen at −80°C for further analysis.

Flow cytometric analysis

The cell pellet recovered from the BAL was resuspended in PBS containing 1% BSA and incubated with antibodies directed against the following cell subsets: T cells were identified as CD4 or CD8, as naïve (CD45RA) or memory (CD45RO), and surface phenotyped for CD28, CD25 or CD30. B cells were identified as CD19+. NK cells were identified as CD56+. Regulatory T cells were identified by staining with CD4, CD25 and FoxP3. Dendritic cells were identified via lineage cocktail negative (CD3/CD14/CD16/CD19/CD20/CD56), HLA-DR high and either CD123+ for plasmacytoid dendritic cells (pDC), or CD11c+ for myeloid dendritic cells (mDC). Myeloid derived suppressor cells (MDSC) were identified as lineage cocktail negative, CD33+ and HLA-DR low. Eosinophils were identified by light scatter properties, CD16 negative and CD11b+. Fluorescently conjugated antibodies were purchased from BD Biosciences (San Jose, CA), BioLegend (San Diego, CA) or eBiosciences (San Diego, CA). In brief, $1-2 \times 10^6$ BAL cells were labeled with fluorescently conjugated antibodies at room temperature for 30 minutes. After labeling, RBC were lysed in 1X RBC lysis buffer (eBioscience) for 1–2 minutes and extensively washed in FACS wash (eBioscience). For FoxP3 staining, after surface labeling, cells were labeled with anti-FoxP3 antibody according to the manufactures protocol (human FoxP3 kit, eBioscience). The labeled cells were then analyzed on a 4-color FACSCalibur flow cytometer using CellQuest software (Becton-Dickinson Corporation, Mountainview, CA). Samples were gated on a lymphocyte gate followed by a second gate relevant for the population being analyzed (i.e., CD4+) and a minimum of 10,000 gated events collected. Data was further analyzed using Winlist v7 software (Verity Software Corporation, Topsham, ME).

Measurement of cytokine and soluble CD30 levels

BAL fluid was analyzed for cytokine content using the Cytokine Bead Array (Th1/Th2/Th17 kit, BD Biosciences) per the manufacturer's instructions. The soluble fragment of CD30 (sCD30) was measured by a standard enzyme-linked immunosorbent assay (ELISA) per the manufacturer's directions (human sCD30 ELISA kit,

Abnova, Walnut, CA). The limit of detection of the CBA is 5 pg/mL while the sCD30 ELISA is 0.3 ng/mL.

Statistical analysis

All data were analyzed using either SAS version 9.3 (SAS Institute, Cary, NC) or Prism version 4 (GraphPad Software Inc., La Jolla, CA). Outcomes are presented as the mean ± standard deviation or graphically as individual subject points. A non-parametric two-tailed Mann–Whitney U test was performed between pre- and post-SAC data. A 1-way ANOVA (Kruskal-Wallis) and Dunn's Multiple Comparison Test for individual means was performed when analyzing groups of 3 or more. A p-value <0.05 was considered significant.

Results

Inflammatory response to allergen

We re-analyzed data from 24 atopic asthmatics that underwent a bronchoscopy and allergen challenge prior to randomization in the parent trial [10]. As indicated in Figure 1, allergen challenge led to an increase in the total cell number present in the BAL fluid ($1.5 \times 10^5 \pm 6.5 \times 10^4$ vs $8.8 \times 10^5 \pm 1.5 \times 10^6$; p < 0.001). There was also a significant change in the cellular composition, with an increase in both eosinophils (28.7% ± 26.2%) and neutrophils (4.5% ± 7.3%), along with a decrease in macrophages detected (−32.1% ± 26.0%) (Figure 1).

We measured the concentrations of pro-inflammatory (IL-6 and TNF) and T cell-derived (IL-10, IL-2, IL-17, IL-4 and IFN-γ) cytokines in the BAL by multi-plex ELISA. IL-6, was significantly induced following allergen challenge (30.8 ± 82.1 vs 311.6 ± 540.0 pg/mL, Figure 1B) while TNF was only detected in a single subject (< 10 pg/mL, data not shown). The T cell-dependent cytokines were not detected pre-allergen; however, IL-2 (4.2 ± 8.8 pg/mL), IFN-γ (6.0 ± 19.3 pg/mL) and IL-10 (5.9 ± 18.2 pg/mL) were detected in some of the subjects (Figure 1B). Neither IL-4 nor IL-17A was observed post-allergen challenge in BAL fluid (data not shown).

Surprisingly, most subjects had no detectable levels of T cell-derived cytokines even after allergen instillation in the lung (Figure 1B). An analysis based upon the type of allergen instilled and/or the dilution of allergen that induced a positive skin test did not yield statistically relevant differences due to the limited number of subjects in each group (Table 1). These data indicate that the instillation of allergen in the lung induces the infiltration of inflammatory cells and the production of both pro-inflammatory and T-cell dependent cytokines.

Allergen challenge results in recruitment of innate and adaptive immune cells to the lung

Multi-color flow cytometry was utilized to provide a more detailed phenotypic analysis of immune cells recovered following allergen challenge. An increase in CD4+ T cells along with a decrease in CD8+ T cells was observed 48 hours following allergen challenge (Figure 2). The innate immune response to allergen has also been recognized as an important component of asthma [5]; therefore, we determined the recruitment of natural killer cells (Nk) and dendritic cells (DC) to the lung. No change in Nk or myeloid dendritic cells (mDC) was observed; however, a small yet significant increase in plasmacytoid dendritic cells (pDC; 0.5% ± 0.5% vs 3.9% ± 6.8%; p < 0.05) was observed in the BAL fluid after allergen challenge (Figure 2).

To further characterize the inflammatory response in the lung following allergen challenge, we enumerated the number of suppressor cells present in the lung. Regulatory T cells (Tregs) and myeloid derived suppressor cells (MDSC) are important mechanisms for down-modulating immune responses to antigen; interestingly, both were recruited to the lung following allergen challenge (Tregs: 4.2% ± 2.1% vs 7.0% ± 4.4% [p < 0.001]; MDSCs: 10.4% ± 8.5% vs 20.6% ± 5.9% [p < 0.01]) (Figure 2). In addition to being present in the BAL, this MDSC population expressed co-stimulatory B7-molecules

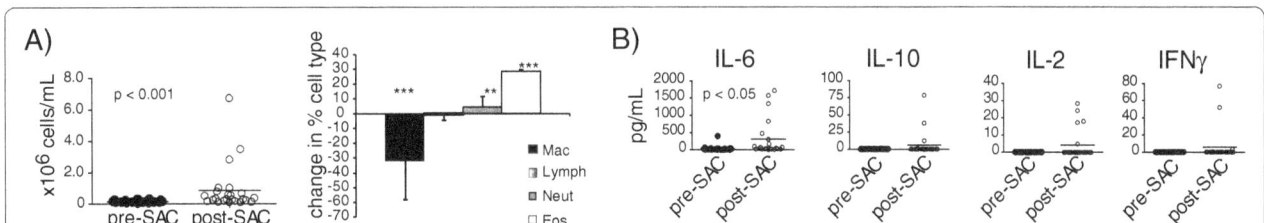

Figure 1 Segmental allergen challenge (SAC) induces an inflammatory response detected in the BAL fluid of atopic asthmatics. In **A)**, total cell counts and differential analysis are presented for BAL fluid obtained pre- and post-SAC. In **B)**, cytokine levels in the BAL fluid were measured by multiplex ELISA using the Cytokine Bead Array (CBA). Shown is the re-analysis performed on the 24 subjects enrolled in the randomized, placebo controlled, double blinded Costimulation Inhibition of Asthma (CIA) trial at pre-randomization. In **A** (right panel), the average (change in percent cell type) is presented with error bars representing ± the standard deviation with an (* = p < 0.05; ** = p <0.01; *** = p < 0.001). Each subject is represented by a single circle in the graphs with p values presented. Due to pre-SAC cytokines being below the detection limit of the assay (5 pg/mL), no statistical analysis was performed for IL-10, IL-2 or IFN-γ.

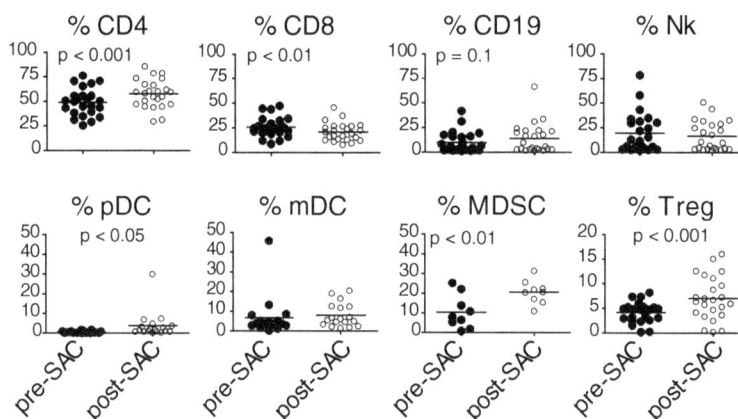

Figure 2 Innate and adaptive immune cells are recruited to the BAL fluid after allergen challenge. Cellular populations in the BAL fluid pre- and post-SAC were labeled with specific fluorophore conjugated antibodies and analyzed by multi-color flow cytometry. The percentages were calculated as a percent of the lymphocyte gate, with the exception of the DC (plasmacytoid [pDC], myeloid [mDC]) and myeloid derived suppressor cell (MDSC) subsets which were calculated as a percentage of the lineage cocktail negative gate. Each subject is represented by a single symbol on the graphs, with p values indicated.

(CD80 12.2% ± 17.4% and CD86 25.7% ± 12.5%, Additional file 1).

In addition to analyzing the percentage of lymphocyte populations, we performed an extensive phenotypic analysis of these cell subsets. An increase in the percentage of CD45RA+ (naïve or effector memory) T cells (1.1% ± 0.6% vs 5.6% ± 5.4%; p < 0.001) CD4+ and CD8+ (13.3% ± 8.7% vs 21.2% ± 13.5%; p < 0.01) T cells was observed post-allergen challenge along with a reduction in memory (76.8% ± 12.4% vs 70.3% ± 14.8%; p < 0.05) CD8+ T cells (Figure 3). We detected an increase in the percentage of cells that expressed the activation marker CD25 (IL-2R) for both CD4+ (16.0% ± 7.4% vs 19.8% ± 6.9%; p < 0.001) and CD8+ (0.7% ± 0.8% vs 1.3% ±

1.3%; p < 0.0001) T cells (Figure 3). These data demonstrate that allergen challenge results in the recruitment of activated CD4+ and CD8+ T cells and innate immune cells along with specific regulatory cell populations.

CD30 expression in BAL fluid after allergen challenge

CD30 has been shown to be expressed on eosinophils [14,15], and is associated with Th2 type T lymphocytes [16] and may correlate with severity of asthma [17,18]; therefore, we analyzed whether CD30 was expressed on BAL cells and present in the BAL fluid after allergen challenge. Contrary to some reports in the literature [14,15], we were unable to detect any CD30 expression

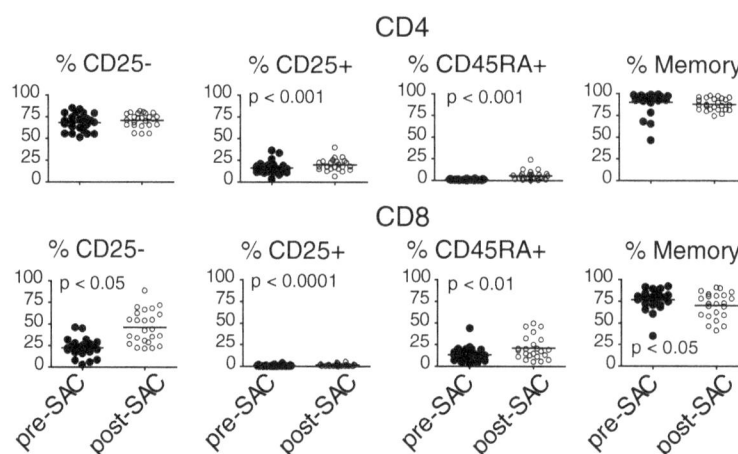

Figure 3 Expansion in both naïve and activated T cells in the BAL fluid after allergen challenge. T cell subsets in the BAL fluid pre- and post-SAC were determined by the expression of CD25 (IL-2R; activated), CD45RA (naïve or effector memory) and CD45RO (memory) by multi-color flow cytometry. The percentages were calculated as a percent of either the CD4+ or CD8+ T cell population. Each subject is represented as a single symbol on the graphs, with p values indicated.

on the surface of BAL eosinophils by multi-color flow cytometry (Figure 4) or by immuno-histochemical staining of cytospins (data not shown) either pre- or post-allergen challenge. However, CD30 expression was detected on a low yet significant percentage of T and B cells (Figure 4) and by immuno-histochemical staining of BAL cytospins (data not shown) obtained following allergen challenge. Of note, the percentage of CD30+ Tregs (22.1% ± 9.1%) was ~10-fold more than detected on either B cells (2.1% ± 2.8%) or T cells (CD4+ 3.2% ± 2.0%; CD8+ 0.3% ± 0.7%) (Figure 4). Soluble CD30 (sCD30), the cleaved fragment of membrane CD30 [19,20], was quantitated by ELISA in the concentrated BAL fluid. There was a 4-fold increase in sCD30 protein in the BAL fluid upon allergen challenge (3.0 ± 1.1 vs 14.1 ± 24.6 in pg/mL; p < 0.05) (Figure 4). These data identify the presence of CD30 positive lymphocytes, especially Tregs, but not eosinophils, and sCD30 in the BAL fluid after allergen challenge of atopic asthmatics.

Discussion

In this study, we took advantage of results originally obtained in an interventional trial designed to test the effects of inhibition of T cell costimulation on the response of mild atopic asthmatics to allergen challenge [10]. Data obtained prior to administration of study drug provided a comprehensive data set describing the inflammatory response to allergen. We found that allergen instillation in the airway results in the recruitment of both innate and adaptive immune cells to the lung, including populations of suppressor cells. We also detected elevated expression of CD30, predominantly on regulatory T cells. Thus, the inflammatory response to allergen is a complex mixture of cell types.

Clinical and animal studies have supported the role of T lymphocytes as controllers of the aberrant Th2 initiated response and eosinophils as predominant effectors that induce asthma symptoms. The most dominant Th2 cytokine in asthma is IL-4 which has a plethora of activity including increasing IgE production, and differentiating T cells from a Th0 to Th2 [21,22]. We detected an increase in eosinophil percentage yet no significant increase in IL-4 after allergen challenge. Batra et al. determined the peak level of IL-4 is reached within 24 hours after allergen challenge [23] potentially explaining the lack of IL-4 detected in our study. In most subjects the majority of cytokines were below the limits of detection. This might reflect the extensive dilution that occurs due to the BAL procedure. Given this limitation, a meaningful biological difference is hard to conclude from these data.

Asthma is a predominate Th2 disease but there is also data for Th1 and Th17 responses. Th2 effector responses in asthma such as eosinophil recruitment, mucus production and AHR are inhibited by IFN-γ which is produced by Th1 T lymphocytes [1]. We detected a significant increase in IFN-γ as well as neutrophils which are recruited by IFN-γ [1] after allergen challenge

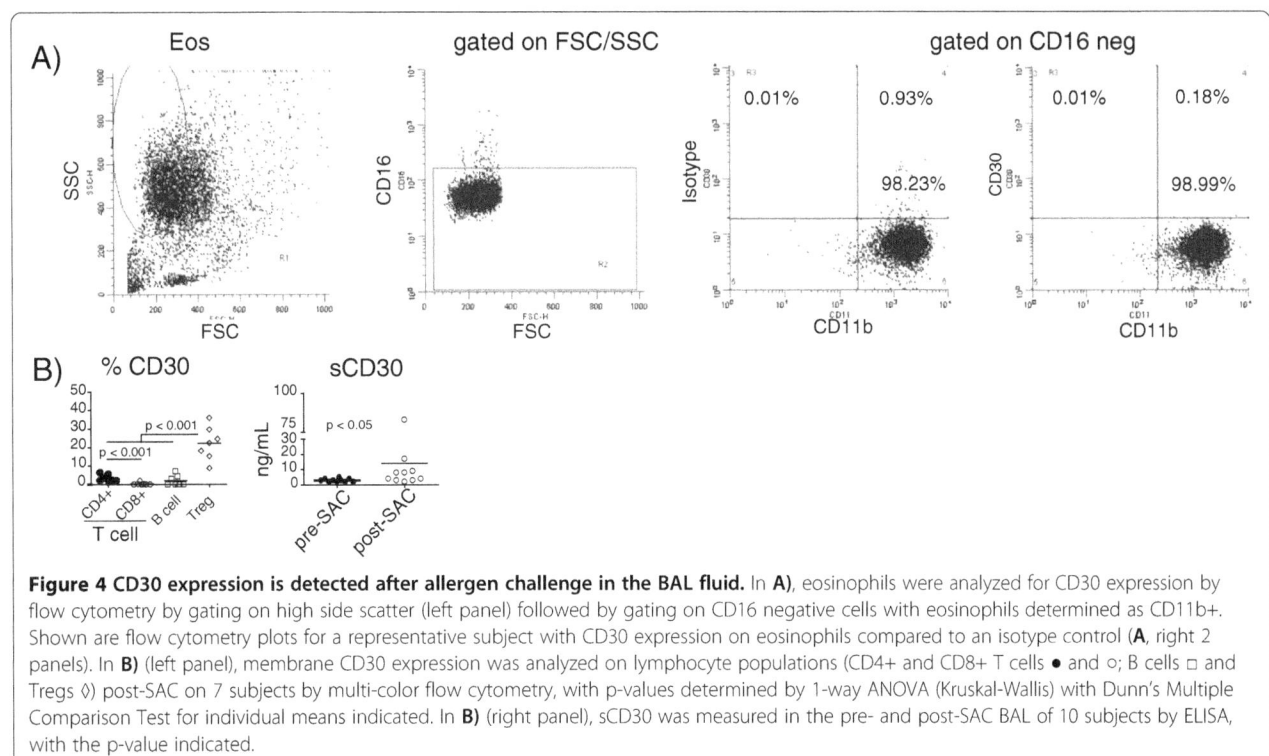

Figure 4 CD30 expression is detected after allergen challenge in the BAL fluid. In **A**), eosinophils were analyzed for CD30 expression by flow cytometry by gating on high side scatter (left panel) followed by gating on CD16 negative cells with eosinophils determined as CD11b+. Shown are flow cytometry plots for a representative subject with CD30 expression on eosinophils compared to an isotype control (**A**, right 2 panels). In **B**) (left panel), membrane CD30 expression was analyzed on lymphocyte populations (CD4+ and CD8+ T cells ● and ○; B cells □ and Tregs ◊) post-SAC on 7 subjects by multi-color flow cytometry, with p-values determined by 1-way ANOVA (Kruskal-Wallis) with Dunn's Multiple Comparison Test for individual means indicated. In **B**) (right panel), sCD30 was measured in the pre- and post-SAC BAL of 10 subjects by ELISA, with the p-value indicated.

(Figure 1A and 1B). Thus, our data supports a role for both Th2 and IFN-γ responses in asthma.

Allergen challenge in asthmatics induces changes in both innate and adaptive cellular populations. Although we did not detect increases in B lymphocytes, a significant increase in CD4+ T lymphocytes while a significant decrease in CD8+ T lymphocytes were observed (Figure 2). Furthermore, we observed alterations in T lymphocyte differentiation including: increases in naïve or effector memory (CD45RA+) percentages, increased CD25 (IL-2R) expression, and a decreased memory CD8+ pool after allergen challenge signifying a T cell response to antigen [1,24]. This is consistent with mouse models of asthma where increased levels of IFN-γ inhibit the generation of memory T cells [25] further contributing to the expansion of an effector T cell pool [26].

We did not observe differences in Nk cells or myeloid dendritic cells (mDC), innate cells important in asthma pathology [5]; however, a significant increase in plasmacytoid dendritic cells (pDC) was detected after allergen challenge. The recruitment of pDC may be part of the anti-inflammatory response in asthma [5,27]. In accordance with this anti-inflammatory response, an increase in regulatory T cells (Treg) as well as increased IL-10 secretion, a regulatory T and pDC effector cytokine, were detected after allergen challenge (Figures 2 and 1B). Regulatory T cells inhibit allergic responses by 1) suppressing myeloid dendritic cells (mDC) important for T lymphocyte activation and differentiation, 2) inhibiting Th1/Th2 and Th17 differentiation, 3) inhibiting IgE production, 4) preventing T lymphocyte migration into the lung and 5) inhibiting effector cell function of mast cells, basophils and eosinophils [5]. Importantly, we further identified an additional innate cell population termed myeloid derived suppressor cells (MDSC) as being increased after allergen challenge in adult atopic asthmatics (Figure 2). Our report is the first to identify MDSC in the BAL fluid of adult atopic asthmatics after allergen challenge. Interestingly in a mouse model of asthma, MDSC were shown to recruit regulatory T cells and down modulate T lymphocyte responses [28]. We also show that MDSC expressed co-stimulatory ligands, both CD80 and CD86, which have been associated with inducing Th2 T cells [3] as well as producing IL-10 [29]. Therefore, multiple suppressor cell types are associated with the anti-inflammatory response detected in the lung after allergen challenge.

Soluble CD30 is increased in the serum of pediatric asthma patients when compared to healthy individuals [18,30] as well as after allergen challenge in our study. We also detected sCD30 in the serum prior to allergen challenge (20.3 ± 8.0 ng/mL; data not shown) in adult atopic asthmatics. The role of soluble CD30 in asthma is not clear but is thought to block CD30-CD153 induced apoptosis and the induction of IgG class switching on B cells [31]. The presence of sCD30 in the BAL after allergen challenge may play a role in either preventing apoptosis of activated lymphocytes or in their differentiation. However, the role of sCD30 in asthma is unknown and requires further study.

Contrary to reports that detected mRNA and low surface expression of CD30 on eosinophils [14,15], we did not observe any CD30 expression on eosinophils by either flow cytometry (Figure 4A) or immunohistochemistry (data not shown). We did however detect membrane CD30 on lymphocytes, especially regulatory T cells, after allergen challenge. CD30 expression on CD4+ T cells has been associated with IL-4 secretion [16] while CD30+ eosinophils undergo apoptosis in asthmatics [14,15]. Memory CD8+ T lymphocytes express CD30 [32], yet in our study the lowest percentage of CD30+ cells were CD8+ T lymphocytes. This may be partly explained by the decreased memory pool of CD8+ T cells after allergen challenge (Figure 3). There are no reports of CD30 expression on regulatory T cells in human asthma. In mouse model systems of allograft tolerance, a Th2 dominated response like asthma, CD30-deficient Tregs failed to reject grafts [33,34]. Due to the low cellularity of pre-allergen BAL sample, we were unable to measure CD30 expression on lymphocytes in most subjects. However, in a single subject, the percentage of CD30+ Tregs in the BAL after allergen challenge increased from 0.04% pre-allergen to 24.6% post-allergen challenge (data not shown). The role of CD30 expression on Tregs in asthma remains unclear; however, interaction between CD30 on the Treg and CD153 on a CD8+ T cell results in apoptosis of the CD8+ T cell [33,34]. Therefore, we speculate that CD30+ regulatory T cells and sCD30 play a role in controlling asthma in a CD30-dependent manner.

Conclusions
Atopic asthmatics increase innate and adaptive immune cell populations after allergen challenge. In particular, alterations in both the activation and memory state of T lymphocytes as well as detection of a novel suppressor cell population termed MDSC. Furthermore, we detected soluble CD30 and identified significant expression of CD30 on immune cells, most notably on regulatory T cells, not eosinophils in atopic asthmatics after allergen challenge.

Abbreviations

MDSC: Myeloid derived suppressor cells; *BAL*: Bronchoalveolar lavage; *sCD30*: Soluble CD30; *SAC*: Segmental allergen challenge; *Th2*: T helper type 2; *Th1*: T helper type 1; *mDC*: Myeloid dendritic cell; *pDC*: Plasmacytoid dendritic cell; *Treg*: Regulatory T cell; *CIA*: Costimulation inhibition of asthma trial.

Competing interests

The authors declare that they have no competing interests.

Authors' contributions

JSB developed and performed the research assays and contributed to the formulation of the manuscript. ADP enrolled subjects, performed SAC protocols, analyzed specimens and data. HYD CMP and SC performed research assays and analyzed data. BMP was the lead research coordinator and was involved in all aspects involving participants. NNJ was the lead investigator at University of Wisconsin, MC and JMG collaboratively designed the study as well as provided oversight over the conduct of the entire study. All authors reviewed and contributed to the writing of the manuscript. All authors read and approved the final manuscript.

Acknowledgements

We thank Chandrika Christie for help with the research assays and Jamie Tarsi for assistance in conducting this study. This study was funded by an investigator initiated grant awarded to JMG by Bristol-Myers Squibb Corporation and Medimmune Corporation.

Author details

[1]Department of Internal Medicine, Washington University School of Medicine, St Louis, MO 63110, USA. [2]Current affiliation: Department of Internal Medicine, Baylor College of Medicine, Houston, TX 77030, USA. [3]Department of Internal Medicine, University of Wisconsin School of Medicine and Public Health, Madison, WI 53792, USA.

References

1. Cohn L, Elias JA, Chupp GL: Asthma: mechanisms of disease persistence and progression. *Annu Rev Immunol* 2004, 22:789–815.
2. Umetsu DT, McIntire JJ, Akbari O, Macaubas C, DeKruyff RH: Asthma: an epidemic of dysregulated immunity. *Nat Immunol* 2002, 3:715–720.
3. Ishmael FT: The inflammatory response in the pathogenesis of asthma. *J Am Osteopath Assoc* 2011, 111:S11–S17.
4. Asquith KL, Ramshaw HS, Hansbro PM, Beagley KW, Lopez AF, Foster PS: The IL-3/IL-5/GM-CSF common receptor plays a pivotal role in the regulation of Th2 immunity and allergic airway inflammation. *J Immunol* 2008, 180:1199–1206.
5. Holgate ST: Innate and adaptive immune responses in asthma. *Nat Med* 2012, 18:673–683.
6. Deppong C, Degnan JM, Murphy TL, Murphy KM, Green JM: B and T lymphocyte attenuator regulates T cell survival in the lung. *J Immunol* 2008, 181:2973–2979.
7. Deppong C, Juehne TI, Hurchla M, Friend LD, Shah DD, Rose CM, Bricker TL, Shornick LP, Crouch EC, Murphy TL, *et al*: Cutting edge: B and T lymphocyte attenuator and programmed death receptor-1 inhibitory receptors are required for termination of acute allergic airway inflammation. *J Immunol* 2006, 176:3909–3913.
8. Deppong CM, Parulekar A, Boomer JS, Bricker TL, Green JM: CTLA4-Ig inhibits allergic airway inflammation by a novel CD28-independent, nitric oxide synthase-dependent mechanism. *Eur J Immunol* 2010, 40:1985–1994.
9. Deppong CM, Xu J, Brody SL, Green JM: Airway epithelial cells suppress T cell proliferation by an IFNgamma/STAT1/TGFbeta-dependent mechanism. *Am J Physiol Lung Cell Mol Physiol* 2012, 302:L167–L173.
10. Parulekar AD, Boomer JS, Patterson BM, Yin-Declue H, Deppong CM, Wilson BS, Jarjour NN, Castro M, Green JM: A randomized, controlled trial to evaluate inhibition of T cell costimulation in allergen induced airway inflammation. *Am J Respir Crit Care Med* 2013.
11. Weiland SK, Bjorksten B, Brunekreef B, Cookson WO, von Mutius E, Strachan DP: Phase II of the International Study of Asthma and Allergies in Childhood (ISAAC II): rationale and methods. *Eur Respir J* 2004, 24:406–412.
12. Romanet-Manent S, Charpin D, Magnan A, Lanteaume A, Vervloet D: Allergic vs nonallergic asthma: what makes the difference? *Allergy* 2002, 57:607–613.
13. Pepys J, Roth A, Carroll KB: RAST, skin and nasal tests and the history in grass pollen allergy. *Clin Allergy* 1975, 5:431–442.
14. Berro AI, Perry GA, Agrawal DK: Increased expression and activation of CD30 induce apoptosis in human blood eosinophils. *J Immunol* 2004, 173:2174–2183.
15. Matsumoto K, Terakawa M, Miura K, Fukuda S, Nakajima T, Saito H: Extremely rapid and intense induction of apoptosis in human eosinophils by anti-CD30 antibody treatment in vitro. *J Immunol* 2004, 172:2186–2193.
16. Rojas-Ramos E, Garfias Y, Jimenez-Martinez Mdel C, Martinez-Jimenez N, Zenteno E, Gorocica P, Lascurain R: Increased expression of CD30 and CD57 molecules on CD4(+) T cells from children with atopic asthma: a preliminary report. *Allergy Asthma Proc* 2007, 28:659–666.
17. Lombardi V, Singh AK, Akbari O: The role of costimulatory molecules in allergic disease and asthma. *Int Arch Allergy Immunol* 2010, 151:179–189.
18. Heshmat NM, El-Hadidi ES: Soluble CD30 serum levels in atopic dermatitis and bronchial asthma and its relationship with disease severity in pediatric age. *Pediatr Allergy Immunol* 2006, 17:297–303.
19. Aizawa S, Nakano H, Ishida T, Horie R, Nagai M, Ito K, Yagita H, Okumura K, Inoue J, Watanabe T: Tumor necrosis factor receptor-associated factor (TRAF) 5 and TRAF2 are involved in CD30-mediated NFkappaB activation. *J Biol Chem* 1997, 272:2042–2045.
20. Ansieau S, Scheffrahn I, Mosialos G, Brand H, Duyster J, Kaye K, Harada J, Dougall B, Hubinger G, Kieff E, *et al*: Tumor necrosis factor receptor-associated factor (TRAF)-1, TRAF-2, and TRAF-3 interact in vivo with the CD30 cytoplasmic domain; TRAF-2 mediates CD30-induced nuclear factor kappa B activation. *Proc Natl Acad Sci U S A* 1996, 93:14053–14058.
21. Barnes PJ: The cytokine network in asthma and chronic obstructive pulmonary disease. *J Clin Invest* 2008, 118:3546–3556.
22. Maes T, Joos GF, Brusselle GG: Targeting interleukin-4 in asthma: lost in translation? *Am J Respir Cell Mol Biol* 2012, 47:261–270.
23. Batra V, Musani AI, Hastie AT, Khurana S, Carpenter KA, Zangrilli JG, Peters SP: Bronchoalveolar lavage fluid concentrations of transforming growth factor (TGF)-beta1, TGF-beta2, interleukin (IL)-4 and IL-13 after segmental allergen challenge and their effects on alpha-smooth muscle actin and collagen III synthesis by primary human lung fibroblasts. *Clin Exp Allergy* 2004, 34:437–444.
24. Wilson JW, Djukanovic R, Howarth PH, Holgate ST: Lymphocyte activation in bronchoalveolar lavage and peripheral blood in atopic asthma. *Am Rev Respir Dis* 1992, 145:958–960.
25. Wu CY, Kirman JR, Rotte MJ, Davey DF, Perfetto SP, Rhee EG, Freidag BL, Hill BJ, Douek DC, Seder RA: Distinct lineages of T(H)1 cells have differential capacities for memory cell generation in vivo. *Nat Immunol* 2002, 3:852–858.
26. Purwar R, Campbell J, Murphy G, Richards WG, Clark RA, Kupper TS: Resident memory T cells (T(RM)) are abundant in human lung: diversity, function, and antigen specificity. *PLoS One* 2011, 6:e16245.
27. Dua B, Watson RM, Gauvreau GM, O'Byrne PM: Myeloid and plasmacytoid dendritic cells in induced sputum after allergen inhalation in subjects with asthma. *J Allergy Clin Immunol* 2010, 126:133–139.
28. Deshane J, Zmijewski JW, Luther R, Gaggar A, Deshane R, Lai JF, Xu X, Spell M, Estell K, Weaver CT, *et al*: Free radical-producing myeloid-derived regulatory cells: potent activators and suppressors of lung inflammation and airway hyperresponsiveness. *Mucosal Immunol* 2011, 4:503–518.

29. Nakajima A, Watanabe N, Yoshino S, Yagita H, Okumura K, Azuma M: **Requirement of CD28-CD86 co-stimulation in the interaction between antigen-primed T helper type 2 and B cells.** *Int Immunol* 1997, **9:**637–644.

30. Remes ST, Delezuch W, Pulkki K, Pekkanen J, Korppi M, Matinlauri IH: **Association of serum-soluble CD26 and CD30 levels with asthma, lung function and bronchial hyper-responsiveness at school age.** *Acta Paediatr* 2011, **100:**e106–e111.

31. Hargreaves PG, Al-Shamkhani A: **Soluble CD30 binds to CD153 with high affinity and blocks transmembrane signaling by CD30.** *Eur J Immunol* 2002, **32:**163–173.

32. Ellis TM, Simms PE, Slivnick DJ, Jack HM, Fisher RI: **CD30 is a signal-transducing molecule that defines a subset of human activated CD45RO + T cells.** *J Immunol* 1993, **151:**2380–2389.

33. Dai Z, Li Q, Wang Y, Gao G, Diggs LS, Tellides G, Lakkis FG: **CD4+CD25+ regulatory T cells suppress allograft rejection mediated by memory CD8+ T cells via a CD30-dependent mechanism.** *J Clin Invest* 2004, **113:**310–317.

34. Zeiser R, Nguyen VH, Hou JZ, Beilhack A, Zambricki E, Buess M, Contag CH, Negrin RS: **Early CD30 signaling is critical for adoptively transferred CD4+CD25+ regulatory T cells in prevention of acute graft-versus-host disease.** *Blood* 2007, **109:**2225–2233.

11

Improper inhaler technique is associated with poor asthma control and frequent emergency department visits

Hamdan AL-Jahdali[1,4*], Anwar Ahmed[2], Abdullah AL-Harbi[1], Mohd Khan[1], Salim Baharoon[1], Salih Bin Salih[1], Rabih Halwani[3] and Saleh Al-Muhsen[3]

Abstract

Background: Uncontrolled asthma remains a frequent cause of emergency department (ED) visits and hospital admissions. Improper asthma inhaler device use is most likely one of the major causes associated with uncontrolled asthma and frequent ED visits.

Objectives: To evaluate the inhaler technique among asthmatic patients seen in ED, and to investigate the characteristics of these patients and factors associated with improper use of inhaler devices and its relationship with asthma control and ED visits.

Methods: A cross-sectional study of all the patients who visited the ED with bronchial asthma attacks over a 9-month period was undertaken at two major academic hospitals in Saudi Arabia. Information was collected about demographic data and asthma management and we assessed the inhaler techniques for each patient using an inhaler technique checklist.

Results: A total of 450 asthma patients were included in the study. Of these, 176(39.1%) were males with a mean age of 42.3 ±16.7 years and the mean duration of asthma was 155.9 ± 127.1 weeks. The improper use of asthma inhaler devices was observed in 203(45%) of the patients and was associated with irregular clinic follow-ups (p = 0.0001), lack of asthma education (p = 0.0009), uncontrolled asthma ACT (score ≤ 15) (p = 0.001), three or more ED visits (p = 0.0497), and duration of asthma of less than 52 weeks (p = 0.005). Multiple logistic regression analysis revealed that a lack of education about asthma disease (OR =1.65; 95% CI: 1.07, 2.54) or a lack of regular follow-up (OR =1.73; 95% CI: 1.08, 2.76) was more likely to lead to the improper use of an asthma inhaler device.

Conclusion: Improper asthma inhaler device use is associated with poor asthma control and more frequent ED visits. We also identified many avoidable risk factors leading to the improper use of inhaler devices among asthma patients visiting the ED.

Keywords: Asthma control, Inhaled corticosteroid, Emergency department, Inhaler devices, Asthma education

* Correspondence: Jahdalih@gmail.com
[1]Department of Medicine, Pulmonary Division-ICU, King Saud bin Abdulaziz University for Health Sciences, Riyadh, Saudi Arabia
[4]King Saud University for Health Sciences, Head of Pulmonary Division, Medical Director of Sleep Disorders Center, King Abdulaziz Medical City, Riyadh, Saudi Arabia
Full list of author information is available at the end of the article

Introduction

Asthma is a chronic inflammatory disease of the airways associated with bronchial hyper-responsiveness and reversible airflow obstruction [1,2]. The incidence and prevalence of asthma have increased during the past 20 years, affecting 5-10% of the global population [3,4]. The prevalence of bronchial asthma among Saudi patients is approximately 20-25% [4,5]. The primary goal of asthma treatment is to control symptoms and to reduce emergency department (ED) use for acute asthma treatment [1,6-8]. One study reported only 5% asthma control among patients seen at tertiary care hospital [9]. Poor asthma control remains a frequent cause of ED presentation and hospital admission [10], and the cost of uncontrolled asthma care is substantial. For example, ED use for asthma management accounts for almost one-third of all asthma costs in the United States [11]. The administration of corticosteroids via inhalation is considered the optimal route for appropriate drug delivery for treatment of bronchial asthma and could reduce asthma hospitalizations by as much as 80% [12]. The most important advantage of inhaled therapy is the direct, localized delivery of a high concentration of drugs to the airways with minimal systematic side effects [13]. However, improper inhaler device use is one of the most common causes that hinder better asthma control [14-18].

The improper use of inhaled devices in the management of bronchial asthma decrease drug delivery, patient's adherence to the treatment regimen and drug effectiveness. This subsequently leads to uncontrolled asthma management and multiple ED visits [14,15,17-22]. The improper inhaler device use as a cause of uncontrolled asthma management and frequent ED visits, to best of our knowledge, had never previously been studied in the Saudi population. The objective of this study was to evaluate the inhaler technique among asthmatic Saudi patients seen in ED and to identify the characteristics of these patients along with factors associated with the improper use of inhaler devices, asthma control and the number of ED visits.

Methods

This cross-sectional study was conducted at the King Abdulaziz Medical City – King Fahad National Guard Hospital in Riyadh (KAMC-KFNGH) and the King Khalid University Hospital (KKUH). We enrolled adult patients (≥ 18 years old) diagnosed with asthma who visited the ED for asthma management between August 2010 and March 2011. The enrolled patients had a documented diagnosis of bronchial asthma as diagnosed by their primary physician and were on a prescribed inhaled corticosteroid (ICS) therapy for at least the last three months. We excluded patients without a documented diagnosis of bronchial asthma and those who were not prescribed ICS according to their medical records.

This study was approved by the Institutional Review Board (IRB) (Ref. IRBC/123/11). During the ED visit, a trained co-investigator collected information about demographic data, the duration of the illness and the medication used for asthma therapy. Additionally, the data were gathered on whether the patient received any formal education about asthma as a disease and, how to use their inhaler devices. The co-investigators also verified this information by reviewing the medical record of the patients and they assessed the asthma control over the last month by administering a validated published Arabic version of the Asthma Control Test (ACT)[23]. The co-investigators also determined whether the patient knew how to use the prescribed inhaler properly following specific steps in the check list (Table 1). All patients were observed for two trials of using their inhalers and proper use was identified if the patient

Table 1 Inhaler device check list

Use of a pressurized metered-dose inhaler

1. Shake the canister
2. Hold the canister upright at opening of mouth
3. Begin a slow breath
4. Actuate the MDI once while continuing with a slow breath
5. Inhale to total lung capacity
6. Hold breath for at least 4 seconds

MDI with spacer

1. Remove the cap of the spacer.
2. Remove the cap of the puffer. Shake the puffer 5 or 6 times.
3. Insert the puffer in the hole at the back of the spacer.
4. Blow all your breath out until lungs are empty.
5. Insert the spacer mouthpiece into the mouth
6. Press the down once on the puffer's canister.
7. Slowly breathe in from the spacer full breath.
8. Hold your breath for at least 4 seconds

Using the turbuhaler

1. Unscrew the cover and remove it.
2. Holding the Turbuhaler upright, turn the colored wheel one way and back the other way until it clicks.
3. Breathe out normally.
4. Put the mouthpiece between your lips and tilt your head back slightly.
5. Breathe in deeply and forcefully.
6. Hold your breath for 10 seconds

Diskus

1. Open the device
2. Slide the lever
3. Exhale away from device, to empty lung
4. Place mouthpiece between teeth and lips
5. Inhale rapidly and fully

fulfilled all of the steps required. The written informed consent was obtained from all participants.

Statistical analysis

The data collected was transferred and analyzed using SAS® versions 9.2 (SAS Institute Inc., Cary, NC). Descriptive statistics, such as the means and standard deviations, were used to summarize the quantitative variables. The frequencies and percentages were used to summarize categorical variables. Chi-squared tests were used to test the association between clinical characteristics across the variables regarding asthma device use and asthma control test. P-values less than 0.05 were considered significant. Multiple logistic models were used to identify the risk factors that were associated with the improper use of asthma inhaler devices. The odds ratios (ORs) with 95% CIs were reported to describe the strength of these associations.

Results

Among the 450 asthma patients, 176 (39.1%) were male (Table 2). The mean age was 42.3 ±16.7 and the mean duration of asthma was 155.9 ± 127.1 weeks. There were 270 (60%) patients with regular physician follow-up. Approximately half of the patients, 232 (51.6%) had no formal asthma education as a disease and 183 (40.7%) had no formal education about the medications or the asthma inhaler devices by any health care professional. Of the patients who received asthma and device education, 200 (44.5%) were educated by physicians, 35 (7.8%) were educated by asthma educators, and 21 (4.7%) were educated by the pharmacists. A total of 165 (36.7%) patients had three or more ED visits per year. Asthma control in the month preceding the ED visit (as per the ACT) was as follows: uncontrolled (ACT ≤ 15) was 105 (23.3%), partial control (16 ≥ ACT ≤ 23) was 335 (74.4%), complete control (ACT ≥ 24) was 8 (1.8%), and missing ACT 2(0.5%).

The improper use of asthma inhaler devices was observed in 203 (45%) of the patients. The improper use had a significant association with irregular clinic follow-ups, lack of education about asthma medication, lack of education about asthma as disease, uncontrolled asthma, and three or more ED visits (See Table 3). The patients with irregular clinic follow-up compared with regular follow-up were more likely to misuse the asthma device (60.9% versus 34.8%, p = 0.0001). Patients who received no education about asthma medication compared with those who did were more likely to use an asthma device improperly (54.6% versus 38.7%, p = 0.0009). Patients with uncontrolled ACT (score ≤ 15) compared to partially/fully controlled ACT (score > 15) were more likely to use asthma device improperly (59.1% versus 40.8%, p =0.001). Patients with 3 or more ED visits

Table 2 Demographics and clinical characteristics about bronchial asthma (N=450)

Characteristics	Levels	N (%) ᵀ
Age, *(Mean ± SD)*		42.3 ± 16.7
Duration of illness in weeks, *(Mean ± SD)*		155.90 ± 127.13
Duration of illness, *n(%)*	> 1 Year	429 (95.97)
Gender, *n(%)*	Female	274 (60.9)
Marital status	Married	371 (83.6)
Improper use of asthma inhaler devices		203 (45.0)
Education level	High school or less	387 (86.0)
	University	62 (13.8)
	Missing	1(0.2)
Follow-up consistently with doctor		270 (60.0)
Follow-up clinic	PHC/FM	208(46.2)
	Pulmonary	46(10.2)
	Internal Medicine	8(1.8)
	Others	8(1.8)
	No follow-up	180(40)
No education about asthma		232(51.6)
No education about medication		183(40.7)
ER visits	≥3	165(36.7)
Asthma control	Uncontrolled	105(23.3)
	Partially controlled	335(74.4)
	Complete control	8(1.8)
	Missing	2(0.5)
Received health education about asthma disease from a physician		200 (44.5)
Received health education about asthma disease from a health educator		35(7.8)
Received health education about asthma disease from a pharmacist		21(4.7)
Knew about asthma disease independently		27(6.0)
Device	MDI	361(80.2)
	Turbuhaler	43 (9.6)
	Diskus	38 (8.4)
	MDI with spacer	3 (0.7)
	Missing	5 (1.1)

ᵀAll percentages were rounded to one decimal place.

because of asthma exacerbations were more likely to improperly use an asthma device compared to those who visited less than 3 times (50.9% versus 41.3%, p =0.0497). Moreover, patients who were diagnosed with asthma for less than 1 year were more likely to use an asthma device

Table 3 The association of asthma device use with demographic and clinical characteristics

Characteristics	Levels	Improper 203 (45%)	Proper 247 (55%)	P-value
Gender	Female	123(44.9)	151(55.1)	0.9066
Age	≥ 45 Years	82(49.7)	83(50.3)	0.1369
Follow up with doctor	Yes	94(34.8)	176(65.2)	0.0001*
	No	109(60.9)	70(39.1)	
Educational level	High school or less	173(44.7)	214(55.3)	0.5884
Education about medication	Yes	103(38.7)	163(61.3)	0.0009*
	No	100(54.6)	83(45.4)	
Education about asthma	Yes	71(32.7)	146(67.3)	0.0001*
	No	132(56.9)	100(43.1)	
ACT	Uncontrolled	62(59.1)	43(41.0)	0.0010*
Full/Partially controlled		140(40.8)	203(59.2)	
ED visits	≥ 3	84(50.9)	81(49.1)	0.0497*
	< 3	114(41.3)	162(58.7)	
Duration of asthma	>1 Year	188(43.8)	241(56.2)	0.0046*
	≤1 Year	14(77.8)	4(22.2)	
Received health education about asthma disease from a physician				
	Yes	60(30.0)	140(70.0)	0.0001*
	No	143(57.4)	106(42.6)	
Received health education about asthma disease from a health educator				
	Yes	14(40.0)	21(60.0)	0.5188
	No	189(45.7)	225(54.4)	
Received health education about asthma disease from a pharmacist				
	Yes	6(28.6)	15(71.4)	0.1166
	No	197(46.0)	231(54.0)	
Knew about asthma disease independently				
	Yes	11(40.7)	16(59.3)	0.6302
	No	192(45.5)	230(54.5)	
Device	MDI	189(45.7)	225(54.4)	0.6958
	Turbuhaler	6(46.2)	7(53.9)	
	MDI with spacer	6(31.9)	13(68.4)	
	Diskus	2(50.0)	2(50.0)	

*The Chi-square/Fisher exact statistic is significant at the .05 level.

improperly compared to those who were diagnosed for more than 1 year (77.8% versus 43.8%, p =0.005). Not receiving health education about asthma disease from a physician is associated with misuse of the device (57.4% versus 30.0%, p =0.0001). Also, our analyses show that this improper use of the device was not associated with gender, age, or education level (p > 0.05). After controlling for all other factors, four risk factors were found to be associated with improper use of the devices: uncontrolled asthma, irregular use of ICS, irregular follow up with clinic and lack of education about asthmatic disease (p < 0.05; Table 4). Additionally, we found patients who lacked asthma education were more likely to use the asthma device improperly compared with the group who received education (OR:

1.65; 95% CI: 1.07, 2.54). Patients who did not follow-up regularly with clinical appointments were also more likely to improperly use asthma devices than those who regularly followed-up (OR: 1.726; 95% CI: 1.081, 2.756). This study also revealed that patients with an uncontrolled ACT (score ≤ 15) were 7 times more likely to use inhaler devices improperly compared with patients with fully controlled ACT (OR: 7.414; 95% CI: 1.345, 40.857).

Discussion
Previous studies have shown that the improper use of inhaler devices decreases drug delivery, patient's regimen adherence and drug effectiveness contributes to uncontrolled asthma and multiple ED visits [14,15,17-22]. In

Table 4 The odds ratios with 95% CIs for risk factors associated with improper use of an asthma device

Variable	Reference	Estimate	SE	P-value	OR	95% CI on OR	
Intercept		−0.5351	0.2924	0.0673			
Uncontrolled ACT	*Full control*	0.8778	0.3177	0.0057*	7.414	1.345	40.857
Partially controlled ACT	*Full control*	0.2477	0.3005	0.4097	3.948	0.743	20.983
ICS regular	*Regular*	0.4322	0.1160	0.0002*	2.374	1.506	3.740
No education about asthma disease	*Education about asthma disease*	0.2514	0.1100	0.0223*	1.653	1.074	2.544
No follow-up with doctor	*Follow-up with doctor*	0.2730	0.1193	0.0221*	1.726	1.081	2.756

* Wald Chi-Square statistic is significant at the .05 level.

this study, we tried to identify the relationship between improper inhaler device use, asthma control and number of ED visits. To the best of our knowledge, this is the first study in Saudi Arabia to examine the factors possibly leading to improper asthma inhaler use. We believe that this study has a sound methodology, being conducted by personal interview, and patient information was confirmed by reviewing medical records for each patient. A trained investigator confirmed the inhaler device use against a standard checklist. Similar to other studies, this study demonstrated that improper inhaler use is common in our population and results from avoidable causes. Furthermore, we demonstrated that improper inhaler device use is associated with poor asthma control and frequent ED visits [17-22]. Interestingly, improper asthma device use is mainly due to a lack of knowledge regarding asthmatic disease.

In this study, a majority (92%) of the patients were using metered-dose inhalers (MDI). This finding is consistent with Saudi Arabian practice for this disease, as most of the patients were seen at primary health care and family medicine clinics where the most common form of inhalers are MDIs. However, this should not be accepted as the cause for improper inhaler use. In fact, studies have shown that newer dry powder inhalers (DPIs) are not associated with an improved inhalation technique. Devices should be selected based on a patient's acceptance and preferences [16]. Selecting a device based on the patients' preference is cost effective in the long term, even if the device is more expensive than the standard devices [24]. However, studies have shown that good educational practice results in the proper use of MDI which will be more cost effective in the long-term [16,25,26].

Importantly, we found that 40% of the patients did not receive any formal education by any health care professionals regarding the proper use of inhaler devices. This was mostly due to a lack of asthma education programs. Almost half of our patients used asthma devices improperly, resulting in more visits to the ED due to subsequently poor asthma control. The major avoidable factors for improper device use were a lack of education regarding asthma as a disease and how the patient use

inhaler device correctly. Therefore, our health care system should emphasize establishing asthma education programs to educate patients on asthma and its management, particularly regarding the use of inhaler devices. These asthma education programs require continuous effort to educate patients and their caregivers. Studies have shown that standardized asthma education programs, education focused on self-management and behavioral change improves inhaler device use, adherence to treatment and asthma control [27,28]. Studies have shown that almost 50% of the patients used the devices correctly and this improved to more than 80% after instruction regardless of the device being used [29,30]. In this study, approximately 59% of the patients received education about how to use the inhaler devices. The education was given by physicians in 44% of cases. However, 30% still improperly used the medication. Furthermore, asthma educators and pharmacists only educated approximately 6-7% of patients about the proper use of inhalers. Similar to other studies, there was no difference in the appropriate use of device stratified by patient age or gender [31].

One limitation of our study was the documentation of specific education that was given to the patients. We had to rely on the patients' recollection of the education, as the education was not documented in the medical records. Additionally, we were not able to evaluate the quality of the teaching and how many educational sessions our patients received by health care professionals. We also had no background information on the psychosocial factors of this group of patients with poor inhaler device use, as this was beyond the scope of our study. Another limitation of this study was that we did not assess the side effects of improper inhaler use and how much this might contribute to poor compliance with medication, asthma control and ED visits. However, studies have shown that trained asthma educators, respiratory therapists and pharmacists are better qualified to teach patients than other health care providers [32,33]. We previously documented that only 5% of our patients seen at tertiary care clinics are completely in control of their asthma [9], and we also documented that many of our patients have a false belief and misconception about asthma pathophysiology and inhaled steroid use [34]. Also, in this study we only assessed the essential steps required for proper drug delivery. We did not score each step separately or count the number of errors or omissions. In addition to our previous studies [9,34], the finding of this study clearly demonstrates some limitations in our health care system. There is an urgent need for a national asthma education program at all level of medical care. We believe that the lack of an appropriate asthma education program in our system leads to improper device use, lack of the patient's knowledge about asthma, false beliefs and misconceptions about ICS. These deficiencies result in poor asthma control and increased ED visits. This study was limited to two academic centers in the Riyadh-central region. Most likely it does not represent the asthma care at the national level; thus, there is a need for national epidemiological studies to assess different aspects of asthma management.

Conclusion

This study shows that improper asthma inhaler technique is common among patients visiting ED in tertiary care centers in Saudi Arabia. This improper technique is associated with poor asthma control and frequent ED visits. The lack of appropriate asthma education is likely a major cause of improper device use. Furthermore, national asthma studies are necessary to explore this problem and to prospectively study the value of an interventional asthma education program to improve asthma inhaler device use and clinical treatment outcomes.

Competing interests
The authors declare that they have no competing interests.
The authors declare that they have no financial competing interests.

Authors' contributions
JH: Reviewed the scientific literature pertinent to the research question. Wrote the proposal and responded to reviewer and IRB comments. Created data collection forms and drafted the first manuscript. AA: Performed all the statistical analysis and wrote the results section. HA: Supervised the data collection at KAMC. SB: Scientifically contributed to writing the proposal. HR: Supervised the data collection at KKUH. KM: Provided scientific expertise and operational guidance for data collection at KAMC and actively precipitated in contributing to writing the manuscript assigned by the PI. MS: Scientifically contributed to writing the proposal and study conduct at KKUH. All authors read and approved the final manuscript.

Acknowledgments
We would like to thank Dr. Ali Al-Farhan and Dr. Raeied Hejaze for facilitating our access to the ED and helping identify potential patients. We also thank King Abdullah International Medical Research Center (KAIMRC) for funding and providing editing support for this research.

Author details
[1]Department of Medicine, Pulmonary Division-ICU, King Saud bin Abdulaziz University for Health Sciences, Riyadh, Saudi Arabia. [2]Department of Epidemiology and Biostatistics, College of Public Health and Health Informatics, King Saud bin Abdulaziz University for Health Sciences, Riyadh, Saudi Arabia. [3]Asthma Research Chair and Prince Naif Center for Immunology Research, Department of Pediatrics, College of Medicine, King Saud University, Riyadh, Saudi Arabia. [4]King Saud University for Health Sciences, Head of Pulmonary Division, Medical Director of Sleep Disorders Center, King Abdulaziz Medical City, Riyadh, Saudi Arabia.

References

1. NIH. National Asthma Education and Prevention Program: *Expert panel report 3: guidelines for the diagnosis and management of asthma.* Bethesda (MD): National Heart, Lung, and Blood Institute. NIH Publication No. 07-4051. NIH Publication No 07-4051; 2007.
2. Turner S, Paton J, Higgins B, Douglas G: **British guidelines on the management of asthma: what's new for 2011?** *Thorax* 2011, **66**(12):1104–5.
3. Gupta RS, Weiss KB: **The 2007 national asthma education and prevention program asthma guidelines: accelerating their implementation and facilitating their impact on children with asthma.** *Pediatrics* 2009, **123**(Suppl 3):S193–8.
4. Al Frayh AR, Shakoor Z, Gad El Rab MO, Hasnain SM: **Increased prevalence of asthma in Saudi Arabia.** *Ann Allergy Asthma Immunol* 2001, **86**(3):292–6.
5. al Frayh AR, Al Nahdi M, Bener AR, Jawadi TQ: **Epidemiology of asthma and allergic rhinitis in two coastal regions of Saudi Arabia.** *Allerg Immunol (Paris)* 1989, **21**(10):389–93.
6. Al-Moamary MS, Al-Hajjaj MS, Idrees MM, Zeitouni MO, Alanezi MO, Al-Jahdal HH, *et al*: **The Saudi initiative for asthma.** *Ann Thorac Med* 2009, **4**(4):216–33.
7. Clancy K: **British guidelines on the management of asthma.** *Thorax* 2004, **59**(1):81–2.
8. Bateman ED, Hurd SS, Barnes PJ, Bousquet J, Drazen JM, FitzGerald M, *et al*: **Global strategy for asthma management and prevention: GINA executive summary.** *Eur Respir J* 2008, **31**(1):143–78.
9. Al-Jahdali HH, Al-Hajjaj MS, Alanezi MO, Zeitoni MO, Al-Tasan TH: **Asthma control assessment using asthma control test among patients attending 5 tertiary care hospitals in Saudi Arabia.** *Saudi Med J* 2008, **29**(5):714–7.
10. Adams RJ, Smith BJ, Ruffin RE: **Factors associated with hospital admissions and repeat emergency department visits for adults with asthma.** *Thorax* 2000, **55**(7):566–73.
11. Weiss KB, Gergen PJ, Hodgson TA: **An economic evaluation of asthma in the United States.** *N Engl J Med* 1992, **326**(13):862–6.
12. Blais L, Suissa S, Boivin JF, Ernst P: **First treatment with inhaled corticosteroids and the prevention of admissions to hospital for asthma.** *Thorax* 1998, **53**(12):1025–9.
13. Broeders ME, Sanchis J, Levy ML, Crompton GK, Dekhuijzen PN: **The ADMIT series--issues in inhalation therapy. 2. Improving technique and clinical effectiveness.** *Prim Care Respir J* 2009, **18**(2):76–82.
14. Giraud V, Roche N: **Misuse of corticosteroid metered-dose inhaler is associated with decreased asthma stability.** *Eur Respir J* 2002, **19**(2):246–51.
15. Melani AS, Bonavia M, Cilenti V, Cinti C, Lodi M, Martucci P, *et al*: **Inhaler mishandling remains common in real life and is associated with reduced disease control.** *Respir Med* 2011, **105**(6):930–8.
16. Lenney J, Innes JA, Crompton GK: **Inappropriate inhaler use: assessment of use and patient preference of seven inhalation devices.** *EDICI Respir Med* 2000, **94**(5):496–500.
17. Molimard M, Le Gros V: **Impact of patient-related factors on asthma control.** *J Asthma* 2008, **45**(2):109–13.
18. Dolovich MB, Ahrens RC, Hess DR, Anderson P, Dhand R, Rau JL, *et al*: **Device selection and outcomes of aerosol therapy: evidence-based guidelines: American college of chest physicians/American college of asthma, allergy, and immunology.** *Chest* 2005, **127**(1):335–71.
19. Cochrane MG, Bala MV, Downs KE, Mauskopf J, Ben-Joseph RH: **Inhaled corticosteroids for asthma therapy: patient compliance, devices, and inhalation technique.** *Chest* 2000, **117**(2):542–50.
20. Coelho AC, Souza-Machado A, Leite M, Almeida P, Castro L, Cruz CS, *et al*: **Use of inhaler devices and asthma control in severe asthma patients at a referral center in the city of Salvador, Brazil.** *J Bras Pneumol* 2011, **37**(6):720–8.
21. Lavorini F, Magnan A, Dubus JC, Voshaar T, Corbetta L, Broeders M, *et al*: **Effect of incorrect use of dry powder inhalers on management of patients with asthma and COPD.** *Respir Med* 2008, **102**(4):593–604.
22. Epstein S, Maidenberg A, Hallett D, Khan K, Chapman KR: **Patient handling of a dry-powder inhaler in clinical practice.** *Chest* 2001, **120**(5):1480–4.

23. Lababidi H, Hijaoui A, Zarzour M: Validation of the Arabic version of the asthma control test. *Ann Thorac Med* 2008, **3**(2):44–7.
24. Sestini P, Cappiello V, Aliani M, Martucci P, Sena A, Vaghi A, *et al*: Prescription bias and factors associated with improper use of inhalers. *J Aerosol Med* 2006, **19**(2):127–36.
25. Brocklebank D, Ram F, Wright J, Barry P, Cates C, Davies L, *et al*: Comparison of the effectiveness of inhaler devices in asthma and chronic obstructive airways disease: a systematic review of the literature. *Health Technol Assess* 2001, **5**(26):1–149.
26. Al Zabadi H, El SN: Factors associated with frequent emergency room attendance by asthma patients in Palestine. *Int J Tuberc Lung Dis* 2007, **11**(8):920–7.
27. Takemura M, Kobayashi M, Kimura K, Mitsui K, Masui H, Koyama M, *et al*: Repeated instruction on inhalation technique improves adherence to the therapeutic regimen in asthma. *J Asthma* 2010, **47**(2):202–8.
28. Giner J, Macian V, Hernandez C: Multicenter prospective study of respiratory patient education and instruction in the use of inhalers (EDEN study). *Arch Bronconeumol* 2002, **38**(7):300–5.
29. Ronmark E, Jogi R, Lindqvist A, Haugen T, Meren M, Loit HM, *et al*: Correct use of three powder inhalers: comparison between Diskus, Turbuhaler, and Easyhaler. *J Asthma* 2005, **42**(3):173–8.
30. van der Palen J, Klein JJ, Kerkhoff AH, van Herwaarden CL, Seydel ER: Evaluation of the long-term effectiveness of three instruction modes for inhaling medicines. *Patient Educ Couns* 1997, **32**(1 Suppl):S87–95.
31. Larsen JS, Hahn M, Ekholm B, Wick KA: Evaluation of conventional press-and-breathe metered-dose inhaler technique in 501 patients. *J Asthma* 1994, **31**(3):193–9.
32. Interiano B, Guntupalli KK: Metered-dose inhalers. Do health care providers know what to teach? *Arch Intern Med* 1993, **153**(1):81–5.
33. Basheti IA, Armour CL, Bosnic-Anticevich SZ, Reddel HK: Evaluation of a novel educational strategy, including inhaler-based reminder labels, to improve asthma inhaler technique. *Patient Educ Couns* 2008, **72**(1):26–33.
34. Al-Jahdali HH, Al-Zahrani AI, Al-Otaibi ST, Hassan IS, Al-Moamary MS, Al-Duhaim AS, *et al*: Perception of the role of inhaled corticosteroids and factors affecting compliance among asthmatic adult patients. *Saudi Med J* 2007, **28**(4):569–73.

12

Effectiveness of montelukast administered as monotherapy or in combination with inhaled corticosteroid in pediatric patients with uncontrolled asthma

Denis Bérubé[1], Michel Djandji[2,3], John S Sampalis[4,5*] and Allan Becker[6]

Abstract

Background: Asthma is the most common chronic disease of childhood and a leading cause of childhood morbidity. The aim of the current study was to assess the effectiveness of montelukast administered as monotherapy or in combination with current inhaled corticosteroids (ICS) in pediatric patients with uncontrolled asthma as per the Canadian Asthma Consensus Guidelines.

Methods: Twelve-week, multicentre, open-label, observational study. Primary effectiveness outcome was the proportion of patients achieving asthma control (Asthma Control Questionnaire (ACQ) score ≤0.75) at weeks 4 and 12.

Results: A total of 328 patients with uncontrolled asthma (ACQ > 0.75) were enrolled with mean ± SD age of 6.9 ± 3.4 years. Among these, 76 (23.2%) were treated with montelukast monotherapy and 252 (76.8%) with montelukast combined with ICS. By 4 weeks of treatment 61.3% and 52.9% of the patients in the monotherapy and combination group, respectively, achieved asthma control. These proportions increased to 75.0% and 70.9%, respectively, at 12 weeks. Within the monotherapy group, clinically significant improvements in the ACQ score (mean ± SD of 1.67 ± 0.69, 0.71 ± 0.70 and 0.50 ± 0.52 at baseline, 4 and 12 weeks, respectively; p < 0.001) and the PACQLQ score (mean ± SD of 5.34 ± 1.14, 6.32 ± 0.89 and 6.51 ± 0.85 at baseline, 4 and 12 weeks, respectively; p < 0.001) were observed. In the combination group, the mean ± SD ACQ score significantly improved from 2.02 ± 0.83 at baseline to 0.90 ± 0.86 at 4 weeks and 0.64 ± 0.86 at 12 weeks (p < 0.001), while the PACQLQ score improved from 4.42 ± 1.35 at baseline to 5.76 ± 1.30 at 4 weeks and 6.21 ± 1.03 at 12 weeks (p < 0.001). After a 12-week montelukast add-on therapy, 22.6% of patients reduced their ICS dosage. Similar results were observed among preschool- and school-aged patients.

Conclusions: Montelukast as monotherapy or in combination with ICS represents an effective treatment strategy for achieving asthma control in pediatric patients and improving caregivers' quality of life.

Trial registration: This study is registered at ClinicalTrial.gov: NCT00832455.

Keywords: Asthma, Montelukast, Inhaled corticosteroids, Pediatric, Preschool age, School age

* Correspondence: jsampalis@jssresearch.com
[4]McGill University, Montréal, Québec, Canada
[5]JSS Medical Research, Montréal, Québec, Canada
Full list of author information is available at the end of the article

Background

Asthma is a chronic inflammatory disorder of the airways with a heterogeneous target age group and an initial diagnosis age of as early as infancy. Its prevalence, especially among children, is increasing worldwide [1,2], including Canada [3,4]. From 2000 to 2001, 13.4% of Canadian children aged up to 11 years old were diagnosed with asthma [3]. Relative to the 1994 to 1995 period, this represents a statistically significant increase in the asthma prevalence of nearly 70,000 diagnoses of asthmatic children [3], rendering asthma one of the most prevalent chronic conditions affecting Canadian children.

Current asthma treatment guidelines recognize the importance of early and aggressive intervention for asthma and recommend low-dose inhaled corticosteroids (ICSs) as first-line treatment in childhood [2,5-8]. However, despite ICS treatment, an important proportion of patients remain with uncontrolled asthmatic symptoms. In addition, the response to asthma therapy appears to be variable since some asthmatic children who do not respond to ICSs may respond to other therapies [9,10]. This further highlights the need to identify alternative treatment strategies that will expand the array of therapeutic options available to physicians who treat pediatric asthma [11].

Leukotriene receptor antagonists (LTRAs), such as montelukast, provide an alternative treatment for asthma patients who are not controlled or satisfied with ICS therapy [2,5-7,12]. Montelukast is an orally administered, once-daily LTRA that can be prescribed as monotherapy or in combination with other asthma medications, including ICSs, for the treatment of asthma.

Although results from controlled randomized clinical trials have provided evidence of the montelukast efficacy in the treatment of asthmatic children [13,14], continuous evaluation of the effectiveness and safety of montelukast in a less controlled real-life setting is essential to help health care professionals bridge the gap between current knowledge and routine practice in the management of asthmatic children. There is currently little information available on montelukast effectiveness in every day practice for children, which could complement the findings of randomized clinical trials. Therefore, the principal aim of this study was to assess the effectiveness of montelukast administered either as monotherapy or in combination with current ICS treatment in pediatric patients with uncontrolled asthma, in a clinical setting emulating real-life.

Methods

Study design

This was a 12-week, open-label, multicenter, prospective study conducted in 58 Canadian clinics between June 2006 and October 2008. Patients were treated with montelukast sodium for 12 weeks, either as a monotherapy or in combination with their current ICS treatment.

Clinical assessments were conducted at baseline, 4 and 12 weeks of treatment at the clinics of their treating physicians. During the course of the study, tapering of ICS dosage was performed at the discretion of the treating physician and on an individual basis when asthma control was achieved. An optional visit after 8 weeks of treatment was performed to determine if an ICS dosage adjustment was necessary and to assess asthma control of patients previously tapered. Parents or legal guardians provided written informed consent prior to the participation of their children in this study. The study was approved by three independent Ethics Review Boards (IRB Services, Aurora, Ontario; the College of Physicians and Surgeons of Alberta, Edmonton; and the *Comité central de l'éthique de la recherche du Ministère de la santé et des services sociaux du Québec*, Montréal, Québec), and was conducted in accordance with ICH Good Clinical Practice Guidelines, the World Medical Association Declaration of Helsinki and all applicable local regulations.

Patients

Eligible patients were between 2 and 14 years of age and had been diagnosed with asthma for at least 6 months. In order to be included in the study, patients had to have a peak expiratory Flow (PEF) $\geq 80\%$ of the predicted value (applicable only for patients older than 7 years old) and they had to be either currently untreated, using a short-acting β_2-agonist (SABA) on an as-needed basis or using an ICS at any dosage. In addition, one of the following conditions had to be satisfied: i) the physician and/or patient was dissatisfied with the current controller therapy; ii) the patient was reluctant to take ICS therapy, or; iii) the patient was insufficiently controlled with the current therapy through the preceding 6 weeks. Finally, eligible patients had to have uncontrolled asthma as per the 2003 Canadian Asthma Consensus Guidelines [6].

Patients were excluded if their asthma symptoms were controlled and if they were treated with montelukast or any of the following treatments at the time of entry into the study: long-acting β_2-agonist (LABA) alone or in a combination product, oral prednisone, regular use of theophylline and/or other asthma medications such as sodium cromoglycate or nedocromil. Patients using an antibiotic for respiratory tract infection at the time of entry into the study or treated with an antibiotic for respiratory tract infection (initiation of antibiotic treatment was permitted during the study) within 30 days were also excluded. A history of cystic fibrosis, immune deficiency requiring specific therapy or any other disease that could influence the evolution of asthma was also a reason for exclusion. Finally, patients with a history of hypersensitivity to any component of montelukast were excluded.

Considering that the primary outcome measure was the proportion of patients achieving asthma control based on the ACQ criteria (ACQ ≤ 0.75), a re-analysis of the data was conducted including only patients with ACQ > 0.75 at baseline the results of which are reported here.

Treatment strategies
All patients were treated with montelukast sodium (SINGULAIR®, Merck & Co. Inc., USA) taken once-daily at bedtime as monotherapy or in addition to their current ICS therapy. Patients aged between 6 and 14 years were treated with 5 mg montelukast sodium chewable tablets, while patients between 2 and less than 6 years of age were treated with 4 mg montelukast chewable tablets. The 4 mg granule formulation was also available for the latter age group on demand. The use of a short-acting β_2-agonist (SABA) as rescue medication was allowed during the study, but patients were asked to refrain from its utilization for 6 hours prior each study visit.

Outcome measures
The primary effectiveness outcome measures was the proportion of patients achieving asthma control, defined as a score ≤ 0.75 [15] in the self-administered Asthma Control Questionnaire (ACQ) (completed by the patient or their caregiver) [16]. Secondary effectiveness outcome measures included: (i) the mean change in ACQ score between baseline and the 4- and 12-week assessments, considering a change of ≥ 0.5 in ACQ score as clinically important [16]; (ii) the change in quality of life of the caregivers between baseline and the 4- and 12-week assessments, as assessed using the Pediatric Asthma Caregivers Quality of Life Questionnaire (PACQLQ) [17], considering changes of ≥ 0.7 in PACQLQ as clinically important [17]; (iii) the patient (completed by the patient or their caregiver) and physician satisfaction with treatment as measured using the 5-point Likert scale ranging from 0 (very dissatisfied) to 4 (very satisfied), upon 4 and 12 weeks of treatment with montelukast; and (iv) the proportion of patients on montelukast combination therapy whose baseline ICS daily dosage was tapered to a lower ICS dose category after 4, 8 and 12 weeks of treatment. The ICS daily doses were categorized according to the 2006 report of the Global Initiative for Asthma (GINA) [18] as follows: (i) low dose, defined as ≤200 µg/day of fluticasone propionate or equivalent (≤200 µg/day of beclomethasone dipropionate and ≤200 µg/day of budesonide); (ii) moderate dose, defined as >200 to ≤500 µg/day of fluticasone propionate or equivalent (>200 to ≤400 µg/day of beclomethasone dipropionate and >200 to ≤400 µg/day of budesonide); and (iii) high dose, defined as >500 µg/day of fluticasone propionate or equivalent (>400 µg/day of beclomethasone dipropionate and >400 µg/day of budesonide).

Compliance with the study medication was assessed by tablet counts, as recorded in the study worksheets. Safety and tolerability were assessed with the incidence of treatment-emergent adverse events, which were coded and reported according to the MedDRA dictionary of terms, version 9.0 [19].

Statistical methods
Descriptive statistics were produced for patient demographics and characteristics at baseline. Comparisons between baseline and follow-up visits were performed with the matched Chi-Square test for categorical scales and the paired Student's t-test for continuous scales. Two-tailed tests were performed using a significance level (α) of 0.05. Subgroup analyses by treatment strategy and stratified analyses for preschool-aged children (less than 6 years old) and school-aged children (6 years of age or older) were performed. There were no imputations for missing data. All analyses were performed using the SPSS version 12.0 for Windows (SPSS Inc., Chicago, IL).

Results
Patient disposition
A total of 420 patients with uncontrolled asthma as per the 2003 Canadian Asthma Consensus Guidelines completed the baseline assessment of whom 92 (21.9%) had an ACQ score of ≤ 0.75 at baseline. Considering that the primary outcome measure was the proportion of patients achieving asthma control based on the ACQ criteria, only the 328 patients with ACQ > 0.75 were included in this analysis. Among these, 320 (97.6%) and 288 (87.8%) patients completed the 4- and 12-week assessment, respectively, while the optional 8-week assessment was performed on 197 (60.1%) patients. There were 40 (12.2%) patients who were discontinued from the study: 10 (3.0%) due to an adverse event, 8 (2.4%) withdrew consent, 9 (2.7%) were lost to follow-up, 4 (1.2%) due to protocol violation, 8 (2.4%) discontinued for other reasons, while the reason of discontinuation was missing for 1 (0.3%) patient.

Patient demographics and baseline characteristics
The demographics and baseline characteristics of the study population are summarized in Table 1. The mean (SD) age was 6.92 (3.35) years, 192 (58.5%) patients were male and 209 (63.7%) were Caucasian. At baseline, 252 patients were on ICS therapy and were therefore included in the montelukast add-on group, the majority of whom were taking moderate doses of ICS (n = 143; 56.7%). The remaining 76 patients were not taking ICS at baseline and comprised the montelukast monotherapy treatment group. Overall, at baseline, 269 (82.0%) patients had nighttime symptoms ≥ 1 night/week, 247 (75.3%) had daytime symptoms ≥ 4 days/week, and 122 (37.2%) reported absenteeism from school in the last week due to asthma.

Table 1 Demographics and baseline characteristics

Characteristics	Montelukast monotherapy			Montelukast + ICS			Total
	Preschool age	School age	All	Preschool age	School age	All	
N	34	42	76	112	140	252	328
Age (years), mean (SD)	4.01 (1.12)	9.19 (2.26)	6.87 (3.19)	3.86 (1.13)	9.54 (2.35)	7.02 (3.41)	6.92 (3.35)
Gender, n (%)							
Male	18 (52.9)	25 (59.5)	43 (56.6)	60 (53.6)	89 (63.6)	149 (59.1)	192 (58.5)
Female	16 (47.1)	17 (40.5)	33 (43.4)	52 (46.4)	51 (36.4)	103 (40.9)	136 (41.5)
Race, n (%)							
Caucasian	25 (73.5)	32 (76.2)	57 (75.0)	66 (58.9)	86 (61.4)	152 (60.3)	209 (63.7)
Black	0 (0.0)	1 (2.4)	1 (1.3)	8 (7.1)	13 (9.3)	21 (8.3)	22 (6.7)
Asian	4 (11.8)	8 (19.0)	12 (15.8)	32 (28.6)	32 (22.9)	64 (25.4)	76 (23.2)
Hispanic	0 (0.0)	1 (2.4)	1 (1.3)	3 (2.7)	3 (2.1)	6 (2.4)	7 (2.1)
Other	3 (8.8)	0 (0.0)	3 (3.9)	2 (1.8)	6 (4.3)	8 (3.2)	11 (3.4)
Missing	2 (5.9)	0 (0.0)	2 (2.6)	1 (0.9)	0 (0.0)	1 (0.4)	3 (0.9)
Duration of asthma since diagnosis (years), mean (SD)	2.06 (1.11)	4.32 (3.25)	3.31 (2.76)	2.11 (1.27)	5.46 (3.08)	3.97 (2.96)	3.82 (2.92)
Smoking history, n (%)							
Patient is a smoker	0 (0.0)	0 (0.0)	0 (0.0)	0 (0.0)	0 (0.0)	0 (0.0)	0 (0.0)
Patient quit smoking	0 (0.0)	0 (0.0)	0 (0.0)	0 (0.0)	1 (0.7)	1 (0.4)	1 (0.3)
Patient never smoked	34 (100.0)	41 (97.6)	75 (98.7)	104 (92.9)	133 (95.0)	237 (94.0)	312 (95.1)
Member of household is a smoker	8 (23.5)	14 (33.3)	22 (28.9)	20 (17.9)	40 (28.6)	60 (23.8)	82 (25.0)
Member of household quit smoking	5 (14.7)	11 (26.2)	16 (21.1)	8 (7.1)	7 (5.0)	15 (6.0)	31 (9.5)
Use of ICS at baseline, n (%)							
Low dose[*]	-	-	-	58 (51.8)	39 (27.9)	97 (38.5)	97 (29.6)
Moderate dose[†]	-	-	-	53 (47.3)	90 (64.3)	143 (56.7)	143 (43.6)
High dose[‡]	-	-	-	1 (0.9)	11 (7.9)	12 (4.8)	12 (3.7)
Profile of asthma symptoms, n (%)							
1. Daytime symptoms ≥ 4 days/week	24 (70.6)	26 (61.9)	50 (65.8)	91 (81.3)	106 (75.7)	197 (78.2)	247 (75.3)
2. Night-time symptoms ≥ 1 night/week	29 (85.3)	30 (71.4)	59 (77.6)	99 (88.4)	111 (79.3)	210 (83.3)	269 (82.0)
3. Absenteeism from school due to asthma in the last week	7 (20.6)	16 (38.1)	23 (30.3)	33 (29.5)	66 (47.1)	99 (39.3)	122 (37.2)
4. SABA ≥ 4 doses in the last week[§]	13 (38.2)	13 (31.0)	26 (34.2)	76 (67.9)	92 (65.7)	168 (66.7)	194 (59.1)
5. FEV in one second or PEF ≥90% of their personal best in the last week	2 (5.9)	9 (21.4)	11 (14.5)	11 (9.8)	41 (29.3)	52 (20.6)	63 (19.2)
6. Diurnal variability in peak expiratory flow >10% to 15% in the last week	2 (5.9)	2 (4.8)	4 (5.3)	8 (7.1)	22 (15.7)	30 (11.9)	34 (10.4)

*Low dose was defined as ≤ 200 μg/day for fluticasone propionate or equivalent (≤200 μg/day for beclomethasone dipropionate and ≤200 μg/day for budesonide).
†Moderate dose was defined as >200 to 500 μg/day for fluticasone propionate or equivalent (>200 to 400 μg/day for beclomethasone dipropionate and >200 to 400 μg/day for budesonide) [18].
‡High dose was defined as > 500 μg/day for fluticasone propionate or equivalent (>400 μg/day for beclomethasone dipropionate and >400 μg/day for budesonide).
§Excluding one dose/day before exercise.

Notably, SABA utilization (≥4 doses in the last week) was reported twice as frequently by patients in the combination therapy compared to the monotherapy group (66.7% vs 34.2%).

Effectiveness outcomes

Table 2 presents the proportions of patients who achieved asthma control after 4 and 12 weeks of treatment with montelukast, administered either as a monotherapy or in addition to ICS therapy, overall and stratified by treatment strategy and age group. The overall proportion of patients who achieved asthma control (ACQ score ≤ 0.75) was 54.9% (n = 175) at 4 weeks and 71.9% (n = 207) at 12 weeks. Among preschool patients, the proportion of patients with controlled asthma increased from 63.3% (n = 88) at 4 weeks to 77.3% (n = 99) at 12 weeks, while among school aged patients, these proportions were 48.3% (n = 87) and 67.5% (n = 108), respectively. This significant rate of asthma control was consistent across both treating strategies; montelukast alone and in combination with ICS.

The mean (SD) ACQ score of the total study sample decreased from 1.94 (0.82) at baseline to 0.85 (0.83) at 4 weeks and 0.61 (0.79) at 12 weeks of treatment, representing statistically and clinically significant absolute mean (SD) changes of –1.08 (1.00) and –1.34 (1.03) from baseline to 4 and 12 weeks, respectively (p < 0.001) (Table 3). Among the patients treated with montelukast monotherapy, the mean (SD) ACQ score significantly decreased from 1.67 (0.69) at baseline to 0.71 (0.70) at 4 weeks and to 0.50 (0.52) 12 weeks (Figure 1A). Among the patients treated with the montelukast add-on treatment strategy,

the mean (SD) ACQ score significantly decreased from 2.02 (0.83) at baseline to 0.90 (0.86) at 4 weeks and to 0.64 (0.86) at 12 weeks (Figure 1B).

The mean ACQ scores throughout the treatment period for the monotherapy and combination therapy patients, stratified by age group are also shown in Figure 1A and B. Among preschool and school-aged patients treated with montelukast monotherapy, the mean (SD) ACQ score significantly decreased from 1.68 (0.75) and 1.66 (0.65) at baseline to 0.79 (0.76) and 0.64 (0.65) at 4 weeks, to 0.54 (0.59) and 0.47 (0.45) at 12 weeks (Figure 1A), representing statistically and clinically significant absolute mean (SD) changes of –1.13 (0.94) and –1.18 (0.64) from baseline to 12 weeks, respectively (Table 3). Similarly, statistically and clinically significant decreases in the ACQ score were also observed among preschool and school aged patients treated with montelukast add-on therapy (Figure 1B and Table 3). Among children 7 years of age or older the PEF assessment showed a statistically significant improvement increasing from 253.9 L/min at baseline to 275.0 L/min at 12 weeks of treatment (P < 0.001).

The mean (SD) PACQLQ score of the total study sample increased from 4.63 (1.36) at baseline to 5.89 (1.24) at 4 weeks (mean (SD) change = 1.55 (1.40); P < 0.001) and 6.28 (1.00) at 12 weeks (mean (SD) change = 1.82 (1.30); P < 0.001). Among the patients who adopted the montelukast monotherapy treatment strategy, the mean (SD) PACQLQ score increased from 5.34 (1.14) at baseline to 6.32 (0.89) at 4 weeks and 6.51 (0.85) at 12 weeks. The absolute mean (SD) change in PACQLQ of 0.98 (1.12) at 4 weeks and 1.13 (1.04) at 12 weeks was both clinically (change in PACQLQ > 0.7) and statistically significant (p < 0.001) (Table 3). Among the patients who adopted the montelukast add-on treatment strategy, the mean (SD) PACQLQ score increased from 4.42 (1.35) at baseline to 5.76 (1.30) at 4 weeks and 6.21 (1.03) at 12 weeks corresponding to a mean (SD) absolute change of 1.34 (1.34) at 4 weeks and 1.78 (1.36) at 12 weeks (p < 0.001) (Table 3). In both treatment strategies, significant changes were observed in both the emotional and activity limitation domains of the PACQLQ questionnaire. Comparable clinically and statistically significant changes in PACQLQ scores were observed among preschool and school aged patients (Figure 2A and B and Table 3).

Figures 3 and 4 summarize the results of the patients and physicians global satisfaction with montelukast, respectively. At baseline, 54.9% of the patients were dissatisfied or very dissatisfied with their current asthma therapy and 12.8% were satisfied or very satisfied. After 4 and 12 weeks of treatment with montelukast, 8.8% and 2.4% of the patients were dissatisfied/very dissatisfied and 73.9% and 85.3% were satisfied/very satisfied, respectively. With regards to the physician's global satisfaction, 74.6% of the treating physicians were dissatisfied or very dissatisfied

Table 2 Proportion of patients with asthma control (ACQ score ≤ 0.75)

Asthma control	4 weeks		12 weeks	
	n	%	n	%
Montelukast monotherapy				
All patients, n (%)	(N = 75)		(N = 68)	
Well controlled	46	61.3	51	75.0
Not controlled	29	38.7	17	25.0
Preschool aged patients, n (%)	(N = 34)		(N =32)	
Well controlled	19	55.9	24	75.0
Not controlled	15	44.1	8	25.0
School aged patients, n (%)	(N =41)		(N = 36)	
Well controlled	27	65.9	27	75.0
Not controlled	14	34.1	9	25.0
Montelukast + ICS				
All patients, n (%)	(N = 244)		(N = 220)	
Well controlled	129	52.9	156	70.9
Not controlled	115	47.1	64	29.1
Preschool aged patients, n (%)	(N = 105)		(N = 96)	
Well controlled	69	65.7	75	78.1
Not controlled	36	34.3	21	21.9
School aged patients, n (%)	(N = 139)		(N = 124)	
Well controlled	60	43.2	81	65.3
Not controlled	79	56.8	43	34.7
Total study sample (Montelukast monotherapy & Montelukast + ICS)				
All patients, n (%)	(N = 319)		(N = 288)	
Well controlled	175	54.9	207	71.9
Not controlled	144	45.1	81	28.1
Preschool aged patients, n (%)	(N = 139)		(N = 128)	
Well controlled	88	63.3	99	77.3
Not controlled	51	36.7	29	22.7
School aged patients, n (%)	(N = 180)		(N = 160)	
Well controlled	87	48.3	108	67.5
Not controlled	93	51.7	52	32.5

Table 3 Mean change in Asthma Control Questionnaire and Pediatric Asthma Caregivers Quality of Life Questionnaire

Age group		Treatment group				Total	
		Montelukast monotherapy		Montelukast + ICS			
		Mean	SD	Mean	SD	Mean	SD
All patients							
ACQ score*	Change between Week 4 and Baseline	−0.95	0.88	−1.12	1.03	−1.08	1.00
	Change between Week 12 and Baseline	−1.15	0.79	−1.40	1.09	−1.34	1.03
PACQLQ score*	Change between Week 4 and Baseline	0.98	1.12	1.34	1.34	1.25	1.30
	Change between Week 12 and Baseline	1.13	1.04	1.78	1.36	1.63	1.32
Emotional function*	Change between Week 4 and Baseline	0.90	1.14	1.25	1.32	1.17	1.29
	Change between Week 12 and Baseline	1.02	1.01	1.71	1.41	1.55	1.36
Activity limitation*	Change between Week 4 and Baseline	1.16	1.32	1.53	1.61	1.44	1.55
	Change between Week 12 and Baseline	1.38	1.34	1.94	1.51	1.81	1.49
Pre-School patients							
ACQ score*	Change between Week 4 and Baseline	−0.89	1.10	−1.38	1.08	−1.26	1.11
	Change between Week 12 and Baseline	−1.13	0.94	−1.56	1.16	−1.45	1.12
PACQLQ score*	Change between Week 4 and Baseline	1.01	1.19	1.73	1.42	1.55	1.40
	Change between Week 12 and Baseline	1.18	1.06	2.03	1.30	1.82	1.30
Emotional function*	Change between Week 4 and Baseline	0.88	1.16	1.60	1.41	1.42	1.39
	Change between Week 12 and Baseline	1.05	0.95	1.94	1.34	1.72	1.31
Activity limitation*	Change between Week 4 and Baseline	1.29	1.40	2.02	1.62	1.84	1.60
	Change between Week 12 and Baseline	1.47	1.47	2.24	1.45	2.05	1.49
School aged patients							
ACQ score*	Change between Week 4 and Baseline	−1.01	0.64	−0.93	0.94	−0.94	0.88
	Change between Week 12 and Baseline	−1.18	0.64	−1.27	1.02	−1.25	0.95
PACQLQ score*	Change between Week 4 and Baseline	0.96	1.08	1.04	1.20	1.02	1.17
	Change between Week 12 and Baseline	1.09	1.03	1.58	1.37	1.47	1.31
Emotional function*	Change between Week 4 and Baseline	0.92	1.14	0.99	1.19	0.97	1.18
	Change between Week 12 and Baseline	1.00	1.08	1.53	1.44	1.41	1.38
Activity limitation*	Change between Week 4 and Baseline	1.04	1.26	1.15	1.49	1.13	1.44
	Change between Week 12 and Baseline	1.29	1.23	1.70	1.52	1.61	1.47

*P < 0.001 for all changes from baseline based on Student's t-test for Paired Observations.

with their patient's current asthma therapy and 4.6% were satisfied or very satisfied at baseline. After 4 and 12 weeks of treatment with montelukast, 8.3% and 4.1% of the physicians were dissatisfied/very dissatisfied while 66.6% and 87.8% were satisfied/very satisfied, respectively. Overall, the changes in patient and physician satisfaction upon treatment with montelukast for 4 and 12 weeks were statistically significant (p < 0.001) without any significant differences between preschool and school aged patients (data not shown).

The proportions of patients who tapered their baseline ICS daily dosage use to a lower ICS dose category after adding montelukast to their treatment regimen are reported in Table 4. There were 45 (18.4%), 40 (25.2) and 44 (20.0) patients who reduced their ICS dosage after the addition of montelukast to their current ICS treatment

regimen at 4, 8 and 12 weeks, respectively. Similar results were observed for preschool and school aged patients.

Treatment compliance and safety

Compliance with the treating regimen was high during the follow-up period with patients taking by average 91.6%, 93.6% and 92.2% of their prescribed doses upon 4, 8 and 12 weeks of treatment, respectively. During the course of the study, there were 182 non-serious adverse events (NSAEs) reported by 112 (34.1%) patients. Of these, 157 (86.3%) were probably or definitely not related to study medication and 15 led to study drug discontinuation in 12 (3.7%) patients. There were 25 (13.7%) NSAEs possibly, probably or definitely related to montelukast. Of these, the most frequent NSAEs related to montelukast were nightmares and sleep terror (n = 6),

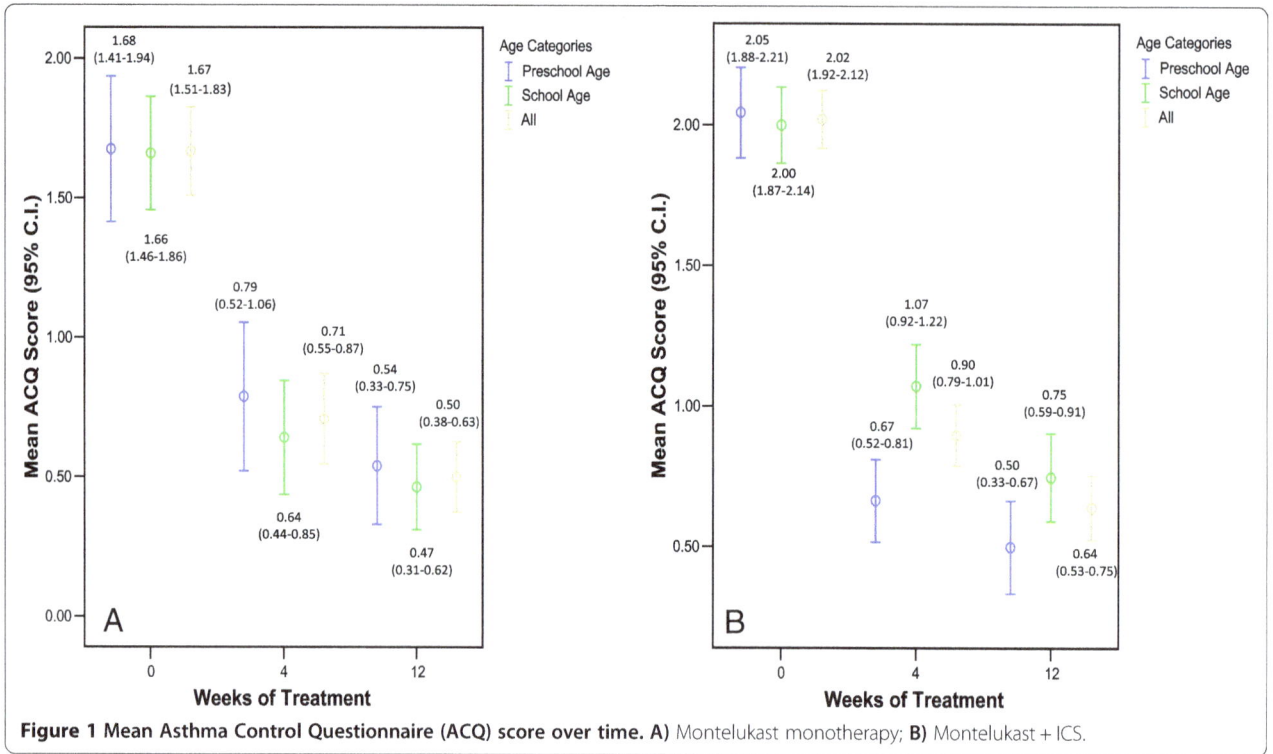

Figure 1 Mean Asthma Control Questionnaire (ACQ) score over time. **A)** Montelukast monotherapy; **B)** Montelukast + ICS.

abdominal pain (n = 5), insomnia (n = 2) and headache (n = 2). A total of 3 serious adverse events (SAEs) were experienced by 3 patients: 1 asthma episode, 1 bronchitis and 1 pneumonia, none of which were judged to be related to the study medication by the treating physicians.

Discussions

Although results from controlled randomized clinical trials indicate that montelukast is efficacious in the treatment of asthmatic children [13,14], continuous evaluation of the effectiveness and safety of montelukast in a less controlled real-life setting is essential in order to help

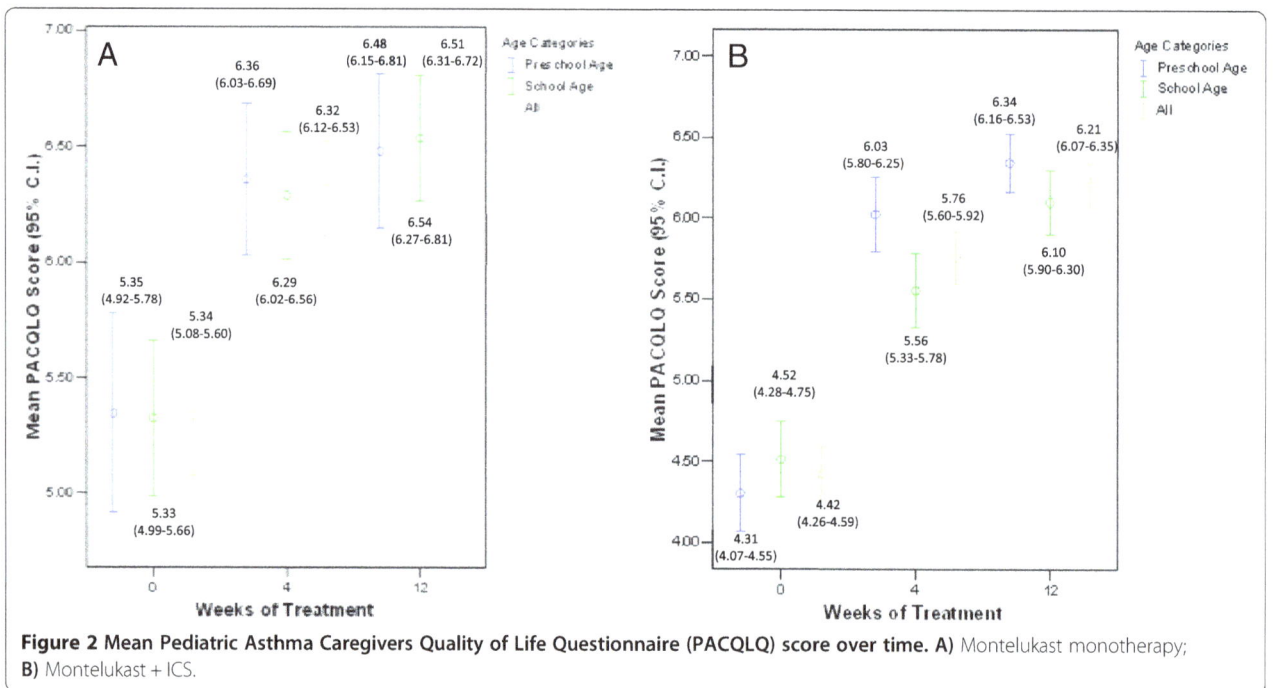

Figure 2 Mean Pediatric Asthma Caregivers Quality of Life Questionnaire (PACQLQ) score over time. **A)** Montelukast monotherapy; **B)** Montelukast + ICS.

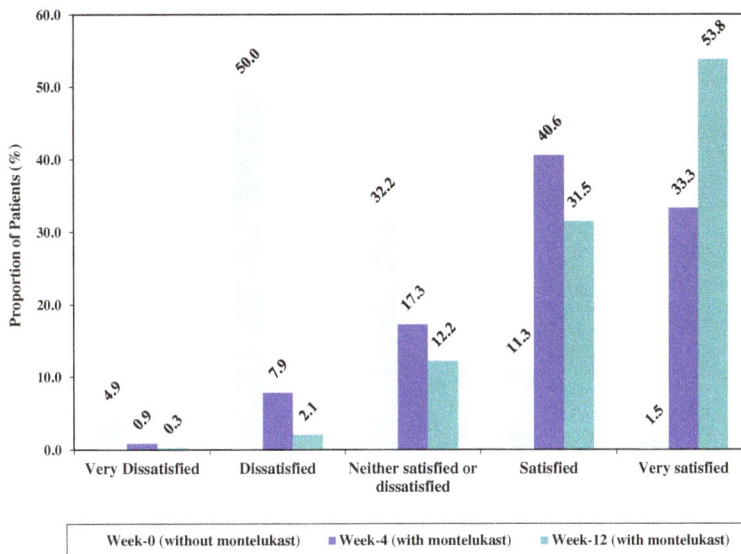

Figure 3 Patient global satisfaction upon treatment with montelukast. *Note: Percentages were calculated on available observations.*

health care professionals bridge the gap between current knowledge and practice in the management of asthmatic children. Accordingly, the principal objective of this study was to assess the effectiveness of montelukast administered either as a monotherapy or in combination with ICS treatment in children with uncontrolled asthma. Furthermore, in line with the fact that recommendations for asthma treatment differ according to children age categories [5,8,20], the effectiveness assessments of montelukast asthma treatment strategies were stratified by preschool and school aged pediatric patients.

The results of this 12-week multicenter observational study support the therapeutic effectiveness of montelukast in pediatric patients with uncontrolled asthma, in a clinical setting emulating real-life. Asthma control was achieved by the majority of patients who received montelukast either as monotherapy or in combination with ICS treatment for 12 weeks. Furthermore, clinically and statistically significant decreases in ACQ scores were observed after 4 and 12 weeks of treatment with montelukast mono- and add-on therapies, among both preschool and school-aged patients.

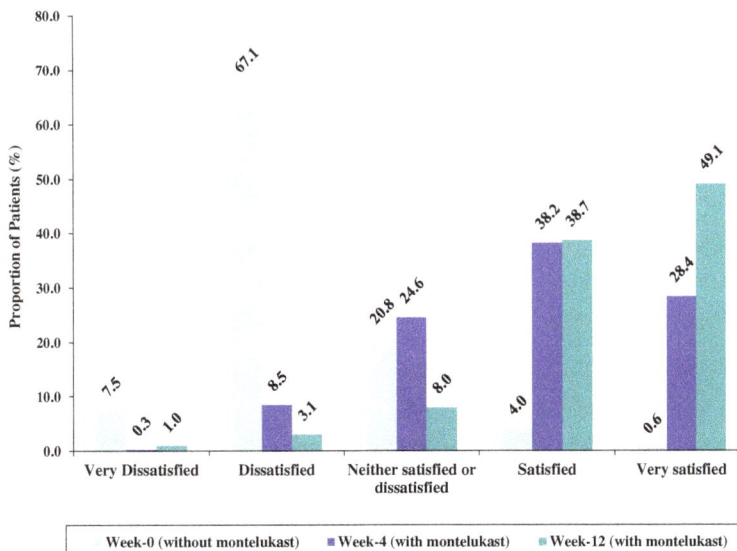

Figure 4 Physician global satisfaction with utilization of montelukast. *Note: Percentages were calculated on available observations.*

Table 4 Proportion of patients who tapered their dosage of inhaled corticosteroids in the montelukast add-on group

	Duration of treatment			
	Baseline	4 weeks	8 weeks	12 weeks
All patients	328	320	197	288
Use of ICS, n				
Yes	252	245	159	220
No	76	75	38	68
Tapered ICS, n (%)				
Yes*	-	45 (18.4)	40 (25.2)	44 (20.0)
No	-	194 (79.2)	117 (73.6)	175 (79.5)
Missing	-	6 (2.4)	2 (1.3)	1 (0.5)
Preschool aged patients	146	140	93	128
Use of ICS, n				
Yes	112	106	72	96
No	34	34	21	32
Tapered ICS, n (%)				
Yes[†]	-	21 (19.8)	20 (27.8)	19 (19.8)
No	-	82 (77.4)	50 (69.4)	76 (79.2)
Missing	-	3 (2.8)	2 (2.8)	1 (1.0)
School aged patients	182	180	104	160
Use of ICS, n				
Yes	140	139	87	124
No	42	41	17	36
Tapered ICS, n (%)				
Yes[‡]	-	24 (17.3)	20 (23.0)	25 (20.2)
No	-	112 (80.6)	67 (77.0)	99 (79.8)
Missing	-	3 (2.2)	0 (0.0)	0 (0.0)

*There were 45 patients who newly tapered their ICS at 4 weeks, 17 at 8 weeks and 9 at 12 weeks.
[†]There were 21 preschool aged patients who newly tapered their ICS at 4 weeks, 8 at 8 weeks and 3 at 12 weeks.
[‡]There were 24 school aged patients who newly tapered their ICS at 4 weeks, 9 at 8 weeks and 6 at 12 weeks.

Although cross-study comparisons are difficult due to differences in study designs and diversity in efficacy outcomes, the results of the current study are consistent with the efficacy profiles of montelukast in childhood asthma that were previously reported in systematic reviews and randomized clinical trials conducted in preschool [11,13,21,22] and school-aged [11,14,22-28] children. Furthermore, the observed ACQ improvement is significantly higher to that observed with placebo in clinical trials with comparable follow-up schedules to the current study [29,30]. In addition, our findings provide further evidence of the benefits of montelukast administered either as monotherapy or in combination with ICS in everyday childhood asthma management and real-life clinical practices.

Asthma is the most common chronic disease of childhood and a leading cause of childhood morbidity. In addition to considerably affecting children's physical, emotional and social lives, uncontrolled asthma also directly correlates with a loss of productivity and quality of life of the children's caregivers [31,32]. Therefore, an effective strategy for the management of pediatric asthma should involve the development of an effective, convenient, safe and well tolerated pharmacologic intervention while improving the quality of life of the children and their caregivers.

The results of this study indicate that both asthmatic children and their caregivers can benefit from montelukast therapy since it is an effective treating option enabling asthma control, while significantly improving the caregivers' quality of life. After 12 weeks of treatment with montelukast administered as monotherapy or in combination with ICS, clinically (mean change of ≥ 0.7 in PACQLQ score) and statistically (p < 0.001) significant improvements in caregivers' quality of life were observed with mean (SD) changes in PACQLQ score of 1.25 (1.30) and 1.63 (1.32) from baseline, respectively.

Furthermore, the vast majority of the patients and physicians were satisfied or very satisfied with montelukast. This high level of satisfaction can be probably attributed to the observed effectiveness of montelukast in controlling asthma symptoms and improving caregivers' quality of life, the ease of medication administration which enhances treatment compliance, and the safety and tolerability profile of montelukast.

The results of previous randomized clinical trials conducted with adult asthmatic patients suggested that montelukast could facilitate a reduction in ICS use [33,34]. However, the evidence on the ICS-sparing effect of montelukast in children is sparse and inconsistent. While Strunk RC et al. [35] reported that montelukast is not an effective ICS-sparing alternative in children, Tamesis GP et al. [36] have shown significantly lower use of supplemental ICS by children when montelukast was added to their ICS treatment. Moreover, although Phipatanakul W et al. [27] reported a non-significant reduction of ICS dose, they observed that children aged between 6 and 14 years experienced by average a 17% decrease in their ICS dose. In the current study the potential ICS-sparing effect of montelukast in children with uncontrolled asthma was also examined. In order to better reflect the everyday clinical practice, ICS tapering guidelines were distributed to treating physicians and the decision of tapering the ICS dosage was left to the discretion of the physician and made on an individual basis. After 12 weeks of treatment with montelukast in combination with ICS, 71 (21.6%) children reduced their ICS daily dosage. These results further reinforce the potential ICS-sparing benefit of montelukast in asthma childhood.

Overall, once-daily administration of montelukast for 12 weeks was well tolerated in the context of this study. The observed safety and tolerability results are consistent with the safety profile of montelukast previously reported in asthma childhood [2,13,14,22,24-26,37-39].

Potential limitations of the current study are related to the open-label and single cohort design without a parallel control group. However, since this study emulated the real-world clinical setting, blinding to the treatment used and comparison to a control group were not appropriate. Furthermore, the primary objective of the study was to assess the real-life effectiveness of treatment with montelukast in achieving asthma control and not the comparison of montelukast treatment with alternate treatment strategies. By conducting within- instead of between-group comparison, possible confounding bias related to disease and lifestyle factors that could affect the effectiveness of montelukast were minimized since each patient provided both control (pre-treatment) and on-treatment data. In light of the heterogeneous response documented for both ICS [39,40] and leukotriene receptor antagonist [39] treatments, and the real-life practice in which physicians often switch treatment in patients who are not responding or adhering to their current therapy, there may be concerns that the selected patients may have been more likely to respond to montelukast treatment. However, treatment response could not have been foreseen as no patient characteristics are currently known to predict response to montelukast [41]. The follow-up schedule recommended in the current study may not be representative of Canadian routine clinical practice which may have resulted in increased adherence with treatment and, thus, treatment effectiveness compared to that observed in real-life. Observational studies are required in order to substantiate this hypothesis. However, frequent assessment of uncontrolled asthma should be encouraged given that uncontrolled asthma has been shown to predict future risk of instability and exacerbations [42]. Finally, in the current analysis 92 (21.9%) patients who had an ACQ score of ≤ 0.75 at baseline were excluded. This was due to the fact that, although the primary outcome measure was the proportion of patients achieving asthma control based on the ACQ criteria, in order to be eligible for the study patients had to have uncontrolled asthma as per the Canadian Asthma Consensus Guidelines. However, it should be noted that both analyses gave comparable results.

An important strength of this study is the generalizability of its results to the Canadian target population. Since this study was conducted in a real-life clinical setting, inclusion and exclusion criteria were less selective and therefore more representative of the general population compared to the highly controlled environment of clinical trials. In addition, as recommended by the Global Initiative for Asthma (GINA), the current study focused on asthma control achievement rather than on asthma severity [2,5,8]. The effectiveness of montelukast in controlling asthma symptoms was assessed with the asthma control questionnaire (ACQ), a cost-effective [43] and validated questionnaire [15,16,43]. Since there are no reliable or validated measures of pulmonary airways function in preschool children younger than 6 years old [44] and given that the omission of the question on the forced expiratory volume from the seven-item ACQ does not alter the validity and the measurement properties of the instrument [45], the use of ACQ for assessing asthma effectiveness outcomes is considered suitable for the real-life clinical management of childhood asthma. Finally, the use of standardized and validated questionnaires to assess asthma control (ACQ) [15,16,43] and caregiver's quality of life (PACQLQ) [17], also enhances the internal validity of the study.

Conclusions
In conclusion, the results of this study indicate that montelukast, administered either as monotherapy or in combination with ICS treatment, is an effective, convenient and well tolerated therapeutic option for the management of asthma in preschool and school aged paediatric patients with uncontrolled asthma symptoms.

Abbreviations
ICS: Inhaled corticosteroids; LTRAs: Leukotriene receptor antagonists; PEF: Peak expiratory force; SABA: Short-acting β2-agonist; LABA: Long-acting β2-agonist; ACQ: Asthma Control Questionnaire; PACQLQ: Pediatric asthma caregivers quality of life questionnaire; GINA: Global initiative for asthma; SD: Standard deviation; NSAEs: Non-serious adverse events; SAEs: Serious adverse events.

Competing interests
DB has received honorariums for consulting (Ad Board) and lecturing (CME) from Abbott, Altana, AstraZenaca, Graceway, GlaxoSmithKline, Merck, Novartis, Nycomed and Pfizer. MD is an employee of Merck Canada Inc. JSS is an employee of JSS Medical Research, the CRO contracted by Merck Canada Inc. to conduct the data management and analysis. AB has received research funding from CIHR, NSERC, AllerGen NCE and unrestricted educational grants from AZ, Graceway, GSK, Merck, Novartis and Nycomed.

Authors' contributions
DB contributed to, interpretation, and the critical revision of the article. MD contributed to study design, interpretation, and the critical revision of the article. JSS contributed to study design, data analysis, interpretation, drafting the manuscript, and the critical revision of the article. AB contributed to data collection, interpretation, and the critical revision of the article. All authors have approved the current version of the manuscript.

Acknowledgement
This study was supported by Merck Canada Inc. The authors would like to acknowledge the study investigators: Howard Langer, Hirotaka Yamashiro, Joel Liem, Jasmin Belle-Isle, Frederick Kruger, Gary Rideout, Ted Jablonski, Michelle Young, Richard Hamat, Mohunlall Soowamber, Jay Patidar, Pierre-Alain Houle, Georges Haddad, Darryl J. Ableman, Ronald Collette, Carla Krochak, Herman Lee, Rebecca Bodok-Nutzati, Julie Fabbro, Lee Ann Gallant, Marvin Gans, Hartley Garfield, Saul Greenberg, Stephen Grodinsky, Mabel Hsin, Pauline Kerr, Sohail Khattak, Vijay Kumar, Kevin Luces, Janette Milne, Susan Morgan, Rasik Morzaria, Santosh Paikatt, George Rogan, Kunwar Singh, Pal Sunerh, Andy Tsang, Richard Wong, Shawn Kao, Elliott Grad, Brian Lyttle, Alan F. Cook, Grouhi Masoud,

Roderick Rabb, Selwyn DeSouza, Nigel Jagan, Douglas Mah, Shawn Kao, Maurice Levy, Cyril Riche, David Hummel, Deepinderjit Dhatt, Kwame Donkor, J. Michael Look, Robert Ames, Danielle Houde, Yolanda Gonzalez, Julius Erdstein.

Research support funding
The study was funded by Merck Frosst Canada Ltd.

Author details
[1]CHU Ste-Justine, Université de Montréal, Montréal, Québec, Canada. [2]Merck Canada Inc., Kirkland, Québec, Canada. [3]Current address: Novartis Canada, Dorval, Québec, Canada. [4]McGill University, Montréal, Québec, Canada. [5]JSS Medical Research, Montréal, Québec, Canada. [6]Section of Allergy and Clinical Immunology, Department of Pediatrics and Child Health, University of Manitoba, Manitoba, Canada.

References

1. Akinbami LJ, Schoendorf KC: Trends in childhood asthma: prevalence, health care utilization, and mortality. *Pediatrics* 2002, **110**(2 Pt 1):315–322.
2. Bateman ED, Hurd SS, Barnes PJ, Bousquest J, Drazen JM, Fitzgerald M, Gibson P, Ohta K, Byrne P, Pedersen SE, Pizzichini E, Sullivan SD, Wenzel SE, Zar J: Global strategy for asthma management and prevention: GINA executive summary. *Eur Respir J* 2008, **31**(1):143–178.
3. Garner R, Kohen D: Changes in the prevalence of asthma among Canadian children. *Health Rep Stat Can Catalogue 82–003* 2008, **19**:1–7.
4. Millar WJ, Gerry BH: Childhood asthma. *Health Rep Stat Can Catalogue 82–003* 1998, **10**:9–21.
5. Global strategy for asthma management and prevention. Global Initiative for Asthma (GINA), 2009. http://www.ginasthma.org (Version current at May 05, 2010).
6. Becker A, Lemière C, Bérubé D, Boulet LP, Ducharme FM, Fitzgerald M, Kovesi T: Summary of recommendations from the Canadian asthma consensus guidelines, 2003. *CMAJ* 2005, **173**(Suppl 6):S3–S11.
7. Becker A, Bérubé D, Chad Z, Dolovich M, Ducharme F, D'Urzo T, Ernst P, Ferguson A, Gillespie C, Kapur S, Kovesi T, Lyttle B, Mazer B, Montgomery M, Pedersen S, Pianosi P, Reisman JJ, Sears M, Simons E, Spier S, Thivierge R, Watson W, Zimmerman B: Canadian pediatric asthma consensus guidelines, 2003 (updated to December 2004): introduction. *CMAJ* 2005, **173**(Suppl 6):S12–S14.
8. Global strategy for the diagnosis and management of asthma in children 5 years and younger. Global Initiative for Asthma (GINA), 2009. http://www.ginasthma.org (Version current at May 05, 2010).
9. Zeiger RS, Szefler SJ, Phillips BR, Schatz M, Martinez FD, Chinchilli VM, Lemanske RF, Strunk RC, Larsen G, Spahn JD, Bacharier LB, Bloomberg GR, Guilbert TW, Heldt G, Morgan WJ, Moss MH, Sorkness CA, Taussig LM: Response profiles to fluticasone and montelukast in mild-to-moderate persistent childhood asthma. *J Allergy Clin Immunol* 2006, **117**(1):45–52.
10. Szefler SJ, Phillips BR, Martinez FD, Chinchilli VM, Lemanske RF, Strunk RC, Zeiger RS, Larsen G, Spahn JD, Bacharier LB, Bloomberg GR, Guilbert TW, Heldt G, Morgan WJ, Moss MH, Sorkness CA, Taussig LM: Characterization of within-subject responses to fluticasone and montelukast in childhood asthma. *J Allergy Clin Immunol* 2005, **115**(2):233–242.
11. Wahn U, Dass SB: Review of recent results of montelukast use as a monotherapy in children with mild asthma. *Clin Ther* 2008, **30**:1026–1035.
12. National Asthma Education and Prevention Program: National Asthma Education and Prevention Program. Expert panel report: guidelines for the diagnosis and management of asthma update on selected topics–2002. *J Allergy Clin Immunol* 2002, **110**(5):S141–S219.
13. Knorr B, Franchi LM, Bisgaard H, Vermeulen JH, LeSouef P, Santanello N, Michele TM, Reiss TF, Ngyen HH, Bratton DL: Montelukast, a leukotriene receptor antagonist, for the treatment of persistent asthma in children aged 2 to 5 years. *Pediatrics* 2001, **108**(3):E48–E58.
14. Knorr B, Matz J, Bernstein JA, Nguyen H, Seidenberg BC, Reiss TF, Becker A: Montelukast for chronic asthma in 6- to 14-year-old children: a randomized, double-blind trial. Pediatric Montelukast Study Group. *JAMA* 1998, **279**(15):1181–1186.
15. Juniper EF, Bousquet J, Abetz L, Bateman ED, GOAL Committee: Identifying 'well-controlled' and 'not well-controlled' asthma using the asthma control questionnaire. *Respir Med* 2006, **100**(4):616–621.
16. Juniper EF, O'Byrne PM, Guyatt GH, Ferrie PJ, King DR: Development and validation of a questionnaire to measure asthma control. *Eur Respir J* 1999, **14**(4):902–907.
17. Juniper EF, Guyatt GH, Feeny DH, Ferrie PJ, Griffith LE, Townsend M: Measuring quality of life in the parents of children with asthma. *Qual Life Res* 1996, **5**(1):27–34.
18. Global strategy for asthma management and prevention. Global Initiative for Asthma (GINA), 2006. http://www.ginasthma.com/Guidelineitem.asp?l1=2&l2=1&intId=1388. 2010.
19. International Conference on Harmonization of Technical Requirements for Registration of Pharmaceuticals for Human Use (ICH): Medical dictionary for regulatory activities terminology. *MedDRA Version 90* 2006.
20. Phillips C, McDonald T: Trends in medication use for asthma among children. *Curr Opin Allergy Clin Immunol* 2008, **8**(3):232–237.
21. Bisgaard H, Zielen S, Garcia-Garcia ML, Johnston SL, Gilles L, Menten J, Tozzi CA, Polos P: Montelukast reduces asthma exacerbations in 2- to 5-year-old children with intermittent asthma. *Am J Respir Crit Care Med* 2005, **171**(4):315–322.
22. Muijsers RB, Noble S: Montelukast: a review of its therapeutic potential in asthma in children 2 to 14 years of age. *Paediatr Drugs* 2002, **4**(2):123–139.
23. Bukstein DA, Luskin AT, Bernstein A: "Real-world" effectiveness of daily controller medicine in children with mild persistent asthma. *Ann Allergy Asthma Immunol* 2003, **90**(5):543–549.
24. Garcia Garcia ML, Wahn U, Gilles L, Swern A, Tozzi CA, Polos P: Montelukast, compared with fluticasone, for control of asthma among 6- to 14-year-old patients with mild asthma: the MOSAIC study. *Pediatrics* 2005, **116**(2):360–369.
25. Joos S, Miksch A, Szecsenyi J, Wieseler B, Grouven U, Kaiser T, Schneider A: Montelukast as add-on therapy to inhaled corticosteroids in the treatment of mild to moderate asthma: a systematic review. *Thorax* 2008, **63**(5):453–462.
26. Kondo N, Katsunuma T, Odajima Y, Morikawa A: A randomized open-label comparative study of montelukast versus theophylline added to inhaled corticosteroid in asthmatic children. *Allergol Int* 2006, **55**(3):287–293.
27. Phipatanakul W, Greene C, Downes SJ, Cronin B, Eller TJ, Schneider LC, Irani AM: Montelukast improves asthma control in asthmatic children maintained on inhaled corticosteroids. *Ann Allergy Asthma Immunol* 2003, **91**(1):49–54.
28. Williams B, Noonan G, Reiss TF, Knorr B, Guerra J, White R, Matz J: Long-term asthma control with oral montelukast and inhaled beclomethasone for adults and children 6 years and older. *Clin Exp Allergy* 2001, **31**(6):845–854.
29. Holbrook JT, Wise RA, Gold BD, Blake K, Brown ED, Castro M, Dozor AJ, Lima JJ, Mastronarde JG, Sockrider MM, Teague WG: Lansoprazole for children with poorly controlled asthma: a randomized controlled trial9. *JAMA* 2012, **307**(4):373–381.
30. Kersten ET, van Leeuwen JC, Brand PL, Duiverman EJ, de Jongh FH, Thio BJ, Driessen JMM: Effect of an intranasal corticosteroid on exercise induced bronchoconstriction in asthmatic children2. *Pediatr Pulmonol* 2012, **47**(1):27–35.
31. Dean BB, Calimlim BM, Kindermann SL, Khandker RK, Tinkelman D: The impact of uncontrolled asthma on absenteeism and health-related quality of life. *J Asthma* 2009, **46**(9):861–866.
32. Halterman JS, Yoos HL, Conn KM, Callahan PM, Montes G, Neely TL, Szilagyi PG: The impact of childhood asthma on parental quality of life. *J Asthma* 2004, **41**(6):645–653.
33. Löfdahl CG, Reiss TF, Leff JA, Israel E, Noonan MJ, Finn AF, Seidenberg BC, Capizzi T, Kundu S, Godard P: Randomised, placebo controlled trial of effect of a leukotriene receptor antagonist, montelukast, on tapering inhaled corticosteroids in asthmatic patients. *BMJ* 1999, **319**(7202):87–90.
34. Riccioni G, Vecchia RD, Castronuovo M, Ilio CD, D'Orazio N: Tapering dose of inhaled budesonide in subjects with mild-to-moderate persistent asthma treated with montelukast: a 16-week single-blind randomized study. *Ann Clin Lab Sci* 2005, **35**(3):285–289.
35. Strunk RC, Bacharier LB, Phillips BR, Szefler SJ, Zeiger RS, Chinchilli VM, Martinez FD, Lemanske RF, Taussig LM, Mauger DT, Morgan WJ, Sorkness CA, Paul IM, Guilbert T, Krawiec M, Covar R, Larsen G: Azithromycin or montelukast as inhaled corticosteroid-sparing agents in moderate-to-severe childhood asthma study. *J Allergy Clin Immunol* 2008, **122**(6):1138–1144.
36. Tamesis GP, Covar RA: Long-term effects of asthma medications in children. *Curr Opin Allergy Clin Immunol* 2008, **8**(2):163–167.

37. Jartti T: Inhaled corticosteroids or montelukast as the preferred primary long-term treatment for pediatric asthma? *Eur J Pediatr* 2008, **167**(7):731–736.

38. Bisgaard H: Leukotriene modifiers in pediatric asthma management. *Pediatrics* 2001, **107**(2):381–390.

39. Malmstorm K, Rodriguez-Gomez G, Guerra J, Villaran C, Pineiro A, Wei LX, Seidengerg BC, Reiss TF: Oral montelukast, inhaled beclomethasone, and placebo for chronic asthma. A randomized, controlled trial. Montelukast/Beclomethasone Study Group. *Ann Intern Med* 1999, **130**(6):487–495.

40. Szefler SJ, Martin RJ, King TS, Boushey HA, Cherniack RM, Chinchilli VM, Craig TJ, Dolovich M, Drazen JM, Fagan JK, Fahy JV, Fish JE, Ford JG, Israel E, Kiley J, Kraft M, Lazarus SC, Lemanske RF, Mauger E, Peters SP, Sorkness CA: Significant variability in response to inhaled corticosteroids for persistent asthma. *J Allergy Clin Immunol* 2002, **109**(3):410–418.

41. Meyer KA, Arduino JM, Santanello NC, Knorr BA, Bisgaard H: Response to montelukast among subgroups of children aged 2 to 14 years with asthma. *J Allergy Clin Immunol* 2003, **111**(4):757–762.

42. Bateman ED, Reddel HK, Eriksson G, Peterson S, Ostlund O, Sears MR, Jenkins C, Humbert M, Buhl R, Harrison TW, Quirce S, O'Byrne PO: Overall asthma control: the relationship between current control and future risk 14. *J Allergy Clin Immunol* 2010, **125**(3):600–608. 608.

43. van den Nieuwenhof L, Schermer T, Eysink P, Halet E, van Weel C, Bindels P, Bottema B: Can the asthma control questionnaire be used to differentiate between patients with controlled and uncontrolled asthma symptoms? A pilot study. *Fam Pract* 2006, **23**(6):674–681.

44. Stocks J, Sly PD, Tepper RS, Morgan WJ: *Infant Respiratory Function Testing.* New York, NY: Wiley-Liss, Inc.; 1996.

45. Juniper EF, O'Byrne PM, Roberts JN: Measuring asthma control in group studies: do we need airway calibre and rescue beta2-agonist use? *Respir Med* 2001, **95**(5):319–323.

13

Encasing bedding in covers made of microfine fibers reduces exposure to house mite allergens and improves disease management in adult atopic asthmatics

Naomi Tsurikisawa[1*], Akemi Saito[2], Chiyako Oshikata[1], Takuya Nakazawa[2], Hiroshi Yasueda[2] and Kazuo Akiyama[1,2]

Abstract

Background: Studies of avoidance of exposure to group 1 allergens of the *Dermatophagoides* group (Der p 1) have not yielded consistent improvements in adult asthma through avoidance. We explored whether the use of pillow and bed covers and allergen-avoidance counseling resulted in Der 1-level reduction, as measured by enzyme-linked immunosorbent assay, and thus improved asthma symptoms in adult patients.

Methods: Twenty-five adult patients with moderate or severe atopic asthma were randomized into intervention and control groups. Intervention patients slept on pillows and mattresses or futons encased in microfine-fiber covers and were counseled in allergen avoidance through bedroom cleaning. Control patients received neither special covers nor counseling. In the period August to October in 2009 (pre-intervention) and 2010 (post-intervention), dust samples were collected in open Petri dishes placed in bedrooms for 2 weeks and by rapid lifting of dust from bedding and skin using adhesive tape on the morning of 1 day of Petri dish placement. We examined the associations between changes in Der 1 level (as measured by enzyme-linked immunosorbent assay) and clinical symptom score, minimum % peak expiratory flow, and fraction of exhaled nitric oxide.

Results: Der 1 allergen levels on the mattress/futon covers and near the floor of the bedrooms of intervention patients, but not controls, were lower in 2010 than in 2009. From 2009 to 2010, asthma symptom scores decreased significantly, and minimum % peak expiratory flow increased significantly, in intervention patients. The fall in Der p 1 concentration was correlated with a reduction in the fraction of exhaled nitric oxide.

Conclusions: Minimization of Der 1 allergen exposure by encasing pillows and mattresses or futons and receiving counseling on avoiding exposure to indoor allergens improved asthma control in adult patients.

Keywords: Adult intervention, Allergen, Atopic asthma, Bed cover, *Dermatophagoides*, Group 1 mite antigen

Background

Exposure of sensitized individuals to allergens, including those associated with house dust mites (HDMs), cats, and fungi, is a risk factor for asthma exacerbation or persistence of asthma symptoms [1-3]. HDMs (i.e., *Dermatophagoides pteronyssinus* and *Dermatophagoides farinae*), are major indoor allergens that can trigger or exacerbate atopic asthma [1-3]. Asthmatic symptoms [4] and bronchial hyper-responsiveness [5] are reduced in children with asthma when exposure to HDMs is minimized by encasing mattresses and using special pillow covers. Individualized, home-based comprehensive environmental intervention can decrease levels of exposure to indoor allergens and reduce asthma-associated morbidity in children [6]. A 90% reduction in allergen levels is feasible and is considered appropriate [1]. However, most studies, including a meta-analysis [7,8], have concluded that reducing levels of exposure to HDMs by using chemical and physical methods does not improve asthma symptoms,

---

* Correspondence: n-tsurikisawa@sagamihara-hosp.gr.jp
[1]Department of Allergy and Respirology, National Hospital Organization Sagamihara National Hospital, 18-1 Sakuradai, Minami-ku, Sagamihara, Kanagawa 252-0392, Japan
Full list of author information is available at the end of the article

levels of medication use, lung function, or the extent of bronchial hyper-responsiveness [7-10]. Particularly in adults, lowering HDM levels does not effectively reduce asthma symptoms [5,11-14]. One report found no clear dose–response relationship between indoor allergen levels and symptom severity [15].

Many factors influence the relationship between exposure to HDM allergens and symptom development or exacerbation. These include the presence of several different allergens on HDMs, the interaction of many factors to enhance the airway inflammatory response, and the existence of several triggers or enhancers of airway narrowing or the perceived severity of symptoms [2]. Such factors include cold air, exercise, passive or active exposure to cigarette smoke and bronchial infection [2]. Unsurprisingly, therefore, several reviews have concluded that avoidance of exposure to HDM allergens is not clinically beneficial for asthma patients and that efforts to avoid these allergens cannot be recommended as part of asthma management [7,8,10]. These results showed that the concentration of D. pteronyssinus allergen 1 (Der p 1) in mattresses did not decrease after an intervention treatment by using bed covers, or that lung function in terms of peak expiratory flow (PEF), bronchial hyperresponsiveness, asthma symptom score, and asthma medication use did not change after the concentration of Der p 1 in mattresses was decreased by intervention treatments. In most studies, the level of Dermatophagoides mite group 1 (Der 1) allergens in reservoir dust is measured by collecting mites from bedding with a vacuum cleaner and is used as an index of allergen exposure [1,2]. Allergen levels in dust samples are typically presented as micrograms of allergen per gram of dust protein. However, allergen levels in reservoir dust are not necessarily good indicators of the amounts of allergens inhaled [16,17]. Yasueda et al. [18] developed a sensitive fluorometric enzyme-linked immunosorbent assay (ELISA) for detecting Der p 1 and D. farinae group 1 (Der f 1) allergens and used it to measure the levels of these components on bedding and human skin. These values were used as indices of exposure and reduced the sensitivity of detection of Der 1 to 1 pg/mL. Earlier, we showed that the levels of Der 1 allergens collected from bedding and skin by using adhesive tape were correlated with those collected from airborne dust through simple dust deposition on plastic Petri dishes [19].

Inhaled corticosteroids (ICS) are the recommended first-line therapy for persistent adult asthma of all grades of severity [20]. In studies of avoidance of mite allergen by intervention using bed covers, almost all adult patients with asthma have been receiving ICS treatment [7].

The above-mentioned earlier measures of allergen levels may not have truly reflected the extent of HDM allergen exposure, and it remains unknown whether measuring Der 1 levels by using the newer, more sensitive, fluorometric ELISA will reveal that exposure avoidance improves clinical symptoms or lung function in adult asthmatics. We explored whether reductions in HDM levels on bedding and in the bedroom, as measured by fluorometric ELISA, affected asthma control in adult patients who were being treated with ICS and other asthma medications.

Methods

Patients

Between August and October 2009, we recruited 25 adult asthma patients at the National Hospital Organization, Sagamihara, National Hospital, Kanagawa, Japan. All patients suffered from moderate or severe atopic asthma, as diagnosed by using the criteria of the American Thoracic Society [21]. Asthma severity was assessed by following the current Global Initiative for Asthma (GINA) guidelines [20] and graded accordingly as follows: Step 1, intermittent asthma; Step 2, mildly persistent asthma; Step 3, moderately persistent asthma; and Step 4, severely persistent asthma. All patients had atopic asthma and were sensitized to dust mites, as revealed by measurement of mite-specific IgE. Other allergic conditions exhibited by the patients included allergic rhinitis (which can worsen asthma [22]), allergic dermatitis (diagnosed as described in [23],) and allergic conjunctivitis (diagnosed by using the 2009 criteria of the Japanese Dermatological Association [24]). Exclusion criteria included the presence of pulmonary diseases other than asthma (chronic obstructive pulmonary disease presenting as pulmonary emphysema, interstitial pulmonary fibrosis, or bronchiectasis).

Study design

Between 1 August and 31 October 2009, each patient collected ambient dust samples in open Petri dishes (plastic, not pre-coated with any protein) (90 × 15 mm; SH90-15; Asahi Glass Co. Ltd., Tokyo, Japan) [19,25,26] that had been left in the bedroom for 2 weeks. Patients also collected bedding and skin dust samples with adhesive tape (Tegaderm Transparent Dressing 1625WJ; 6 × 7 cm; 3 M Health Care, St Paul, MN) [20] on the morning of one day in this period before cleaning the bed room. The patients were randomized into intervention and control groups. Intervention and control patients were classified in two groups composed of odd number and even number in accordance with the highest amount of Der 1 in the bedroom. During February or March 2010, patients in the intervention group were counseled one-on-one once for 30 min in regard to methods of allergen avoidance; the protocol was modified from that of Nishioka et al. [4,27]. In February or March 2010, intervention patients placed covers made of microfine fibers (Microgard; Yasaka Co., Chiba, Japan) over their pillows and futons or mattresses to minimize contact with HDMs. The following recommendations were made. First, all family members' bedding and futon/mattress covers were to be washed at least monthly at room temperature. Second, the surfaces of mattresses or futons of all family members were to be vacuumed at least weekly with a powerful (>900 W) appliance. Third, wooden floors or tatami matting were to be wiped with a wet cloth before being vacuumed. Fourth, all rooms, including bedrooms, were to be vacuumed at least weekly. Fifth, all carpets were to be removed or (if this was not possible) vacuumed with a powerful appliance at least weekly. Sixth, no stuffed dolls or soft toys were to be kept in the house. Finally, no furred pets were kept in the house. Patients in the control group received neither the special covers nor any hygiene guidelines. In the 2010 sampling period from August to October, a researcher confirmed by interview that all patients in the intervention group were in fact following most of the seven recommended practices described above. All patients collected house dust samples in the period 1 August to 31 October 2010 for follow-up clinical measurement. The start time of the 2-week interval in which each patient collected the 2010 samples differed by less than 1 month from the start time of the sampling interval used by the patient in 2009. Airborne dust was collected in four plastic Petri dishes. Two were placed side by side on the bedroom floor and two were placed side by side at a height of 100 cm above floor level. Both sets of dishes were placed within 2 m of the bed or futon and left undisturbed for 2 weeks before collection. Two adhesive tapes were used to obtain dust samples from the surface of the center of the futon or mattress microfiber cover, where the patient's back would have been positioned in bed. Similarly, subjects sampled dust on the skin once, on a morning within the sampling period when the bedroom was due to be cleaned, by applying tape to the skin of the right and left neck for a few seconds. All patients continued taking daily ICS; doses, particle sizes, and delivery devices were not changed from 1 August 2009 to 31 October 2010. Other medications taken during the study included long-acting β2 agonists (LABAs), leukotriene receptor antagonists (LTRAs), and long-acting muscarinic antagonists (LAMAs). Clinical symptoms were assessed and used to derive total clinical scores. We documented the presence of cough, sputum production, wheezing, dyspnea caused by an asthma attack, sneezing or nasal discharge attributable to exposure to mites, use of short-acting β stimulants, and emergency hospital visits for asthma treatment for whole period from August 1 to October 31 each year. Symptoms were scored as follows: 0, no occurrence within a month; 1, some occurrences (more than one a month but fewer than two a week); and 2, frequent occurrences (more than once a week).

Our hospital ethics committee approved the study. All relevant tenets of the Helsinki Declaration were followed. Written informed consent was obtained from each patient. The study was supported by Health and Labor Science Research Grants for Research on Allergic Disease and Immunology, awarded by the Ministry of Health, Labor, and Welfare of Japan.

Measurement of peak expiratory flow
Patients measured PEF three times every morning and evening before bronchodilator use during the 2-week dust collection period each year with an ASSESS PEF meter (CHEST, Tokyo, Japan) [20]; measurements with an error of less than 10% variance among PEF measured three times were recorded by the patient in a diary. After collecting the patients' diaries we noted the minimum pre-bronchodilator PEF level (as a percentage of the predicted value) obtained within each 2-week test period.

Measurement of exhaled nitric oxide
NO was measured only once in each test period, on the day on which the Petri dishes were placed in the bedroom. Exhaled air was collected in a Sievers bag that formed part of an NO collection kit (Tsuburai et al. [28]). Each subject took a deep breath of room air through the NO-scavenging filter and exhaled through a mouthpiece with a flow rate of 70 mL/s against an expiratory resistance of 10 cm H_2O. Five seconds later, the exhaled air was collected into the 1.5-L Mylar bag from the kit. This air was stored at room temperature and the NO concentration measured within 12 h. Air was drawn out of each bag at 200 mL/min into an NO chemiluminescence analyzer (NOA model 280A; Sievers Instruments, Boulder CO) that had a response time of 200 ms. The fraction of expired NO (FeNO) measured by this method was within 80% of that measured by using direct methods [28].

Eosinophil levels in peripheral blood
We quantified eosinophils and white blood cells (WBCs) in the peripheral blood of all patients by hemocytometry at first hospital visit and at study entry before the intervention.

Measurement of total IgE, DER F-specific IgE, and DER P 1–specific IgE
Several enzymatic assays employing anti-immunoglobulin E (IgE) antibodies have supplanted the radioallergosorbent test (RAST) [29]. Total IgE levels in serum (IU/mL) were measured by using a radioimmunosorbent test (RIST). Der f–specific IgE (IU/mL) was measured by using crude mite allergen and a RAST that featured the use of ELISA; a nephelometric method was employed (BN II; Dade Behring Inc., Deerfield, IL) [30]. Der p 1–specific IgE levels (UA/mL) were measured with component allergen made

by using recombinant antigen and the CAP system (Pharmacia, Uppsala, Sweden).

Measurement of DER 1 levels

Airborne dust that had settled in the Petri dishes was suspended in 1 mL of phosphate-buffered saline (PBS) with 0.05% (v/v) Tween 20, 0.2% (w/v) bovine serum albumin (BSA), and 0.1% (w/v) sodium azide and then stored at 4°C until analysis of Der p 1 or Der f 1 levels [25]. Samples on adhesive tapes were placed on paper tissue (one sample per tissue) (Kimwipe S-200; Crecia, Tokyo, Japan), placed into polystyrene tubes (10 × 70 mm), and extracted with 2 mL of PBS containing 0.2% (v/v) Tween 20, 0.2% (w/v) BSA, and 0.05% (w/v) sodium azide (PBS-T-BSA) by orbital rotation overnight at room temperature. Dust samples on adhesive tapes at 1:100 w/v (20 mg in 2 mL of PBS-T-BSA) were extracted for 4 h at room temperature. Der p 1 or Der f 1 was quantified by using the fluorometric ELISA developed by Yasueda et al. [18]. Polystyrene microplates were coated for 30 min at 37°C with 200 ng of anti-Der p 1 or anti-Der f 1 monoclonal antibody (P1A03), prepared as described by Yasueda et al. [31]. The plates were incubated overnight at 25°C with 5 ng of biotinylated rabbit anti-Der p 1 or anti-Der f 1 in 100 μL of PBS-T-BSA containing 1 mg/mL normal rabbit γ-globulin. After termination of the reaction with glycin–NaOH, the fluorescence intensity was read with a microplate fluorescence reader (Spectra Fluor; TECAN GmbH, Salzburg, Austria). The excitation wavelength was 360 nm and the emission wavelength 465 nm [18]. Results were expressed as nanograms of allergen per square meter. The Der p 1 or Der f 1 detection limit was 1 pg/mL [18]. Der 1 level was calculated as the total amount Der p 1 and Der f 1.

Statistical analysis

All values are expressed as means ± 1 SD (with ranges), unless otherwise specified. Statistical comparisons among groups were achieved by using two-way analysis of variance (ANOVA) with a repeated-measures algorithm, followed by post-hoc comparisons using the Newman-Keuls test. The mean values obtained by this process were compared by using the Wilcoxon matched-pairs T-test. Correlation coefficients were obtained by using Spearman's rank correlation test. P values of <0.05 were considered statistically significant. Statistical analysis was performed with SPSS for Windows, version 20 (SPSS Inc., Chicago, IL).

Results

The two groups did not differ significantly in terms of age at entry into the study, sex ratio, age of onset of asthma, duration of asthma, severity of asthma, atopy status, or presence of other atopic disease. All patients were treated with ICS. The groups did not differ significantly in use of the medications LABA, LTRA, LAMA, or theophylline (Table 1). Patients in the intervention group washed their bedding or futon covers, cleaned their mattresses or futons, and wiped surfaces with wet towels before vacuuming more significantly frequently than did controls (data not shown). In the intervention group, one patient kept a cat and three kept dogs; in the control group two kept cats and one kept a dog. No significant between-group differences were evident in terms of serum IgE level (measured by using RIST), IgE RAST for Der f 1, or eosinophil count, either at the time of the first hospital visit or at the time of study entry (Table 2). The eosinophil count in both groups was not higher than the normal range (less than 6% of WBCs). The levels of Der 1 allergen collected from the futon/mattress covers by using tape (Figure 1(a); $P < 0.01$) and from Petri dishes placed on the floor in the bedrooms (Figure 1(b); $P < 0.01$) were significantly lower after intervention; the levels did not differ significantly between pre- and postintervention in the control group. The levels of Der 1 allergen on the skin tape (data not shown) and in Petri dishes placed 100 cm above the bedroom floor (Figure 1(c)) did not change in either group. The levels of Der 1 on the futon/mattress covers or on skin samples taken with adhesive tape were each significantly correlated with those in the Petri dishes on the floor or 100 cm high ($P < 0.01$; data not shown). The clinical symptom score at the time of assay of Der 1 allergen levels in patients in the intervention group fell after the 2010 intervention (Figure 2(a); $P < 0.01$). The minimum % PEF value in patients in the intervention group increased in 2010 after intervention (Figure 2(b); $P < 0.05$). Neither the clinical symptom score nor the % PEF value differed between 2009 and 2010 in the control patients (Figure 2). FeNO levels did not change between 2009 and 2010 in either group (data not shown). In all patients, the change in Der 1 level in the bedroom in the Petri dishes on the floor between the time of study entry (2009) and the same time in 2010 was inversely correlated with the change in minimum % PEF ($P < 0.01$) (Figure 3(a)) and positively correlated with the change in FeNO level ($P < 0.05$) (Figure 3(b)). However, the change between 2009 and 2010 in Der 1 levels on adhesive tape samples from the skin or bedding was not correlated with the change in minimum % PEF or FeNO level (data not shown). In the intervention group in 2010, Der 1 levels on tape samples from the futon/mattress covers of 10 of 16 patients (Figure 4(a)) ($P = 0.16$) and in the bedroom air of 10 of 14 patients (Figure 4(b)) ($P < 0.05$) fell to lower than the levels before intervention. The levels of Der p 1–specific IgE decreased in patients in both the intervention (Figure 5(a)) ($P < 0.05$) and control (Figure 5(b)) ($P < 0.01$) groups between 2009 and 2010.

Discussion

Levels of Der 1 allergen exposure were decreased in adult patients by encasing pillows and mattresses or futons and

Table 1 Baseline data on the intervention and control groups

	Intervention group N = 13	Control group N = 12	P-value
Age (years) at time of study entry; mean ± SD	47.8 ± 11.0	46.5 ± 16.1	NS[1]
Sex (M/F)	5/8	4/8	NS[2]
Atopic rhinitis (yes/no)	9/4	9/3	NS[2]
Atopic conjunctivitis (yes/no)	7/6	10/2	NS[2]
Atopic dermatitis (yes/no)	4/9	5/7	NS[2]
Age at onset of asthma (years); mean ± SD	23.4 ± 19.7	35.5 ± 17.0	NS[1]
Duration of asthma (from time of onset to time of study entry) (years)	25.2 ± 19.9	12.3 ± 13.7	NS[1]
Step 1/2/3/4 asthma severity*	0/2/4/7	0/3/5/4	NS[2]
Daily dose of ICS (µg; converted to CFC-BDP equivalents)	753.8 ± 489.2	566.7 ± 302.5	NS[1]
Use of LABA; n (%)	8 (61.5)	7 (58.3)	NS[2]
Use of LTRA; n (%)	6 (46.2)	5 (41.7)	NS[2]
Use of LAMA; n (%)	2 (15.4)	2 (16.7)	NS[2]
Use of theophylline; n (%)	6 (46.2)	6 (50.0)	NS[2]

Data are presented as means ± SD or means (ranges).
NS, not significant.
[1] Two-way ANOVA with repeated measures among the two groups.
[2] Chi-squared testing revealed no significant differences between the values of the two groups.
Values of $P < 0.05$ were considered to be statistically significant.
* According to GINA guidelines.
CFC-BDP, chlorofluorocarbon-propelled beclomethasone dipropionate; LABA, long-acting β2 agonist; LAMA, long-acting muscarinic antagonist; LTRA.

giving counseling on avoiding exposure to indoor allergens; asthma control was also increased. Factors that exacerbate asthma in adult patients include not only exposure to indoor allergens derived from HDMs, cockroaches, cats, dog, and fungi, but also respiratory infections [32], development of allergic rhinitis [33], high levels of airborne pollutants [34,35], changes in the weather [36], and exercise [37]. No clear evidence of a dose–response relationship between HDM levels and asthma severity has yet been found [2].

Cockroach allergen (Bla g 1) levels greater than 8 U/g dust are associated with asthma exacerbation. Cockroach allergen avoidance by cleaning, vacuuming, dishes, and sealing food does not reduce asthma exacerbation related to the levels cockroach allergen. Similarly, there is no relationship between cat allergen (Fel d 1) sensitization or symptoms and the current level of cat allergen in the home. Moreover, cat allergen levels in the home for several years are maintained after the cat has been removed [2].

Table 2 Serum IgE and eosinophil levels in peripheral blood at the first hospital visit and at study entry

	Intervention group N = 13	Control group N = 12	P-value
At first hospital visit			
Serum IgE RIST (UA/mL)	1718.9 ± 4164.8	928.6 ± 1258.0	NS[1]
Log serum IgE RIST (UA/mL)	2.61 ± 0.69	2.57 ± 0.66	NS[1]
Serum IgE RAST for Der f (IU/mL)	25.3 ± 34.0	28.9 ± 41.4	NS[1]
Log serum IgE RAST for Der f (IU/mL)	1.00 ± 0.72	0.95 ± 0.75	NS[1]
No. of eosinophils (/µL)	430.7 ± 231.4	437.4 ± 315.5	NS[1]
At study entry			
Serum IgE RIST (UA/mL)	1169.6 ± 1559.9	589.3 ± 640.0	NS[1]
Log serum IgE RIST (UA/mL)	2.67 ± 0.65	2.57 ± 0.45	NS[1]
Serum IgE RAST for Der f (IU/mL)	24.7 ± 26.2	33.9 ± 48.1	NS[1]
Log serum IgE RAST for Der f (IU/mL)	0.95 ± 0.60	0.89 ± 1.00	NS[1]
No. of eosinophils (/µL)	215.6 ± 149.4	323.8 ± 221.5	NS[1]

Data are presented as means ± SD.
NS, not significant.
[1] Two-way ANOVA with repeated measures among two groups.
Values of $P < 0.05$ were considered statistically significant.

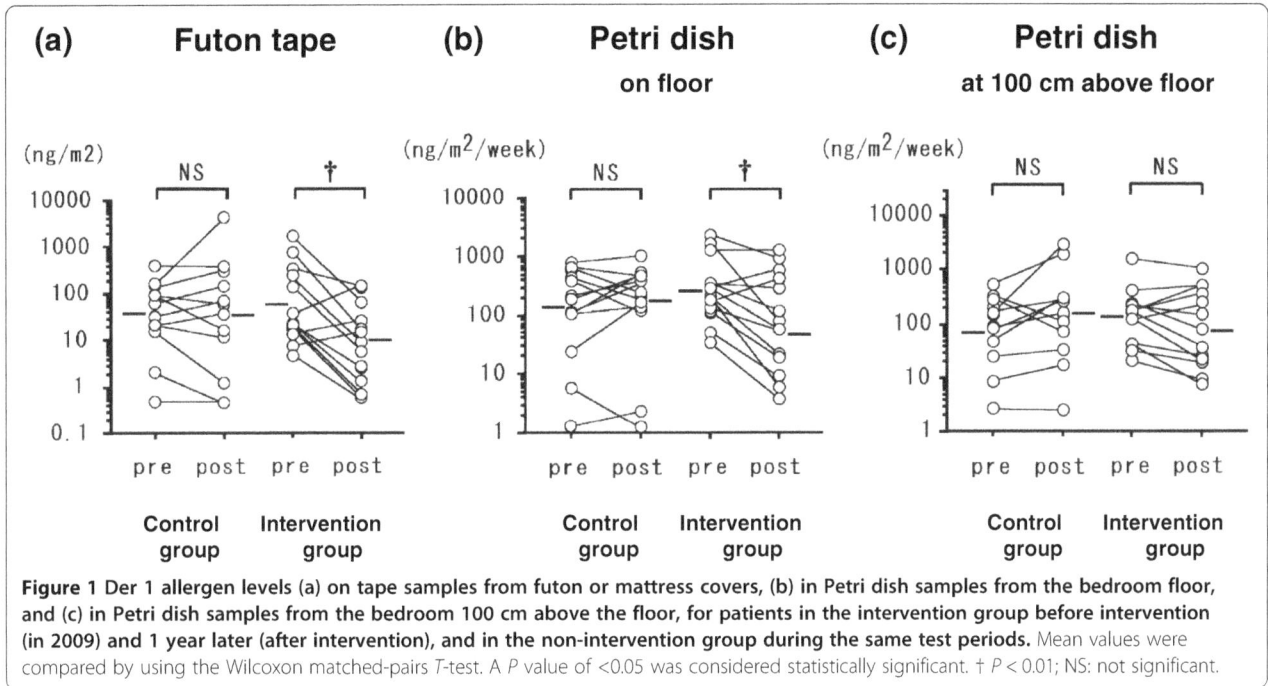

Figure 1 Der 1 allergen levels (a) on tape samples from futon or mattress covers, (b) in Petri dish samples from the bedroom floor, and (c) in Petri dish samples from the bedroom 100 cm above the floor, for patients in the intervention group before intervention (in 2009) and 1 year later (after intervention), and in the non-intervention group during the same test periods. Mean values were compared by using the Wilcoxon matched-pairs T-test. A P value of <0.05 was considered statistically significant. † P < 0.01; NS: not significant.

Despite these negative findings, it is possible that reducing Der 1 levels by covering mattresses or futons and cleaning thoroughly in the bedroom may improve the clinical symptoms of asthma [38,39]. In our study, we confirmed that there was no relationship between bedroom Petri dish Fel d 1 levels and asthma exacerbation in three patients with asthma and cat allergen sensitivity (data not shown).

Here, we showed that, by avoiding exposure to HDMs in bedding and the bedroom, adult patients with atopic asthma who were sensitive to HDMs achieved total asthma control (as defined by the GINA guidelines [20]), unlike the controls. The levels of Der 1 on the futon or mattress covers of intervention-group patients did not fall upon intervention in 2010 after covers made of microfine fibers were employed, unless these patients followed the directions for allergen avoidance (Figure 4(a)). Thus for a decrease in Der 1 allergen levels the patients needed to not only encase the pillows and futon or mattress cover but also to clean the bedroom as instructed.

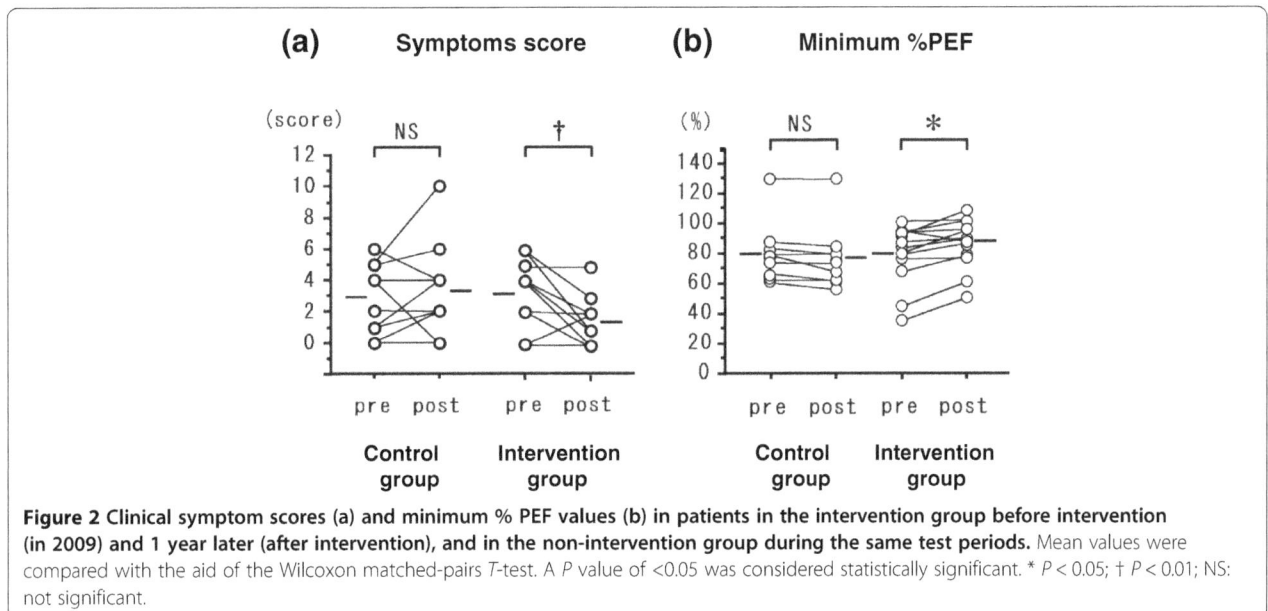

Figure 2 Clinical symptom scores (a) and minimum % PEF values (b) in patients in the intervention group before intervention (in 2009) and 1 year later (after intervention), and in the non-intervention group during the same test periods. Mean values were compared with the aid of the Wilcoxon matched-pairs T-test. A P value of <0.05 was considered statistically significant. * P < 0.05; † P < 0.01; NS: not significant.

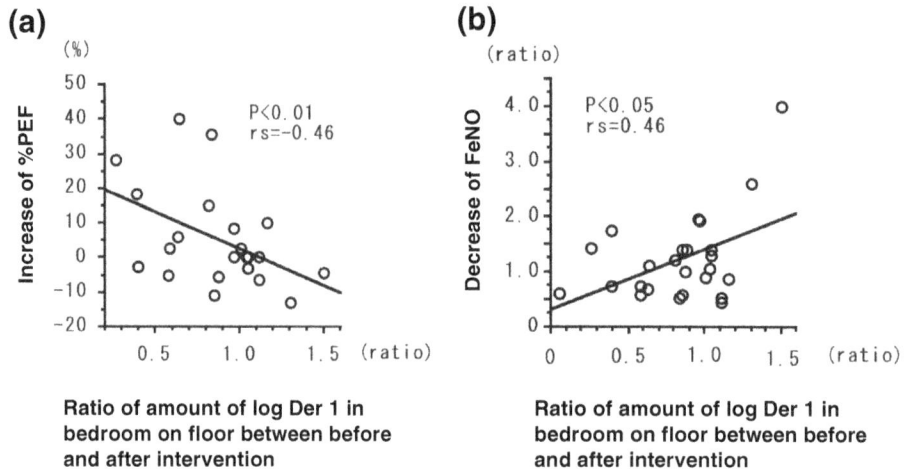

Figure 3 Correlations between log Der 1 ratio and changes in minimum % PEF value (a) and FeNO level (b) in intervention-group patients before intervention (in 2009) and 1 year later (after intervention), and in the non-intervention group during the same test periods. Each ratio is [log Der 1 level in 2010 / log Der 1 level in 2009]. The change in minimum % PEF was calculated as (2010% PEF–2009% PEF)/2009% PEF × 100 (%). Each change in FeNO level was calculated as 2010 FeNO value/2009 FeNO value. Twenty-two of the 25 patients recorded their PEF measurements daily, and 23 of 25 performed FeNO measurements. Correlation coefficients (r values) were obtained by using Spearman's rank correlation test.

Placing bedding in impermeable covers to avoid exposure to indoor allergens has not previously been shown to be of clinical benefit in adult patients [20]. However, such an approach effectively controls asthma in children [40,41]. We found that Der 1 levels in bedrooms were only slightly (but likely valuably) reduced when microfine bedding covers were used (Figure 4(b)). However, the small size of our groups may have influenced the significance of our findings.

Futon or mattress cover levels of Der 1 (sampled by using adhesive tape) were significantly correlated with those in airborne dust (sampled by using Petri dishes) in this study

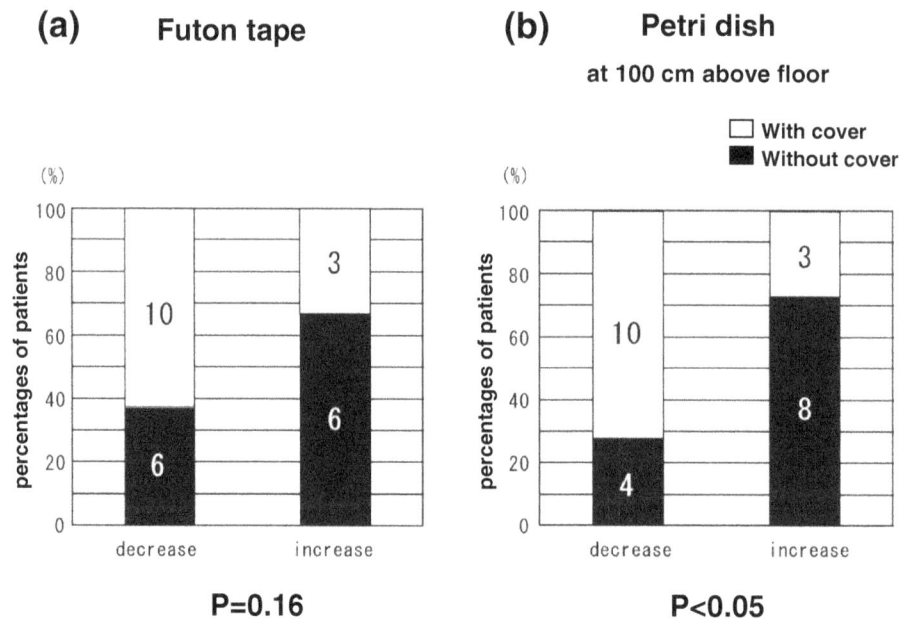

Figure 4 Decreases or increases in Der 1 levels on (a) tape samples from futon or mattress covers and (b) Petri dish samples from 100 cm above the bedroom floor. The "increase" and "decrease" groups respectively include data from patients whose 2010 Der 1 levels rose or fell by more than the 2009 Der 1 levels (intervention group = "With cover"; control = "Without cover"). Numbers in boxes are numbers of patients, and y-axes show percentages of patients. The chi-squared test was used to explore the significance of differences between the two groups. A P value of <0.05 indicates statistical significance.

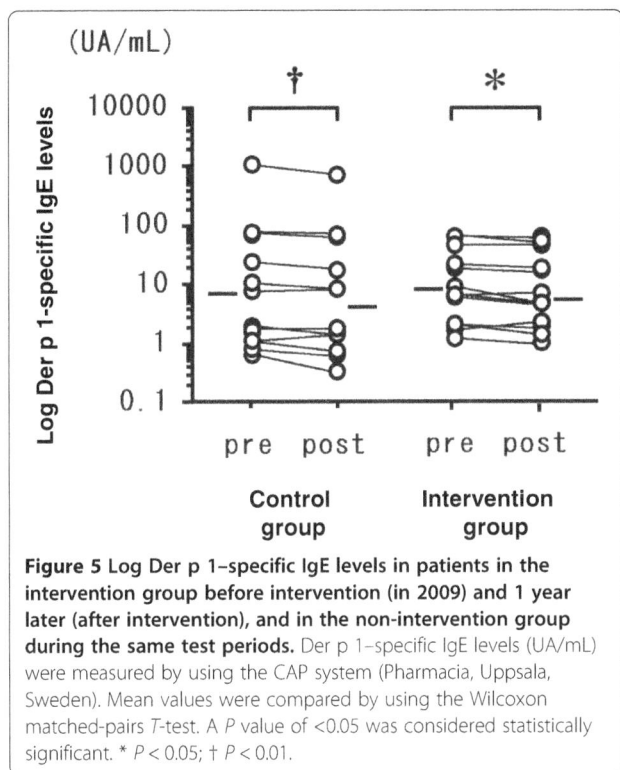

Figure 5 Log Der p 1–specific IgE levels in patients in the intervention group before intervention (in 2009) and 1 year later (after intervention), and in the non-intervention group during the same test periods. Der p 1–specific IgE levels (UA/mL) were measured by using the CAP system (Pharmacia, Uppsala, Sweden). Mean values were compared by using the Wilcoxon matched-pairs T-test. A P value of <0.05 was considered statistically significant. * $P < 0.05$; † $P < 0.01$.

and in another study of ours [19]. The counseling offered to the intervention group likely contributed to the observed reduction in Der 1 levels, because the reduced bedroom air Der 1 level (achieved by applying the recommended cleaning protocols and house hygiene) may have been resulted from the observed reduction in futon or mattress cover Der 1 concentrations. We surmised that the concentration of Der 1 rising up into the bedroom air was decreased not only by the addition of covers but also by vacuuming of the futon or mattress and wiping of the floor with a damp cloth.

Reductions in Der 1 levels on tape samples from futon or mattress covers and in bedroom air samples collected from near the floor over the 2 weeks were associated with improvements in symptom scores and increases in minimum % PEF levels after intervention. However, in the control group neither the ambient level of Der 1 allergen nor the clinical score changed between 2009 and 2010. Reducing levels of exposure to HDM allergens reportedly improves forced expiratory volume in 1 s in asthmatic children [42,43]. However, another study has found that respiratory parameters improve in some, but not all, adult patients [7,44].

FeNO levels did not change between 2009 and 2010 in any of the patients (data not shown). We consider that this was not an artifact caused by the large variation in FeNO levels measured by using our off-line method. Because the observed change in FeNO level after intervention was correlated with the change in bedroom

Der 1 level. Reduced exposure to Der 1 caused the FeNO level to fall and the minimum % PEF to improve. Moreover, the extent of airway eosinophilic inflammation may have fallen after intervention, as this is reflected in a drop in mean FeNO values in adult patients with asthma [45].

Most reports and meta-analyses of asthma management have suggested that avoidance of indoor allergen exposure is not of benefit and should not be recommended as a component of asthma management [2,7,10]. However, here we measured Der 1 levels by using a sensitive (1 pg/mL) fluorometric ELISA. Also, it is usual to collect dust samples by vacuuming and to calculate Der 1 levels as micrograms of allergen per gram of dust [1,2,4,27,46]. Instead, we collected dust samples in open Petri dishes and on adhesive tape and detected a few Der 1 level by ELISA above described. We consider that our assay and collection modes were superior to those used in earlier studies; this is likely the reason why reductions in allergen levels were reflected in improved clinical outcomes.

Der p and Der f–specific IgE levels are correlated with allergen exposure among sensitized participants [47]. Interventions that reduce exposure of child asthmatics to HDMs cause the levels of both specific [44,48] and total IgE [49] to fall.

We found, however, that the levels of Der p 1–specific IgE measured with the CAP system fell between 2009 and 2010 in both the intervention and the control group. Thus, reducing the level of exposure to Der 1 did not affect the serum concentration of Der p 1–specific IgE. We consider that the observed fall in reactive IgE levels was attributable to the fact that all patients were treated more intensively (including with ICS) in the interval between the two test periods than was the case before the 2009 test period.

We conclude that precise measurement of ambient Der 1 levels by using a sensitive fluorometric ELISA may be useful in the clinical management of asthma. Also, encasing pillows and mattresses or futons in covers made of microfine fibers and avoiding Der 1 exposure by using an indoor hygiene protocol [4,27] may be of value in adult asthma management.

Abbreviations
Der 1: *Dermatophagoides* mite antigen group 1; Der p 1: *D. pteronyssinus* allergen 1; Der f 1: *D. farinae* allergen 1; ELISA: Enzyme-linked immunosorbent assay; FeNO: Fraction of exhaled nitric oxide; GINA: Global Initiative for Asthma; HDM: House dust mite; ICS: Inhaled corticosteroids; IgE: Immunoglobulin E; LABA: Long-acting β2 agonist; LAMA: Long-acting muscarinic antagonist; LTRA: Leukotriene receptor antagonist; PEF: Peak expiratory flow.

Competing interests
The authors declared that they have no competing interest.

Authors' contributions
NT examined the patients, analyzed data and statistics, was the main contributor to manuscript preparation, and was involved in manuscript

preparation and editing. CO and TN examined the patients and contributed to discussions about the patients. AS assayed the levels of Der 1 on the skin and futon or mattress covers in the bedrooms. YH and KA contributed to discussions about the manuscript. All authors read and approved the final manuscript.

Acknowledgements
We thank Ms. Yumiko Takeuchi and Ms. Masayo Morie for performing the FeNO measurements.

Author details
[1]Department of Allergy and Respirology, National Hospital Organization Sagamihara National Hospital, 18-1 Sakuradai, Minami-ku, Sagamihara, Kanagawa 252-0392, Japan. [2]Clinical Research Center for Allergy and Rheumatology, National Hospital Organization Sagamihara National Hospital, 18-1 Sakuradai, Minami-ku, Sagamihara, Kanagawa 252-0392, Japan.

References
1. Platts-Mills TA, Thomas WR, Aalberse RC, Vervloet D, Champman MD: **Dust mite allergens and asthma: report of a second international workshop.** *J Allergy Clin Immunol* 1992, **89:**1046–1060.
2. Platts-Mills AE, Platts-Mills TA, Vervloet D, Thomas WR, Aalberse RC, Chapman MD: **Indoor allergens and asthma: report of the Third International Workshop.** *J Allergy Clin Immunol* 1997, **100:**S2–S24.
3. Salo PM, Arbes SJ Jr, Crockett PW, Thorne PS, Cohn RD, Zeldin DC: **Exposure to multiple indoor allergens in US homes and its relationship to asthma.** *J Allergy Clin Immunol* 2008, **121:**678–684.
4. Nishioka K, Saito A, Akiyama K, Yasueda H: **Effect of home environment control on children with atopic or non-atopic asthma.** *Allergol Int* 2006, **55:**141–148.
5. Halken S, Høst A, Niklassen U, Hansen LG, Nielsen F, Pedersen S, Osterballe O, Veggerby C, Poulsen LK: **Effect of mattress and pillow encasings on children with asthma and house dust mite allergy.** *J Allergy Clin Immunol* 2003, **111:**169–176.
6. Morgan WJ, Crain EF, Gruchalla RS, O'Connor GT, Kattan M, Evans R 3rd, Stout J, Malindzak G, Smartt E, Plaut M, Walter M, Vaughn B, Mitchell H, Inner-City Asthma Study Group: **Results of a home-based environmental intervention among urban children with asthma.** *N Engl J Med* 2004, **351:**1068–1080.
7. Gøtzsche PC, Johansen HK: **House dust mite control measures for asthma: systematic review.** *Allergy* 2008, **63:**646–659.
8. MacDonald C, Sternberg A, Hunter PR: **A systematic review and meta-analysis of interventions used to reduce exposure to house dust and their effect on the development and severity of asthma.** *Environ Health Perspect* 2007, **115:**1691–1695.
9. Postma J, Karr C, Kieckhefer G: **Community health workers and environmental interventions for children with asthma: a systematic review.** *J Asthma* 2009, **46:**564–576.
10. Tovey ER, Marks GB: **It's time to rethink mite allergen avoidance.** *J Allergy Clin Immunol* 2011, **128:**723–727.
11. Gøtzsche PC, Johansen HK: **House dust mite control measures for asthma.** *Cochrane Database Syst Rev* 2008, **16**, CD001187.
12. Custovic A, Wijk RG: **The effectiveness of measures to change the indoor environment in the treatment of allergic rhinitis and asthma: ARIA update (in collaboration with GA(2)LEN).** *Allergy* 2005, **60:**1112–1115.
13. Luczynska C, Tredwell E, Smeeton N, Burney P: **A randomized controlled trial of mite allergen-impermeable bed covers in adult mite-sensitized asthmatics.** *Clin Exp Allergy* 2003, **33:**1648–1653.
14. Woodcock A, Forster L, Matthews E, Martin J, Letley L, Vickers M, Britton J, Strachan D, Howarth P, Altmann D, Frost C, Custovic A, Medical Research Council General Practice Research Framework: **Control of exposure to mite allergen and allergen-impermeable bed covers for adults with asthma.** *N Engl J Med* 2003, **349:**225–236.
15. Platts-Mills TA, Sporik RB, Wheatley LM, Heymann PW: **Is there a dose–response relationship between exposure to indoor allergens and symptoms of asthma?** *J Allergy Clin Immunol* 1995, **96:**435–440.
16. Tovey ER, Marks GB: **Methods and effectiveness of environmental control.** *J Allergy Clin Immunol* 1999, **103:**179–191.
17. Gore RB, Custovic A: **Is allergen avoidance effective?** *Clin Exp Allergy* 2002, **32:**662–666.
18. Yasueda H, Saito A, Nishioka K, Kutsuwada K, Akiyama K: **Measurement of Dermatophagoides mite allergens on bedding and human skin surfaces.** *Clin Exp Allergy* 2003, **33:**1654–1658.
19. Saito A, Tsurikisawa N, Oshikata C, Nakazawa T, Yasueda H, Akiyama K: **Evaluation of Petri dish sampling for assessment of airborne dust mite allergen in JAPAN.** *Arerugi* 2012, **61:**1657–1664.
20. GINA: *Global Strategy for Asthma Management and Prevention.* Global Initiative for Asthma; 2012. Available from: www.ginasthma.org/.
21. American Thoracic Society: **Standards for the diagnosis and care of patients with chronic obstructive pulmonary disease (COPD) and asthma.** *Am Rev Respir Dis* 1987, **136:**225–244.
22. Bousquet J, Schünemann HJ, Samolinski B, Demoly P, Baena-Cagnani CE, Bachert C, Bonini S, et al: **Allergic Rhinitis and its Impact on Asthma (ARIA): achievements in 10 years and future needs.** *J Allergy Clin Immunol* 2012, **130:**1049–1062.
23. Bousquet J, Heinzerling L, Bachert C, Papadopoulos NG, Bousquet PJ, Burney PG, Canonica GW, Carlsen KH, Global Allergy and Asthma European Network, Allergic Rhinitis and its Impact on Asthma, et al: **Practical guide to skin prick tests in allergy to aeroallergens.** *Allergy* 2012, **67:**18–24.
24. Terada Y, Nagata M, Murayama N, Nanko H, Furue M: **Clinical comparison of human and canine atopic dermatitis using human diagnostic criteria (Japanese Dermatological Association, 2009): proposal of provisional diagnostic criteria for canine atopic dermatitis.** *J Dermatol* 2011, **38:**784–790.
25. Tovey ER, Marks GB, Matthews M, Green WF, Woolcock A: **Changes in mite allergen Der p I in house dust following a spraying with a tannic acid/acaricide solution.** *Clin Exp Allergy* 1992, **22:**67–74.
26. Oliver J, Birmingham K, Crewes A, Weeks J, Carswell F: **Allergen levels in airborne and surface dust.** *Int Arch Allergy Immunol* 1995, **107:**452–453.
27. Nishioka K, Yasueda H, Saito H: **Preventive effect of bedding encasement with microfine fibers on mite sensitization.** *J Allergy Clin Immunol* 1998, **101:**28–32.
28. Tsuburai T, Tsurikisawa N, Taniguchi M, et al: **The relationship between exhaled nitric oxide measured with an off-line method and airway reversible obstruction in Japanese adults with asthma.** *Allergol Int* 2007, **56:**37–43.
29. Hamilton RG, Williams PB: **Specific IgE Testing Task Force of the American Academy of Allergy, Asthma & Immunology; American College of Allergy, Asthma and Immunology. Allergy diagnostic testing: an updated practice parameter.** *Ann Allergy Asthma Immunol* 2008, **100:**S1–S148.
30. Hargreave FE, Dolovich J, Boulet LP: **Inhalation provocation tests.** *Semin Respir Med* 1983, **4:**224–236.
31. Yasueda H, Saito A, Akiyama K, Maeda Y, Shida M, Sakaguchi M, Inouye S: **Estimation of Der p and Der f 1 quantities in the reference preparations of Dermatophagoides mite extracts.** *Clin Exp Allergy* 1994, **19:**1030–1035.
32. Jackson DJ, Johnston SL: **The role of viruses in acute exacerbations of asthma.** *J Allergy Clin Immunol* 2010, **125:**1178–1187.
33. Boulay ME, Morin A, Laprise C, Boulet LP: **Asthma and rhinitis: what is the relationship?** *Curr Opin Allergy Clin Immunol* 2012, **12:**449–454.
34. Jacquemin B, Schikowski T, Carsin AE, Hansell A, Krämer U, Sunyer J, Probst-Hensch N, Kauffmann F, et al: **The role of air pollution in adult-onset asthma: a review of the current evidence.** *Semin Respir Crit Care Med* 2012, **33:**606–619.
35. Goldsmith CA, Kobzik L: **Particulate air pollution and asthma: a review of epidemiological and biological studies.** *Rev Environ Health* 1999, **14:**121–134.
36. Moseholm L, Taudorf E, Frøsig A: **Pulmonary function changes in asthmatics associated with low-level SO2 and NO2 air pollution, weather, and medicine intake. An 8-month prospective study analyzed by neural networks.** *Allergy* 1993, **48:**334–344.
37. Koh MS, Tee A, Lasserson TJ, Irving LB: **Inhaled corticosteroids compared to placebo for prevention of exercise induced bronchoconstriction.** *Cochrane Database Syst Rev* 2007, **18:**CD002739.
38. Custovic A, Simpson A: **The role of inhalamt allergens in allergic airways disease.** *J Investig Allergol Clin Immunol* 2012, **22:**393–401.
39. Gold DR: **Environmental tobacco smoke, indoor allergens, and childhood asthma.** *Environ Health Perspect* 2000, **108:**643–651.
40. Carswell F, Birmingham K, Oliver J, Crewes A, Weeks J: **The respiratory effects of reduction of mite allergen in the bedrooms of asthmatic children–a double-blind controlled trial.** *Clin Exp Allergy* 1996, **26:**386–396.
41. Ehnert B, Lau-Schadendorf S, Weber A, Buettner P, Schou C, Wahn U: **Reducing domestic exposure to dust mite allergen reduces bronchial hyperreactivity in sensitive children with asthma.** *J Allergy Clin Immunol* 1992, **90:**135–138.

42. Peroni DG, Boner AL, Vallone G, Antolini I, Warner JO: **Effective allergen avoidance at high altitude reduces allergen-induced bronchial hyperresponsiveness.** *Am J Respir Crit Care Med* 1994, **149**:1442–1446.

43. Simon HU, Grotzer M, Nikolaizik WH, Blaser K, Schöni MH: **High altitude climate therapy reduces peripheral blood T lymphocyte activation, eosinophilia, and bronchial obstruction in children with house-dust mite allergic asthma.** *Pediatr Pulmonol* 1994, **17**:304–311.

44. Piacentini GL, Martinati L, Fornari A, Comis A, Carcereri L, Boccagni P, Boner AL: **Antigen avoidance in a mountain environment: influence on basophil releasability in children with allergic asthma.** *J Allergy Clin Immunol* 1993, **92**:644–650.

45. Ricciardolo FL, Di Stefano A, Silvestri M, Van Schadewijk AM, Malerba M, Hiemstra PS, Sterk PJ: **Exhaled nitric oxide is related to bronchial eosinophilia and airway hyperresponsiveness to bradykinin in allergen-induced asthma exacerbation.** *Int J Immunopathol Pharmacol* 2012, **25**:175–182.

46. Sakaguchi M, Inouye S, Yasueda H, Irie T, Yoshizawa S, Shida T: **Measurement of allergens associated with dust mite allergy. II. Concentrations of airborne mite allergens (Der I and Der II) in the house.** *Int Arch Allergy Appl Immunol* 1989, **90**:190–193.

47. Matsui EC, Sampson HA, Bahnson HT, Gruchalla RS, Pongracic JA, Teach SJ, Gergen PJ, Bloomberg GR, *et al*: **Allergen-specific IgE as a biomarker of exposure puls sensitization in inner-city adolescents with asthma.** *Allergy* 2010, **65**:1414–1422.

48. Sensi LG, Piacentini GL, Nobile E, Ghebregzabher M, Brunori R, Zanolla L, Boner AL, Marcucci F: **Changes in nasal specific IgE to mites after periods of allergen exposure-avoidance: a comparison with serum levels.** *Clin Exp Allergy* 1994, **24**:377–382.

49. Zedan M, Attia G, Zedan MM, Osman A, Abo-Elkheir N, Maysara N, Barakat T, Gamil N: **Clinical asthma phenotypes and therapeutic responses.** *ISRN Pediatr* 2013:824781. doi: 10.1155/2013/824781.

14

Conducting retrospective impact analysis to inform a medical research charity's funding strategies: the case of Asthma UK

Stephen R Hanney[1*], Amanda Watt[2], Teresa H Jones[1] and Leanne Metcalf[3]

Abstract

Background: Debate is intensifying about how to assess the full range of impacts from medical research. Complexity increases when assessing the diverse funding streams of funders such as Asthma UK, a charitable patient organisation supporting medical research to benefit people with asthma. This paper aims to describe the various impacts identified from a range of Asthma UK research, and explore how Asthma UK utilised the characteristics of successful funding approaches to inform future research strategies.

Methods: We adapted the Payback Framework, using it both in a survey and to help structure interviews, documentary analysis, and case studies. We sent surveys to 153 lead researchers of projects, plus 10 past research fellows, and also conducted 14 detailed case studies. These covered nine projects and two fellowships, in addition to the innovative case studies on the professorial chairs (funded since 1988) and the MRC-Asthma UK Centre in Allergic Mechanisms of Asthma (the 'Centre') which together facilitated a comprehensive analysis of the whole funding portfolio. We organised each case study to capture whatever academic and wider societal impacts (or payback) might have arisen given the diverse timescales, size of funding involved, and extent to which Asthma UK funding contributed to the impacts.

Results: Projects recorded an average of four peer-reviewed journal articles. Together the chairs reported over 500 papers. All streams of funding attracted follow-on funding. Each of the various categories of societal impacts arose from only a minority of individual projects and fellowships. Some of the research portfolio is influencing asthma-related clinical guidelines, and some contributing to product development. The latter includes potentially major breakthroughs in asthma therapies (in immunotherapy, and new inhaled drugs) trialled by university spin-out companies. Such research-informed guidelines and medicines can, in turn, contribute to health improvements. The role of the chairs and the pioneering collaborative Centre is shown as being particularly important.

Conclusions: We systematically demonstrate that all types of Asthma UK's research funding assessed are making impacts at different levels, but the main societal impacts from projects and fellowships come from a minority of those funded. Asthma UK used the study's findings, especially in relation to the Centre, to inform research funding strategies to promote the achievement of impact.

Keywords: Asthma, Asthma UK, Research impacts, Societal impacts, Clinical guidelines, University spin-out companies, Product development, Immunotherapy, Payback Framework, Research funding strategy

* Correspondence: stephen.hanney@brunel.ac.uk
[1]Health Economics Research Group, Brunel University, Uxbridge UB8 3PH, UK
Full list of author information is available at the end of the article

Background

Globally research funders are under growing pressure to demonstrate the returns or impacts that arise from their research funding [1-4]. In 2006, the UK Evaluation Forum, which brought together the Academy of Medical Sciences, the Medical Research Council (MRC) and the Wellcome Trust, considered ways of assessing the benefits of medical research and called for further studies [2].

For charitable patient organisations that fund medical research it is increasingly important to demonstrate that the money they have invested is leading to improvements in the healthcare and quality of life of the patients they exist to support [5]. Charities are accountable for this in a formal way (for example, to regulators, funders or members) and in a moral way (for example, to beneficiaries, service users, partner charities, staff, volunteers and the general public).

Asthma UK (under its current and previous names) has been funding research since 1927. Since the formation of the National Asthma Campaign in 1989, the charity has spent over £50 million on research to understand more about asthma, its causes and treatments. It has been spending up to £3 million and funding between ten and twenty new projects each year. Asthma UK has historically provided various types of funding for research, including long-term support for two professorial chairs over the last twenty years, medium-term support through a research fellowship scheme, and project support through an annual grant round. Since 2005 the charity has jointly funded the pioneering collaborative MRC-Asthma UK Centre in Allergic Mechanisms of Asthma (the 'Centre') based at both King's College London and Imperial College London. Asthma UK has more recently introduced funding for PhD studentships, initially linked to the Centre.

Asthma UK has a relatively limited budget and so has long engaged with the scientific community to help identify the areas of research that would be most likely to achieve its objectives [6]. However, in response to the charity's wider range of accountabilities, Asthma UK decided to review various aspects of its role as a research funder. These included, firstly, increasingly ensuring people affected with asthma were meaningfully involved in reviewing all proposals for funding, and, secondly, building greater understanding of what had been achieved through the breadth of its previous research funding activities, so as to help inform an enhanced research strategy. This article focuses primarily on the latter, but provides some evidence related to the former.

Although the importance of charities being able to demonstrate the impact of their research funding is widely recognised, attempts to assess rigorously the impact of research funding have been limited, and not just for charitable research funders. This is largely due to the huge difficulties of demonstrating impact in research, attributable to the fact that many pieces of research might contribute to achieving some impacts, and a huge time lag can be involved before tangible benefits are realised [7].

Of the relatively small number of impact studies reported in the literature, the Payback Framework developed by the Health Economics Research Group (HERG) is described as the approach used most often [8-10]. It constitutes a framework for addressing the conceptual issues, and collecting, analysing and reporting data in a reasonably consistent manner to capture the impacts and outputs of research [8]. As such, the Payback Framework has been used as a tool to help funders and stakeholders in research to think about what the likely impacts from research can or might be.

For a research funder there could be clear benefits in having an assessment made of their full portfolio of research funding. Yet, attempts to assess the impact of a wide-ranging research funder's full portfolio of research are even rarer than assessment of selected case studies or specific programmes. This is because they require the combination of two different approaches:

- achieving breadth of coverage to give a reasonable picture of the impacts from the full portfolio;
- conducting the detailed analyses needed to address issues such as how far impacts can be attributed to the specific research being examined.

Doing this rigorously requires the research instruments (surveys and case studies adopting triangulation techniques etc.) to be able to tackle issues such as responders' bias and selective recall.

In 2008, Asthma UK approached HERG to apply their Payback Framework to identify the benefits that have arisen from the charity's various forms of research support and thereby help Asthma UK to continue to use its funds to best effect in terms of maximising benefits for people with asthma in its future research strategy. The team from HERG and RAND Europe conducting the independent retrospective impact analysis provided a complete report to Asthma UK, and an additional 300 page volume of supporting case studies.[a]

The objectives of this article are to describe the methods and results of this evaluation of the impacts from Asthma UK's research (including how the difficulties in assessing the range of impacts from such a comprehensive portfolio were addressed), and then to discuss how the findings have been used by Asthma UK to inform its research funding strategy.

Methods

Assessing the impacts of the full portfolio of a health research funder requires a combination of methods. Those applied in this study included a review of the data already gathered by Asthma UK, a survey sent to the researchers, and detailed case studies. However, such methods are enhanced when informed by a conceptual framework that can help organise the data collection, analysis and reporting in as consistent a manner as possible [8], in contrast to being a collection of one-off case studies.

We therefore organised this project around an adaptation of the HERG Payback Framework [5,11]. The framework combines two aspects: a multi-dimensional categorisation of benefits from health research and the payback logic model. The multi-dimensional categorisation of benefits includes traditional categories such as the knowledge production represented by publications, research capacity building and the targeting of future research. But it also incorporates wider impacts that are increasingly viewed as important by research funders, especially charitable patient organisations, including: informing policy and product development (which includes clinical policies such as guidelines); health and health sector benefits; and broader economic benefits. The logic model is shown in Figure 1 and presents a simplified version of the processes involved in commissioning and undertaking the research, and in generating the full range of impacts. It helps identify where the various categories of impacts themselves might arise, but recognises there is often considerable feedback between the different stages.

Pursuing the analysis through the various stages of the logic model helps address attribution issues. The early stages of the model focus on the context in which the

research was undertaken, and the motivations behind it. Analysis here increases opportunities for identifying impacts in the later payback categories, and attributing them (at least partially) to the specific research funded. Similarly, analysis at the interfaces between researchers and research users can be important in understanding how far impacts have been achieved. Previous studies provide fuller accounts of the Payback Framework and how it is applied to inform the methods used for data collection, analysis and reporting when the focus has been on selected case studies or on specific programmes [5,8,11-13]. The study received appropriate ethical approval from the University Research Ethics Committee at Brunel University.

Survey

We adapted a survey used previously to examine the impacts from the research funded by the Health Technology Assessment programme in England [8], but amended it to increase its relevance to Asthma UK. The full survey can be seen as an additional file [see Additional file 1]. For each project we identified publications already on Asthma UK's database and inserted them into the relevant survey. Respondents were then asked to make any necessary amendments. Many of the survey questions not only asked about whether certain developments had occurred (for example, whether the research led to any follow-on projects) but also asked about the degree of influence on such decisions made by the original research funded by the charity. This was in recognition of the fact that just because Asthma UK funding had been used to create scientific evidence, it

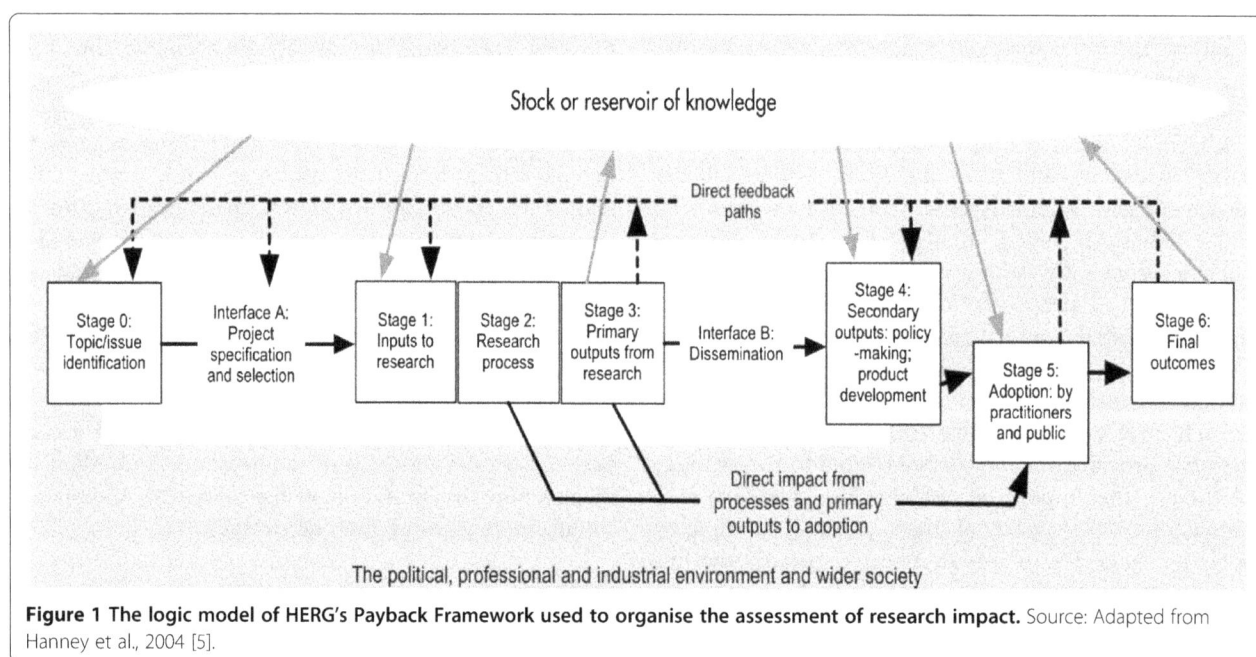

Figure 1 The logic model of HERG's Payback Framework used to organise the assessment of research impact. Source: Adapted from Hanney et al., 2004 [5].

did not guarantee that impact had been achieved in a simple and linear manner, and it was desirable to attempt to identify the level of the charity's contribution.

We also wanted to make some calculation of the amount of follow-on funding that might reasonably be thought to have come from the original projects. Therefore, we not only asked grant-holders to record the funder of the follow-on research and the amount, but also asked the responders to use one of three categories (considerable/moderate/small) to describe the contribution to securing or informing the follow-on funding made by the original Asthma UK funding.

We piloted the survey before sending it to all 153 lead researchers (or principal investigators – PIs) awarded project grants from 1996 (a date from which Asthma UK held reasonable archival data) that had been completed by 2006, and to the ten researchers whose fellowships had been completed. We recorded the survey responses in an Access database, and developed innovative analysis techniques for various issues. For example, previous studies had just totalled the recorded amount of follow-on funding but this was criticised as exaggerating the role of just one funder when several should probably share the credit. Therefore, we not only asked PIs to make an estimate of the contribution to the follow-on funding made by the original Asthma UK-

funded research, but also made a best estimate of what the categories 'considerable', 'moderate' and 'small' might mean in quantitative terms. We took the amount of follow-on funding recorded for projects and multiplied it by the following proportions: considerable: 0.9; moderate: 0.5; small: 0.1. This gave us a total of adjusted follow-on funding for all the projects for which a survey had been completed. We then calculated the total funding supplied by Asthma UK for all the projects that completed a survey, irrespective of whether or not the PI reported any follow-on funding. Finally we calculated the ratio of total follow-on funding (adjusted for the contributions made and excluding the follow-on funding that came from Asthma UK itself) to original Asthma UK funding.

Case studies

The project's research team, in conjunction with the project's Advisory Committee, used information obtained from the survey about claims for impact in the various categories to inform the selection of nine projects and two fellowships on which to undertake case studies – these are listed on Table 1. We also wanted to conduct case studies on the work of the two Asthma UK professorial chairs who had been funded since 1988, and had, therefore been a key element in Asthma UK's funding strategy, and on

Table 1 Case studies on nine project grants and two fellowships

Project grants		
Researcher: title and location at time of proposal	Title of research (and ID)	Duration in months
Bradding, Dr. Peter. Glenfield Hospital, University of Leicester	Human mast cell adhesion to bronchial epithelium and airway smooth muscle (02/014)	24 (2003–05)
Britton, Professor John. University of Nottingham	Study of the role of parasites, dust mite exposure and other environmental factors in the aetiology of asthma and atopy in urban and rural Ethiopia (98/014)	12 (1998–00)
Bush, Dr. Andrew. Imperial College, London	Pathology of severe asthma in children (01/037)	23 (2001–03)
Durham, Professor Stephen. Imperial College, London	Influence of grass pollen immunotherapy (IT) on allergen-specific peripheral blood T-cell lines: allergy or immune deviation? (97/069)	24 (1997–99)
Hawrylowicz, Dr. Catherine. King's College, London	IL-10: A critical regulator of inflammation and glucocorticoid responsiveness in asthma (00/023)	36 (2000–03)
Hubbard, Dr. Richard. University of Nottingham	A birth cohort study of the impact of asthma, acute exacerbations of asthma and asthma therapies on the risk of pregnancy complications and adverse perinatal and paediatric outcomes (04/019)	24 (2004–06)
Johnston, Dr. Sebastian. University of Southampton	Rhinovirus-induced regulation of adhesion molecule expression in asthma exacerbations (332)	24 (1996–98)
Pavord, Professor Ian. Glenfield Hospital, University of Leicester	The immunopathology and corticosteroid responsiveness of non-eosinophilic asthma (02/036)	24 (2002–05)
Sutton, Professor Brian. King's College, London	Structure based design of inhibitors of IgE binding to the mast cell receptor (97/033)	36 (1997–01)
Fellowships		
Custovic, Dr. Adnan. University of Manchester	Gene-environment interaction in the development of atopy, asthma and other allergic diseases (RF01C)	60 (2000–04)
Thomas, Dr Mike. University of Aberdeen	Primary care asthma management: diagnosis, assessments and effective therapy (RF09T)	60 (2005–10)

the MRC-Asthma UK Centre which was a major recent development.

In total, therefore, we undertook 14 case studies using archival and documentary review, interviews and bibliometric analysis. There is inevitably a bias introduced into the study by concentrating on case studies that are thought likely to be positive examples. However, where the main purpose of the case studies is to inform long-term strategy through a richer analysis of the range of impacts that arise - and how they manifest in different payback categories over time - such cases need to have sufficient content with which to explore what has happened to Asthma UK-funded research.

For the project and fellowship case studies we interviewed the PIs and also, where possible, one or two further members of the relevant research team. As in previous studies, we used a semi-structured interview schedule informed by the Payback Framework. For all the case studies we adopted a 'rolling triangulation' approach [14] in which we used the data gathered from documentary and archival review, plus that from earlier interviews, to inform the creation of a specific schedule for each interview [see Additional file 2]. The Payback Framework provided a conceptual framework to organise not only the data collection but also the analysis of the data and its presentation in each case study.

For the case studies on the two professorial chairs and the Centre, the Payback Framework again informed the interview schedules and write-up. In these cases, however, we applied it in an innovative way to take account of the breadth of topics covered, and to allow analysis of how the nature of the funding (long-term in the case of the chairs, and collaborative in the case of the Centre) might facilitate the production of a range of impacts. Various interviews were conducted for each of these three case studies. In total, 15 interviewees helped inform the Centre case study. They were: the two professorial chairs, who became respectively Director and Deputy Director of the Centre upon its creation in 2005; nine other members of the Centre; and four independent experts.

As part of the case study analysis we searched major national and international clinical guidelines related to asthma[b] to see how far the Asthma UK-funded research had influenced the clinical guidelines, which are regarded as a form of clinical policy [14]. To obtain a fuller idea of the contribution made by the Asthma UK-funded research we took the analysis further than in previous studies and on this occasion examined the number of times the relevant articles were cited in the guideline, the importance of specific points being supported by Asthma UK-funded research, and how far the Asthma UK-funded paper was the only, or key, evidence supporting the relevant points. We also used a triangulation approach as far as possible to inform the write-up

of the case studies. A starting point for each case study was the survey, but the archival and documentary review and the interviews allowed claims made in the survey to be checked and the issues further explored.

Case studies such as these on specific pieces of research refer explicitly, and unavoidably, to the work of identified individuals and teams. We therefore obtained clearance for the text of each case study from the PI of the project (fellowship or chair), and also from any other interviewee whose interview evidence is used in an identifiable manner. This is not just a matter of courtesy, but is an important aspect of ensuring the scientific quality of the reported findings and ethical conduct of the study.

Analysis of use of the report's findings
The report was considered by Asthma UK as part of its review of its research strategy. For this article the way in which the report has been drawn upon by Asthma UK was analysed by LM, using her position from within the organisation.

Results
Ninety six surveys were returned (90 projects and six fellowships) giving a response of 59% and we successfully completed the full complement of 14 case studies. The findings of both the survey and case studies are presented according to the categories of impact from the Payback Framework, and then briefly summarised to demonstrate the impact from each type of funding.

Impacts relating to each impact category
Knowledge production
The 90 projects recorded an average of four peer-reviewed journal articles per project, but four of these projects did not record producing any articles. There is a possible bias in the results as there is some evidence from Asthma UK's database of publications, as described in the full report (see End Note[a]), showing that the average number of publications already known to Asthma UK is slightly higher for the projects on which surveys were returned, than for those that were not. The research fellows who completed the survey recorded an average figure of 11 peer-reviewed articles. This higher average figure reflects the view of some fellows that because their career at that time was being funded by Asthma UK, all, or at least most, of their resulting publications could be counted as having some link with the fellowship. Since their appointments in 1988, the two Asthma UK professorial chairs, Tak Lee at King's College London, and Tim Williams, at Imperial College London, published a total of over 500 publications.

For example, Tim Williams, conducted a major stream of research in the search for the chemoattractants for eosinophils, a type of white blood cell regarded as being as of considerable importance. Williams and his colleagues identified a potent endogenous chemoattractant with high specificity for eosinophils. Williams named this chemokine Eotaxin; the main paper describing it was published in the *Journal of Experimental Medicine* (Jose, 1994) [15] and has been cited over 600 times. It has helped target considerable further research including by Williams and his colleagues. They also successfully sought patents on their work that they have been granted worldwide on Eotaxin and antibodies to it. Further examples of key publications from Asthma UK-funded chairs, projects and fellowships [16-18] are described in the case studies summarized in Additional files 3, 4 and 5.

Research training and capacity building

The 90 PIs who completed surveys claimed that at least 62 higher degrees have been obtained or were expected at least in part as a result of Asthma UK's project funding. An additional 15 are linked to the six fellowships covered in this analysis. These 77 higher degrees include 45 PhDs and 21 MDs. Asthma UK has now funded PhD studentships at the MRC-Asthma UK Centre (and several elsewhere jointly with the MRC). According to the case study analysis, this is making an important contribution to the substantial advances in research training in asthma coming from the Centre.

In addition, the researchers from 64% of the funded projects that participated in the survey reported details of career development for at least one team member as a result of the Asthma UK project funding. This included assisting promotion for PIs, and also project researchers moving forward to gain fellowships from major funders and continue their research in the asthma field.

Targeting further research and attracting further income for asthma research

In total Asthma UK invested some £9.2 million in the 90 projects included in the analysis. The PIs claimed that such investment helped to target, i.e. identify relevant research questions for, 99 follow-on projects conducted by themselves or members of their team. These follow-on projects received almost £25 million in funding from funders other than Asthma UK. However in the survey, the PIs indicated that the intellectual contribution from the original Asthma UK project to some of the largest follow-on grants was often only moderate, or sometimes small. Taking this into account, in the manner described above, the £25 million of total follow-on funding could, at a best estimate, be counted as equivalent to £12.9 million follow-on funding linked to Asthma UK's £9.2 million original investment, So, every pound invested by Asthma UK in the research projects funded between 1996 and 2006 is likely to have attracted at least £1.40 in

follow-on research funding from sources other than Asthma UK. In addition, in at least 35 cases, other researchers were reported to have built on the findings from the Asthma UK funded projects.

In some instances Asthma UK funding played a 'pump-priming' role, enabling the researcher to leverage larger sums from other health research funding bodies, a major example of which is described in the case study on peptide-based immunotherapy research [18] [See Additional file 5]. On occasions where Asthma UK itself funded the follow-on research this has, at least in retrospect, amounted to a programme of work according to survey and case study data. Sometimes these major streams of work, involving a succession of project grants from Asthma UK undertaken over many years (including some dating back before 1996), have been important in helping to move towards the wider impacts (policy or product development, and health gains), often supplemented by funding from other sources. Examples include the research that started with an Asthma UK-funded project on IL-10 and glucocorticoid responsiveness in asthma which was outlined on Asthma UK's web site as follows: 'A series of Asthma UK funded projects led by Professor Catherine Hawrylowicz in Professor Lee's department has attracted particular interest, as the work has resulted in a clinical trial to explore whether vitamin D can improve the effectiveness of steroid treatments for asthma in those who are normally resistant to their benefits' [19].

In a similar manner, the chairs directly brought in additional funding for asthma research. Since 1995, Tak Lee successfully applied for grants from the MRC, Wellcome Trust and NHS R&D Programme alone worth about £6 million, in addition to the £2.7 million from the MRC to the MRC-Asthma UK Centre. King's College also made considerable infrastructural investment into Lee's department and the Centre. Overall Lee built up a substantial research division. Similarly, Tim Williams secured three major programme grants from the Wellcome Trust to support his streams of asthma related research and has secured university funding for various posts. Those interviewed for the case study consistently claimed that the creation of the MRC-Asthma UK Centre has helped secure additional funding for asthma research. This is both in terms of the core funding provided by the MRC for additional facilities at the Centre, and the various other ways in which PIs at the Centre are successfully applying for funding (including through Asthma UK), partly by demonstrating the strength of the environment within which the research would be undertaken.

Informing policy development

In the survey just 13% of projects claimed to have made an impact on policy already, and 17% expected such an impact in the future. As part of the triangulation process, checks were made of the impacts on guidelines claimed in surveys by PIs of projects on which case studies were later conducted. Generally exaggerated claims had not been made. Indeed, the case studies often identified additional examples of the research having been cited on guidelines. On the basis of this analysis, we broadly accepted the claims made in the surveys on which case studies were not conducted.

According to the survey and case studies, three of the six fellows claimed already to have made an impact on policies and/or guidelines - longer-term salary funding can allow fellows to develop a distinct role or focus which lends itself more to policy development. For example, a key paper by Mike Thomas [20] is already being used in recent guidelines from the British Thoracic Society/ Association of Chartered Physiotherapists in Respiratory Care [21] to support the use of breathing exercises for improved control of asthma and quality of life.

Using the methods described above we were able to establish that not only were papers from some Asthma UK-funded research cited on international and national guidelines, and other policy statements, but we also identified some examples when they supported key points and were either the only evidence used to support the point, or an important part of it. Some examples are given in the case study on research on immunotherapy that was part funded by Asthma UK [22,23] [see Additional file 4]. Other examples of national and/or international guidelines (or specific sections) influenced by Asthma UK-funded research, along with the Asthma UK-funded paper cited in the guideline, include ones on: cough [24,25]; asthma diagnosis in children [26,27]; and inhaled corticosteroid resistance [26,28].

Whilst there are often time lags involved in achieving an impact on policy, Asthma UK also supported some explicit and successful attempts to provide evidence for guidelines in areas in which there were gaps. In such situations there could be a rapid uptake of the findings. For example, Richard Hubbard specifically applied to Asthma UK for funding to develop stronger evidence on the safety of asthma medicines during pregnancy, an area where expert analysis of existing guidelines indicated the evidence was weak [29]. The findings from this project were published in late 2008 [30], and were almost immediately incorporated into an update of the 2008 guidelines from the British Thoracic Society and Scottish Intercollegiate Guidelines Network published in June 2009 [31].

Informing product development
In the survey only a small minority of projects – just 17% - included in this research claim an impact on product development already, and 31% claim to expect some future impact. The impact on product development

from Asthma UK projects and from chair funding takes various forms, including helping to identify new roles for existing products, contributing to the evidence base for the development and application of major new drugs, and contributing to new therapies being developed by university spin-off companies.

In the stream of Asthma UK-funded projects on IL-10 and glucocorticoid responsiveness in asthma described above, the important new therapy being tested – vitamin D for steroid resistant asthma [32] – might involve using existing products in a new way. The background and significance of a stream of work in supporting the development of anti-leukotriene medicines [16,33,34] is explained in more detail in an additional file taken from the case study on Tak Lee's work as an Asthma UK professorial chair [see Additional file 3].

Based on the projects included in this analysis, Asthma UK-funded research has also contributed to product development now being trialled by university spin-out companies founded by the researchers in several cases. The stream of research that showed T cell peptides have potential in the treatment of cat allergies led to the establishment of Circassia, an Imperial College London spin-out company. The progress made, including successful phase II trials, is described in an additional file which provides further details about the research and contains updates on the important findings published from a subsequent joint Canadian/UK study that is continuing this stream of work [see Additional file 5].

Many years of research by Stephen Holgate and colleagues led to the ideas behind the development of Interferon-beta treatment for rhinoviruses (common cold infections) that cause many asthma exacerbations. At a crucial time Asthma UK provided project funding for Holgate that contributed to key advances, although the MRC had supported much of the stream of work [35]. The spin-out company, Synairgen, successfully completed Phase 1 trials of the treatment and started Phase II in March 2010 [36]. The significant further progress made after the formal end of the retrospective impact analysis is described in the Discussion.

Health gain and broader economic benefits
Of the funded projects included in this research, again only a small minority (10%) claim to have already made an impact in any of the various forms this could take, with 6% of projects believing they had made an impact specifically in relation to health gains. Thirty-one percent of projects suggested that they expected to make some impact on health in the future, though it is recognised that the time lags, and their unpredictable nature, means a real impact on health gain can take many years to materialise and is extremely difficult to measure. Nevertheless, many of the examples described

previously in which Asthma UK-funded research is making an impact on clinical policies, and on product development, are likely already, or in future, to be leading to health benefits. This is described in detail in the full report on this impact analysis but a few key examples are contained in Additional files 3, 4, and 5 which respectively describe the health gains that have arisen from the Asthma UK-funded contributions to research on leukotriene receptor antagonists [37] and on immunotherapy for allergic rhinitis, and the potential health gains from the research on peptide immunotherapy.

Health gains resulting from improved therapies are likely to have broader economic benefits in terms of reducing the working days lost through ill-health [2]. In addition, school children sitting exams during the hay fever season can suffer [38]; they might benefit from immunotherapy.

There have also been broader economic benefits to the UK from some of the cases of product development, including from the work of Tim Williams, because UK companies have been involved in undertaking some of the development. Furthermore, the two spin-out companies described above, Circassia and Synairgen, are UK based.

A summary of impacts from each type of funding

The long-term funding for the professorial chairs has resulted in many impacts across the full range of payback categories, and the establishment of the MRC-Asthma UK Centre is a major additional benefit that can be at least partially attributed to the professorial chairs. Interview and case study evidence suggests both chairs showed considerable leadership in building up their multi-disciplinary departments that formed core elements of the Centre.

The case study approach identified the success of the MRC-Asthma UK Centre in Allergic Mechanisms of Asthma in making scientific and medical breakthroughs, training the next generation of scientists and doctors focused on asthma research, promoting collaboration, and attracting funding from other sources and increasing the funds available for asthma research. Interview evidence confirmed the documentary evidence from the House of Lords Science and Technology Committee which stated: 'We visited a striking example of effective collaboration at the MRC-Asthma UK Centre in Allergic Mechanisms of Asthma' [39]. Asthma UK's strategy documents [6] help inform the Centre's strategies. These successes and the pioneering nature of the collaborative Centre are further analysed in an additional file which summarises key points from the case study based on the Centre [see Additional file 6]. The creation of the Centre reflects current thinking on the importance of both translational health research, and the collaborations

between researchers and service providers and across institutions and disciplines [40-42].

The medium-term funding for the fellowships enabled some of them to develop a strand of research that made a range of impacts. Various individual projects and fellowships provided a very small return according to the survey, but others contributed considerably according to both the surveys and the case studies.

Discussion

As the only national charity dedicated to asthma in the UK, Asthma UK commissioned HERG/RAND Europe to apply the Payback Framework to a comprehensive analysis of the various types of research funding traditionally provided by the charity in order to shape the charity's future research funding to maximise benefits for people with asthma. Based on the funded projects included in this research, it appears that Asthma UK's previous research funding approaches have made some important contributions to research returns in the full range of categories. Whilst there are generally fewer impacts identified in the difficult to measure, and time lag dependent, categories such as impact on healthcare, some examples have been described. Various individual projects and fellowships provided a very small return according to the survey (and, for example the 13% of projects claiming to have made an impact on policies is much lower than the 60% figure claimed by primary studies funded in the English HTA programme, which admittedly is much more oriented to meeting the expressed needs of the NHS). Nevertheless, some Asthma UK-funded projects contributed considerably and the long-term funding of the professorial chairs has led to many and varied impacts, including in part to the establishment of the MRC-Asthma UK Centre.

The limitations of the study include the nature of the survey which attempted to be comprehensive, but some respondents thought it was too long and overall the response was less than 60%. As noted, there is a possible bias in the results as the average number of publications already known to Asthma UK prior to the surveys was slightly higher for the projects on which surveys were returned, than for those that were not. Inevitably there are also gaps in the data that can be collected, especially through surveys. A possible limitation in the other direction is that if PIs have not fully answered all the questions there could be some underestimation of the impacts, for example of the amount of follow-on funding. Furthermore, there are variations in the extent to which impacts have been demonstrated to result from the specific funding provided by Asthma UK. Whilst relying on PIs to complete surveys about their own research is clearly a potential limitation, the limited amount of evidence available from this study is in line with that from previous studies which appears to indicate that, at least in studies where there is no clear correlation between the replies given and future funding, researchers do not routinely exaggerate the impacts of their research [8]. Important impacts have been reported from the funding of professorial chairs, and also fellowships, but it is difficult to assess how much of these impacts should be attributed to Asthma UK funding.

Strengths of the study include the wide coverage of Asthma UK research, which was achieved by sending a survey to all fellows and to the PIs of projects funded and completed over a 10 year time period. In addition, the case studies provide detailed analysis of some of the research funded by the charity. Some of the case studies provide not only more detailed information than comes from the surveys, but also examples of whole categories of impact that had not been mentioned in the survey response from the project. All aspects of the data collection, analysis and detailed write-up in the full report are informed by the well-established Payback Framework which is reported to be the most widely used approach to assess the impacts from health research [8-10]. Previous reviews of studies assessing the impact from programmes of health research [8] do not seem to report a study that has combined such comprehensive coverage of the work of diverse streams of funding from one research funder with an analysis of the organisational mechanisms contributing to achieving the impacts; given the overall objective of the study, this is significant.

Use of the findings to inform Asthma UK's strategy

Overall this analysis has given Asthma UK a unique insight into its research and provided information to guide its future strategy. It has also shown that a medical research charity, even one with relatively modest funds, can make some significant contributions - not just in traditional areas such as knowledge production, but also in health policies, product development and improved healthcare. In particular, the analysis has highlighted to Asthma UK:

- the importance of offering a diverse approach to research funding to create a range of returns on investment;
- the merits in terms of impacts of funding up-and-coming scientists to establish them in their careers, and of providing more costly long-term support to exceptional senior research leaders who can pioneer large-scale developments in a particular research field;
- the niche role that charitable patient organisations have in providing key pump-priming funding to enable leading researchers to make major breakthroughs that they can then take to the larger general medical research funders for more substantial support, which is

particularly important given the relatively small budget available to Asthma UK to fund research;
- that Asthma UK's investment into medical research directly to improve the quality of life of people with asthma, though important, has been relatively small; and
- that the success of the MRC-Asthma UK Centre in Allergic Mechanisms of Asthma builds partly on Asthma UK's series of strategy documents, starting with that from 2002 [6], which helped inform the Centre's strategies, and the creation of the Centre reflects, and contributed to, current thinking on the importance of translational health research and how best to organise health research systems to meet the needs of patients [40-42].

The findings of HERG's evaluation placed Asthma UK in a strong position to re-focus its efforts, define the future vision for Asthma UK research, and publish its 2011–2016 research strategy. This strategy was informed at an underpinning level by the results of HERG's analysis in terms of the mechanisms the charity will employ to fund research. One of the key features of the new research strategy is the establishment of a second research centre focused on improving the quality of life of people with asthma, which will become known as the Asthma UK Centre for Applied Research. Asthma UK wishes to take the collaborative approach which worked so well with the MRC-Asthma UK Centre and create a similar network of leading researchers to develop large scale clinical trials and other investigative studies across the UK.

Whilst the retrospective impact analysis was completed in time to feed into the revised research strategy reported here, Asthma UK continues to monitor the progress of, and be associated with, some of the most successful developments. In the case of Synairgen the findings from the Phase II trials received significant media coverage in April 2012 because the inhaled drug (SNG001) significantly reduced asthma symptoms during the critical first week of infection and reduced the number of exacerbations. According to Stephen Holgate, quoted in the company's press release: 'This is a really promising breakthrough for the future treatment of asthma.... This trial is an important milestone in the development of our SNG001 programme from its origins in research supported by the MRC, Asthma UK, the British Lung Foundation, the National Institute of Health Research and the University of Southampton, to today's exciting results in this 'real world' asthma study' [43].

The progress made by some of the examples of research since the completion of the retrospective impact analysis conducted for Asthma UK illustrates that the relationship between analysing impact and revising the research funding strategy is likely to be a continuing process. The findings of such a retrospective impact analysis can, of course, be used to justify past expenditure, but as demonstrated here the retrospective analysis can also inform the strategies for organisation of health research with the aim of enhancing the level of wider impacts achieved. Some previous applications of the Payback Framework have examined the research impacts from various streams of funding from the same research funding organisation [12,44], and there is growing international interest in applying such approaches [45]. This current application of the Framework to the research funded by Asthma UK is more comprehensive in scope, and, in relation to the professorial chairs, provides for the first time, as far as the authors are aware, a detailed analysis of how long-term chair funding can successfully lead to the creation of an innovative Centre that aims to translate research into improved patient care.

Conclusions

Research funders will continue to be interested in systematically analysing the full range of impacts from the health research they fund. Through this piece of research, we have demonstrated that adapted versions of the Payback Framework can be used to conduct an assessment of the outputs and societal impacts from a portfolio of health research in a comprehensive way and, more significantly, that these can be used not only to help justify research expenditure but also to help inform the strategy of health research funders.

We systematically show all types of Asthma UK's research funding assessed are making impacts at different levels, with the chairs and pioneering collaborative Centre being particularly significant. Whilst inevitably only a minority of individual projects and fellowships directly contributed to societal impacts, some of the research portfolio is influencing asthma-related clinical guidelines, and some contributing to product development. The study's findings, especially in relation to the Centre, are being used to inform research funding strategies to promote the achievement of impact.

Endnotes

[a]The full report and volume of case studies describing the retrospective impact analysis of Asthma UK-funded research will eventually be made available on the charity's web site.

[b]Major clinical guidelines reviewed included: British Thoracic Society/Scottish Intercollegiate Guidelines Network: British Guideline on the Management of Asthma (2008, revised 2009); BSACI guidelines for the management of allergic and non-allergic rhinitis (2008); The European Pediatric Asthma Group: Diagnosis and treatment of asthma in childhood: a PRACTALL consensus report (2008); Chronic cough due to asthma: ACCP evidence-based clinical practice guidelines (2006); Allergen

immunotherapy: A practice parameter (several editions produced by the Joint Task Force on Practice Parameters representing the American Academy of Allergy, Asthma and Immunology; the American College of Allergy, Asthma and Immunology; and the Joint Council of Allergy, Asthma and Immunology); Allergic Rhinitis and its Impact on Asthma (ARIA) 2008 Update (in collaboration with the Word Health Organization, GA^2LEN and AllerGen); Global Strategy for the Diagnosis and Management of Asthma in Children 5 Years and Younger, Global Inititative for Asthma (2009).

Additional files

Additional file 1: Assessment of returns from research funded by Asthma UK. Description: Survey used to gather data about Asthma UK-funded projects and fellowships.

Additional file 2: Evaluating the returns from research funded by Asthma UK. Basic semi-structured schedule for case study interview with Principal Investigators that was amended to meet the circumstances of each individual interview.

Additional file 3: Extract from case study on the impacts from Tak Lee's Asthma UK's Professorial Chair funding: contribution to the development of anti-leukotriene medicines and the treatment of aspirin-sensitive asthma. Description: This is an extract from the full case study on the range of impacts from Tak Lee's Asthma UK's Professorial Chair funding, and focuses on just one of the areas in which he made an important contribution - contribution to the development of anti-leukotriene medicines and the treatment of aspirin-sensitive asthma.

Additional file 4: Asthma UK's project funding: summary of case study on contribution of Stephen Durham's projects to the evidence base supporting the use of immunotherapy. Description: This is a summary of the full case study based on Asthma UK's project funding to support the research of Stephen Durham that made a major contribution to the evidence base supporting the use of grass-pollen immunotherapy.

Additional file 5: Asthma UK's project/fellowship funding: account of pump-priming research leading to successful early trials of peptide immunotherapy and potential health gains. Description: This is a version of the account in the main Impact analysis report to Asthma UK that describes how Asthma UK's project/fellowship funding played a key pump-priming role in funding research that is leading to successful early trials of peptide immunotherapy that has the potential to produce health gains.

Additional file 6: Summary of case study on the emerging impacts from the MRC-Asthma UK Centre in Allergic Mechanisms of Asthma. Description: This is a summary of a few of the key points from the full case study on the emerging impacts from the MRC-Asthma UK Centre in Allergic Mechanisms of Asthma.

Abbreviations

HERG: Health Economics Research Group; LTE_4: Leukotriene E_4; LTRAs1: Leukotriene receptor antagonists; MRC: Medical Research Council; NHS: National Health Service.

Competing interests

The research team from the Health Economic Research Group (HERG) (Stephen Hanney (SH), Teresa Jones (TJ)) and RAND Europe (Amanda Watt (AW)) received funding for Asthma UK to conduct this study. This was a collaborative project between Asthma UK and the research team, but the research team was given independence in the key aspects of the project. Given the nature of the study project it was desirable for the research team from the Health Economics Research Group, Brunel University, and RAND Europe to work with Asthma UK on various matters. Asthma UK conceived the original project, but the research team led on all the remaining aspects, including the design of the project. Asthma UK used their access to researchers to distribute the surveys that had been designed by the research team. The case studies and all the data analysis and interpretation, and preparation of the findings were undertaken independently by the research team, with advice from Asthma UK.

Leanne Metcalf (LM) is Assistant Director, Research & Practice at Asthma UK.

Authors' contributions

LM conceived the project and assisted SH in designing it. SH led the data gathering assisted by AW. SH led the analysis and interpretation of the data, assisted by AW and TJ, with advice from LM. SH drafted the article, with support from LM regarding the links to Asthma UK's strategy, and LM, AW and TJ suggested revisions. All authors approved the final version.

Acknowledgements

We also thank colleagues who contributed in various ways. From Brunel University, Martin Buxton contributed to the design of the project and provided advice throughout, Elisa Garimberti contributed to data gathering and analysis, and Haitao Dan contributed to the data analysis. From RAND Europe, Steve Wooding provided advice throughout and Sue Guthrie contributed to data gathering. From Asthma UK, Malayka Rahman contributed extensively to data gathering, and Elaine Vickers provided advice throughout. We also thank the members of the Advisory Committee who provided a range of expert advice and input, and we thank all the researchers who participated in the project by completing surveys and through case studies.

This study was funded by Asthma UK.

Author details

[1]Health Economics Research Group, Brunel University, Uxbridge UB8 3PH, UK.
[2]RAND Europe, Westbrook Centre, Milton Road, Cambridge CB4 1YG, UK.
[3]Asthma UK, Summit House, 70 Wilson Street, London EC2A 2DB, UK.

References

1. Editorial: Unknown quantities. *Nature* 2010, **465**:665–666.
2. UK Evaluation Forum: *Medical research: assessing the benefits to society.* London: Academy of Medical Sciences; 2006.
3. Smith R: Measuring the social impact of research. *BMJ* 2001, **323**:528.
4. Pang T, Terry RF, The PloS Medicine editors: WHO/PloS collection "No health without research": a call for papers. *PloS Medicine* 2011, **8**:1.
5. Hanney S, Grant J, Wooding S, Buxton M: Proposed methods for reviewing the outcomes of health research: the impact of funding by the UK's 'Arthritis Research Campaign'. *Health Res Policy Syst* 2004, **2**:4.
6. Lee TH, Barnes J: Where next in basic allergy? *Clin Exp Allergy* 2002, **32**:499–506.
7. Buxton M, Hanney S, Morris S, Sundmacher L, Mestre-Ferrandiz J, Garau M, Sussex J, Grant J, Ismail S, Nason E, Wooding S: *Medical research - What's it worth? estimating the economic benefits from medical research in the UK.* London: UK Evaluation Forum (Academy of Medical Sciences, MRC, Wellcome Trust); 2008.
8. Hanney S, Buxton M, Green C, Coulson D, Raftery J: An assessment of the impact of the NHS health technology assessment programme. *Health Technol Assess* 2007, **11**:53.
9. Canadian Academy of Medical Sciences: *Making an impact: a preferred framework and indicators to measure returns on investment in health research.* Ottowa: Canadian Academy of Medical Sciences; 2009.
10. Banzi R, Moja L, Pistotti V, Facchini A, Liberati A: Conceptual frameworks and empirical approaches used to assess the impact of health research: an overview of reviews. *Health Res Policy Syst* 2011, **9**:26.
11. Buxton M, Hanney S: How can payback from health services research be assessed? *J Health Serv Res Policy* 1996, **1**:35–43.
12. Wooding S, Hanney S, Buxton M, Grant J: Payback arising from research funding: evaluation of the arthritis research campaign. *Rheumatology (Oxford)* 2005, **44**:1145–1156.
13. Oortwijn WJ, Hanney SR, Ligtvoet A, Hoorens S, Wooding S, Grant J, Buxton M, Bouter L: Assessing the impact of health technology assessment in The Netherlands. *Int J Technol Assess Health Care* 2008, **24**:259–269.
14. Hanney S, Gonzalez-Block M, Buxton M, Kogan M: The utilisation of health research in policy-making: concepts, examples and methods of assessment. *Health Res Policy Syst* 2003, **1**:2.
15. Jose PJ, Griffiths-Johnson DA, Collins PD, Walsh DT, Moqbel R, Totty NF, Truong O, Hsuan JJ, Williams TJ: Eotaxin: a potent eosinophil chemoattractant cytokine detected in a guinea-pig model of allergic airways inflammation. *J Exp Med* 1994, **179**:881–887.
16. Christie PE, Tagari P, Ford-Hutchinson AW, Charlesson S, Chee P, Arm JP, Lee TH: Urinary leukotriene-e4 concentrations increase after aspirin challenge in aspirin-sensitive asthmatic subjects. *Am Rev Respir Dis* 1991, **143**:1025–1029.
17. Durham SR, Walker SM, Varga EM, O'Brien F, Noble W, Till SJ, Hamid QA, Nouria-Aria KT: Long-term clinical efficacy of grass-pollen immunotherapy. *N Engl J Med* 1999, **341**:468–475.
18. Oldfield WL, Larche M, Kay AB: Effect of T-cell peptides derived from Fel d 1 on allergic reactions and cytokine production in patients sensitive to cats: a randomised controlled trial. *Lancet* 2002, **360**:47–53.
19. Asthma UK: *Asthma UK says farewell to world-leading professor.* http://www.asthma.org.uk/news-centre/latest-news/2012/01/asthma-uk-says-farewell-to-world-leading-professor
20. Thomas M, McKinley RK, Mellor S, Watkin G, Holloway E, Scullion J, Shaw DE, Warlaw A, Price D, Pavord I: Breathing exercises for asthma: a randomised controlled trial. *Thorax* 2009, **64**:55–61.
21. Bott J, Blumenthal S, Buxton M, Ellum S, Falconer C, Garrod R, *et al*: Guidelines for the physiotherapy management of the adult, medical, spontaneously breathing patient. *Thorax* 2009, **64**(Suppl 1):i1–i51.
22. Scadding GK, Durham SR, Mirakian R, Jones NS, Leech SC, Farooque S, *et al*: BSACI guidelines for the management of allergic and non-allergic rhinitis. *Clin Exp Allergy* 2008, **38**:19–42.
23. Bacharier LB, Boner A, Carlsen KH, Eigenmann PA, Frischer T, Gotz M, Helms PJ, Hunt J, Liu A, Papadopoulos N, Platts-Mills T, Pohunek P, Simons FER, Valovirta E, Wahn U, Wildhaber J, The European Pediatric Asthma Group: Diagnosis and treatment of asthma in childhood: a PRACTALL consensus report. *Allergy* 2008, **63**:5–34.
24. Dicpinigaitis PV: Chronic cough due to asthma: ACCP evidence-based clinical practice guidelines. *Chest* 2006, **129**(1 Suppl):75S–79S.
25. Brightling CE, Bradding P, Symon FA, Holgate ST, Wardlaw AJ, Pavord ID: Mast-cell infiltration of airway smooth muscle in asthma. *N Engl J Med* 2002, **346**:1699–1705.
26. British Thoracic Society Scottish Intercollegiate Guidelines Network: *British guideline on the management of asthma.* England; 2008. http://www.brit-thoracic.org.uk/Portals/0/Guidelines/AsthmaGuidelines/PreviousAsthmaGuidelines/asthma_final2008.pdf.
27. Saglani S, Nicholson AG, Scallan M, Balfour-Lynn I, Rosenthal M, Payne DN, Bush A: Investigation of young children with severe recurrent wheeze: any clinical benefit? *Eur Respir J* 2006, **27**:29–35.
28. Berry MA, Shaw DE, Green RH, Brightling CE, Wardlaw AJ, Pavord ID: The use of exhaled nitric oxide concentration to identify eosinophilic airway inflammation: an observational study in adults with asthma. *Clin Exp Allergy* 2005, **35**:1175–1179.
29. Jadad AR, Sigouin C, Mohide PT, Levine M, Fuentes M: Risk of congenital malformations associated with treatment of asthma during early pregnancy. *Lancet* 2000, **355**:119.
30. Tata LJ, Lewis SA, McKeever TM, Smith CJ, Doyle P, Smeeth L, Gibson JE, Hubbard RH: Effect of maternal asthma, exacerbations and asthma medication use on congenital malformations in offspring: a UK population-based study. *Thorax* 2008, **63**:981–987.
31. British Thoracic Society and Scottish Intercollegiate Guidelines Network: *British Guideline on the Management of Asthma: a national clinical guideline. May 2008. Revised June 2009.* http://www.brit-thoracic.org.uk/Portals/0/Guidelines/AsthmaGuidelines/sign101%20revised%20June%2009.pdf.
32. Xystrakis E, Kusumakar S, Boswell S, Peek E, Urry Z, Richards DF, Adikibi T, Pridgeon C, Dallman M, Loke TK, Robinson DS, Barrat FJ, O'Garra A, Lavender P, Lee TH, Corrigan C, Hawrylowicz CM: Reversing the defective induction of IL-10-secreting regulatory T cells in glucocorticoid-resistant asthma patients. *J Clin Invest* 2006, **116**:146–155.
33. Christie PE, Smith CM, Lee TH: The potent and selective sulfidopeptide leukotriene antagonist, SK&F 104353, inhibits aspirin-induced asthma. *Am Rev Respir Dis* 1991, **144**:957–958.
34. Laitinen LA, Laitinen A, Haahtela T, Vikka V, Spur BW, Lee TH: Leukotriene E and granulocytic infiltration into asthmatic airways. *The Lancet* 1993, **341**:989–990.

35. Wark PA, Johnston SL, Bucchieri F, Powell R, Puddicombe S, Laza-Stanca V, Holgate ST, Davies DE: **Asthmatic bronchial epithelial cells have a deficient innate immune response to infection with rhinovirus.** *J Exp Med* 2005, **201:**937–947.

36. Synairgen: *IFNβ in Asthma.* http://www.synairgen.com/programmes/ifn-β-in-asthma.aspx.

37. O'Byrne PM, Gauvreau GM, Murphy DM: **Efficacy of leukotriene receptor antagonists and synthesis inhibitors in asthma.** *J Allergy Clin Immunol* 2009, **124:**397–403.

38. Walker S, Khan-Wasti S, Fletcher M, Cullinan P, Harris J, Sheikh A: **Seasonal allergic rhinitis is associated with a detrimental effect on examination performance in united kingdom teenagers: case-controlled study.** *J Allergy Clin Immunol* 2007, **120:**381–387.

39. House of Lords Science and Technology Committee: *Allergy. Volume 1: Report. HL Paper 166-1.* London: The Stationery Office; 2007.

40. Cooksey D: *A review of UK health research funding.* London: HM Treasury; 2006.

41. Hanney S, Kuruvilla S, Soper B, Mays N: **Who needs what from a national health research system: lessons from reforms to the English department of Health's R&D system.** *Health Res Policy Syst* 2010, **8:**11.

42. National Institute for Health Research: *Delivering health research: national institute for health research progress report 2008/9.* London: Department of Health; 2009.

43. Synairgen: *Positive Phase II asthma clinical trial data.* http://www.synairgen.com/media/1536/19%20april%202012%20Phase%20II%20press%20release%20final.pdf

44. Nason E, Curran B, Hanney S, Janta B, Hastings G, O'Driscoll M, Wooding S: **Evaluating health research funding in Ireland: assessing the impacts of the Health Research Board of Ireland's funding activities.** *Res Eval* 2011, **20:**193–200.

45. Adam P, Solans-Domènech M, Pons JMV, Aymerich M, Berra S, Guillamon I, Sánchez E, Permanyer-Miralda G: **Assessment of the impact of a clinical and health services research call in Catalonia.** *Res Eval* 2012, **21:**319–328.

15

Post-hospital syndrome in adults with asthma

Mohsen Sadatsafavi[1,2*], Larry D Lynd[2,3] and J Mark FitzGerald[1]

Abstract

Background: Post-hospital syndrome refers to the period of generalized risk of adverse health outcomes among patients who are recently discharged from hospital. This period is associated with a short-term increased risk of readmission which may not be related to the original condition. While the majority of studies of post-hospital syndrome have focused on all-cause readmissions, whether and to what extent such a phenomenon exists within discrete medical conditions is not yet known.

Objective: To investigate whether the risk of admission due to asthma is increased in individuals who are discharged following any-cause hospital admission.

Methods: Using administrative health data for the period 1997 to 2007 from the province of British Columbia, Canada, we created a cohort of adults with asthma. Using a case-crossover design, we assessed the association between discharge from a hospital (exposure) within 30 days before an asthma-related hospitalization (the outcome), using two 30-day control periods within the same subject. Conditional logistic regression was performed to calculate the relative risk (RR) of the outcome in association with exposure. We performed several sensitivity and subgroup analyses.

Results: The final cohort included 3,852 patients experiencing 6,333 instances of the outcome. Mean age at the time of the outcome was 43.7 (SD 14.2), 69.0% of such outcomes belonged to females. The RR of the outcome within the next 30 days of a previous any-cause discharge was 1.40 (95% CI 1.22 - 1.59). However, the association was mainly caused by discharge from asthma-related admission [RR = 1.99 (95% CI 1.65 - 2.39)]. The RR associated with non-asthma-related discharge was 0.88 (95% CI 0.74 - 1.04) and was not statistically significant. Similar results were obtained in a range of sensitivity analyses.

Discussion: Our results indicate that in patients with asthma, the 30-day risk of asthma-related admission is increased after an episode of asthma-related hospitalization, but not after an episode of non-asthma-related hospitalization.

Introduction

Post-hospital syndrome refers to the acquired, transient period of generalized increased risk for a broad range of health conditions after discharge from hospital [1]. An important manifestation of this syndrome is the high rate of readmission in the critical 30 days after discharge, which is not necessarily due to the same condition. A recent study showed that nearly 20% of patients covered by a US national insurance program (Medicare, consisting of individuals aged 65 and older as well as those with disabilities or end stage renal disease) discharged from a hospital had another acute medical problem within the subsequent 30 days that necessitated re-hospitalization [2]. Reasons for readmissions often include heart failure, pneumonia, COPD, infection, gastrointestinal conditions, mental illness, metabolic derangements, and trauma [2]. Various etiological reasons are postulated for this phenomenon, including disturbances of sleep, nutritional issues, pain and discomfort, and psychological confusion [1].

While the typical post-hospital syndrome affects mostly elderly patients with co-morbid conditions, the potential etiologic factors exist regardless of age. In addition, potential causal factors might have differential effects across different medical conditions. As such,

* Correspondence: msafavi@mail.ubc.ca
[1]Department of Medicine, Institute for Heart and Lung Health, The University of British Columbia, 7th Floor, 828 West 10th Avenue, Research Pavilion, Vancouver V5Z 1 M9, Vancouver, BC, Canada
[2]Collaboration for Outcomes Research and Evaluation, Faculty of Pharmaceutical Sciences, the University of British Columbia, Vancouver, Canada
Full list of author information is available at the end of the article

studying post-hospital syndrome within the realm of specific diseases can be informative from a patho-physiological
perspective, and is also important from a clinical perspective as it can help risk-stratify individuals at the time of
discharge from hospital.

To our knowledge, no previous study has examined
the risk of an asthma-related hospitalization after discharge
from a previous hospitalization. Any hospitalization independent of the cause might affect the risk of a subsequent
asthma exacerbation in complex ways. Some of the postulated factors for the post-hospital syndrome can increase
the risk of worsening of asthma symptoms and asthma
exacerbations. For example, psychological stress is known
to be associated with asthma attacks [3], and changes in
the immune system and malnutrition are all associated
with an increased risk of the worsening of asthma [4].
In addition, medications that patients receive during
admission (e.g., non-steroidal anti-inflammatory drugs or
beta-blockers) might cause drug-induced exacerbations
[5]. On the other hand, patients with asthma who are
hospitalized for other reasons will most likely also be
managed for their asthma during the inpatient period,
and at times receive potent anti-inflammatory medications
which can reduce the risk of an asthma attack. Combining
all these factors, there seems to be different potential
mechanisms for post-hospital syndrome affecting the
risk of an asthma-related admission that has not hitherto
been evaluated.

Using administrative health data from the province
of British Columbia, Canada, we set out to evaluate
whether individuals with asthma are at higher risk of an
episode of asthma-related hospitalization after discharge
from hospitalization due to any cause. We also evaluated
such a risk across different subgroups of patients, and
evaluated the risk according to the cause of the original
admission as being asthma-related, non-asthma respiratory-
related, or non-respiratory-related.

Methods
Data
Records of the utilization of all billed services for the
fiscal years 1997 to 2007 were obtained from the British
Columbia Ministry of Health (http://www.popdata.bc.
ca/data) [6]. This study was approved by University of
British Columbia-Providence Health Care Research Ethics
Board (#H08-01287). No consent was required as the
data consisted of anonymized health records released to
investigators in accordance with the Provincial Freedom
of Information and Protection of Privacy Act. We had
access to consolidation files [7] and all records of inpatient
[8] and outpatient [9] encounters, as well as medication
dispensations (the PharmaNET database [10]) during this
period. Hospitalization and outpatient service use records
contain encounter dates and International Classification of

Diseases (ICD, 9th and 10th revisions) codes for the reason
for the encounter. For hospitalization records, up to 25
ICD codes are recorded, one of which is designated as the
'most responsible' diagnosis; i.e., the diagnosis responsible
for the greatest portion of the patient's stay in the hospital.
The length of stay in the hospital as well as admission type
(urgent versus elective) is also available. The medication
dispensation database includes variables such as the
unique drug identifier and date of dispensation [11].

Study cohort
Adults (age 18 years and older) were considered as having
asthma if during a rolling time window of 12 months they
filled prescriptions for at least three asthma-related medications (list of such medications is available in Additional
file 1). The date of the first of the three prescriptions was
considered the cohort *entry date*. The date of the last
resource use of any type was considered the *exit date*.

Design
We chose a case-crossover design for this study in which
each individual subject acts as their own control [12]. In
the study of the association of transient exposures with
acute outcomes, such as this study, the case-crossover
design is an attractive option as it inherently removes the
potential biasing effects of unmeasured, time-invariant
confounding factors [13]. Adjusting for such unmeasured
confounding factors is particularly important in the
present context as both the exposure and outcome in this
study are hospitalization events, and many factors might
affect the overall person-specific rate of hospitalization
(e.g., the patient's and care provider's threshold for
inpatient care, the availability of hospital beds in the
local health area, and co-morbid conditions). This design
is similar to the classic case–control design, with the main
difference that the case and control periods belong to
the same subject, albeit at different times. In a sensitivity
analysis we also performed a conventional nested case–
control study to evaluate the robustness of the results to
the design specifications. A schematic illustration of the
case-crossover design is provided in Figure 1.

Exposure
The primary exposure in this analysis was discharge
from an episode of hospital admission with at least one
full day of stay, regardless of the cause. We further categorized such admissions to be due to asthma-related
versus non-asthma-related as well as respiratory-related
versus non-respiratory-related. Asthma-related admissions
were those with the most responsible diagnosis being
for asthma (ICD-9 493.xx, ICD-10 J45/J46). Respiratory-
related admissions were those with the most responsible
diagnosis being for a respiratory condition (ICD-9 codes
460–519, ICD-10 codes Jxx).

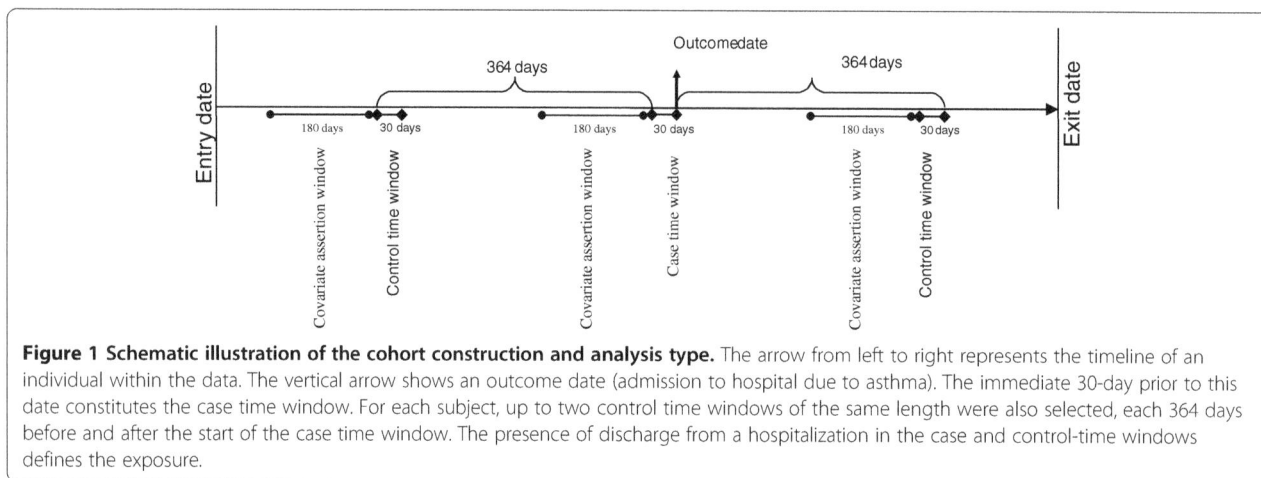

Figure 1 Schematic illustration of the cohort construction and analysis type. The arrow from left to right represents the timeline of an individual within the data. The vertical arrow shows an outcome date (admission to hospital due to asthma). The immediate 30-day prior to this date constitutes the case time window. For each subject, up to two control time windows of the same length were also selected, each 364 days before and after the start of the case time window. The presence of discharge from a hospitalization in the case and control-time windows defines the exposure.

Outcome

The outcome of interest was a non-elective admission to hospital with the main diagnosis being asthma (as described above). A national chart review of the data for the 2005–2006 fiscal year showed that the main diagnosis of asthma in a discharge record had a sensitivity of 87% (95% CI 79%–95%) and a positive predictive value of 90% (95% CI 85%–95%) [14]. In addition, restricting the study population to those who satisfied a case definition of asthma means that the subset of hospitalizations included in the analysis were even more likely to be truly asthma-related. In line with the general definition of post-hospital syndrome, readmissions that counted towards the outcome did not include elective admissions or emergency room visits that did not result in inpatient admissions.

Case and control time windows

The 30-day period immediately before each asthma-related hospitalization was considered as the case time window (see Figure 1). For each case time window, we considered up to two control time windows ending exactly 364 days before and after the index date. The choice of the timing of control time windows was to adjust for the effect of seasonality as well as day of the week as such factors might be potentially correlated with the risk of hospitalizations. We specifically avoided using control time windows that are adjacent to case time windows because first, the individual is protected from experiencing a hospitalization event in the time period immediately after the case time window (due to the length-of-stay of the index hospitalization associated with the case time window); second, the time adjacent to the case time window would belong to different month and potentially season which is an important factor affecting the risk of asthma-related hospitalization.

Eligible control windows were those that fit entirely within the interval between the entry and exit date of the individual. Control time windows that did not satisfy

such criteria were removed. Case time windows for which both control time windows were excluded were also excluded as they could not contribute to the statistical inference. Each individual could contribute several cases and associated control time windows.

Analysis

We calculated the rates of the occurrence of exposure in both the case and control time windows. In doing so, and in line with basic principles, we weighted each control time window according to the reciprocal of the number of control time windows for the corresponding case time window [15]. In the main analysis, using conditional logistic regression we calculated the adjusted relative risk (RR) of the asthma-related hospitalization (outcome) in association with exposure. We controlled for potentially time-varying measures of asthma severity (number of asthma-related admissions, outpatient service use, medication dispensation, as well the number of dispensed canisters of short-acting beta-agonists (SABA), inhaled corticosteroids (ICS), and combined ICS and long-acting beta-agonists (ICS + LABA)) and general measures of co-morbidity (Charlson co-morbidity index [16], total number of admissions, outpatient services use and medication dispensations), all measured in the 180 days prior to the (Case and control) time window (Figure 1). Robust variance estimators were used for inference to account for within-subject clustering of events (as outcomes that belong to the same person cannot be considered as independent observations) [17].

Subgroup, sensitivity, and alternative analyses

Subgroup analysis involved separately performing the analysis by sex and age groups. We performed several sensitivity analyses. These included an unadjusted analysis as well as performing the analysis using a conventional nested case–control design. The nested case control design followed the same principles as the main study

Table 1 Characteristics of individuals in the final data set

Number of outcomes per person	
Mean (S D)	1.64 (1.81)
[1,2,3,4+]	[2804,575,212,261]
Entry time	
(In years since 1/1/1997)	1.5 (2.2)
Event time	
(In years since 1/1/1997)	5.8 (3.0)
Event time	
(Since entry)	4.3 (2.8)
Age at entry date	
Mean (SD)	39.4 (14.1)
Age at outcome date	
Mean (SD)	43.7 (14.2)
Sex	
Female	69.0%
Male	31.0%

(cohort definition, inclusion criteria, case and control time windows) with the difference being that the control time windows were selected from other individuals in the risk set, and no 364-day-interval rule was applied. For a given case time window, the risk set was defined as those individuals who were at the risk of experiencing the outcome (that is, the follow-up day of the index case they was between the entry and exit date of the controls) and had the same sex, year of birth, and similar entry date (within 180 days) as the case. The nested-case control analysis was further adjusted for all covariates that were controlled for in the main case-crossover design. Other sensitivity analyses included choosing control time windows at different distances from the case time window. We performed two alternative analyses exploring the association between discharge from hospital and 60-day and 90-day risk of asthma-related admission. Finally,

to evaluate the potential impact of treatment in the post-discharge period in the association between the exposure and outcome, we performed an additional sensitivity analysis in which the regression model was further controlled for whether the individual received any controller medication (systemic corticosteroids, inhaled corticosteroids with or without long-acting beta-agonists, or leukotriene receptor antagonists) during the exposure (case or control) time window.

Results

The study cohort constituted 178,192 individuals with asthma among whom there were 6,333 asthma-related hospitalizations (outcome) experienced by 3,852 unique individuals. The associated case time windows for these events were matched to 10,737 control time windows (1.70 control time windows per event). Table 1 provides the basic demographics characteristics of the individuals in the final analysis.

Results of the conditional logistic regression are provided in Table 2. In 10.8% of case time windows there was a discharge from hospital. In comparison, in 7.9% of control time windows there was a discharge from hospital, resulting in a RR of asthma-related re-hospitalization following a hospital admission from any cause of 1.40 (95% CI 1.22 - 1.59), $P < 0.001$. Nevertheless, such an increased risk of the outcome was mainly due to the asthma-related discharge, with an RR of 1.99 (95% CI 1.65 - 2.39). Non-asthma-related discharges were not associated with 30-day asthma-related readmissions (RR = 0.88 (95% CI 0.74 - 1.04), $P = 0.14$). 81% of all respiratory-related discharges were due to asthma. As such, and expectedly, they were associated with an increased risk of the outcome (RR = 1.89 (95% CI 1.60 - 2.22)). Respiratory-related, non-asthma discharges were not associated with the risk of the outcome (RR = 1.23 (95% CI 0.90 - 1.68), $P = 0.20$). Non-respiratory-related

Table 2 Association between exposure (discharge from hospital) and outcome (asthma-related admission in the next 30 days)

Exposure	Frequency		Adjusted RR	P-value
	Case window	(95% CI)†Control window		
	N = 6,333	N = 10,737		
Any discharge	687 (10.8%)	849 (7.9%)	1.40 (1.22 – 1.59)	<0.001*
Asthma-related discharge	442 (7.0%)	389 (3.6%)	1.99 (1.65 – 2.39)	<0.001*
Non-asthma-related discharge	273 (4.3%)	495 (4.6%)	0.88 (0.74 – 1.04)	0.141
Respiratory-related discharge	523 (8.3%)	497 (4.6%)	1.89 (1.60 – 2.22)	<0.001*
Respiratory-related, non-asthma discharge	89 (1.4%)	124 (1.2%)	1.23 (0.90 – 1.68)	0.199
Non-respiratory-related discharge	189 (3.0%)	381 (3.5%)	0.78 (0.63 – 0.96)	0.017*

*Significant at 0.05 level.

†All RRs are adjusted for the following variables estimated in the 180 days prior to the start of the time window: number of asthma-related hospital admissions, outpatient services use, medication dispensations, number of dispensations of short-acting beta-agonists, inhaled corticosteroids, and combined inhaled corticosteroids and long-acting beta-agonists, as well as total number of hospital admissions, outpatient services use, medication dispensations, and the Charlson co-morbidity index.

Any discharge

Main results	1.40 (1.22-1.59)
Female	1.31 (1.12-1.53)
Male	1.62 (1.27-2.05)
18-34 y/o	1.74 (1.35-2.26)
35-54 y/o	1.21 (1.02-1.44)
55+y/o	1.56 (1.16-2.09)

Asthma-related discharge

Main results	1.99 (1.65-2.39)
Female	2.10 (1.66-2.67)
Male	1.73 (1.30-2.30)
18-34 y/o	2.43 (1.71-3.44)
35-54 y/o	1.69 (1.33-2.14)
55+y/o	2.52 (1.60-3.96)

Non-asthma-related discharge

Main results	0.88 (0.74-1.04)
Female	0.78 (0.64-0.95)
Male	1.22 (0.85-1.73)
18-34 y/o	1.00 (0.69-1.44)
35-54 y/o	0.79 (0.63-1.00)
55+y/o	1.00 (0.70-1.43)

Respiratory-related discharge

Main results	1.89 (1.60-2.22)
Female	1.93 (1.57-2.37)
Male	1.78 (1.36-2.33)
18-34 y/o	2.41 (1.77-3.29)
35-54 y/o	1.64 (1.33-2.02)
55+y/o	2.09 (1.41-3.08)

Respiratory-related, non-asthma discharge

Main results	1.23 (0.90-1.68)
Female	1.13 (0.78-1.64)
Male	1.49 (0.85-2.60)
18-34 y/o	2.00(0.87 -4.59)
35-54 y/o	1.17 (0.78-1.75)
55+y/o	1.01 (0.52-1.94)

None-respiratory-related discharge

Main results	0.78 (0.63-0.96)
Female	0.70 (0.56-0.89)
Male	1.05 (0.68-1.62)
18-34 y/o	0.83 (0.54-1.30)
35-54 y/o	0.66 (0.50-0.88)
55+y/o	1.03 (0.69-1.52)

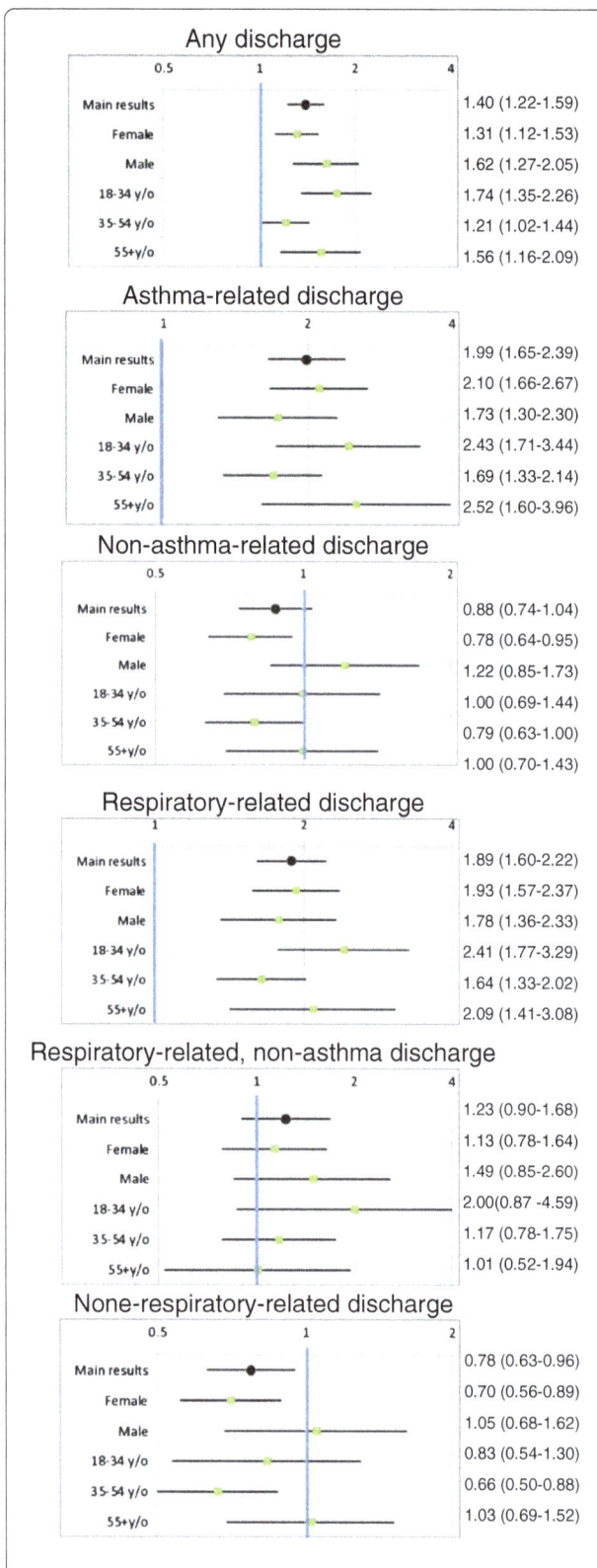

Figure 2 Subgroup analysis*. *All RRs are adjusted for the following variables estimated in the 180 days prior to the start of the time window: number of asthma-related hospital admissions, outpatient services use, medication dispensations, number of dispensations of short-acting beta-agonists, inhaled corticosteroids, and combined inhaled corticosteroids and long-acting beta-agonists, as well as total number of hospital admissions, outpatient services use, medication dispensations, and the Charlson co-morbidity index.

admissions were associated with a lower risk of the outcome (RR = 0.78 (95% CI 0.63 - 0.96)).

Subgroup analyses

Results of the subgroup analysis are provided in Figure 2. No obvious trend could be observed for the RRs across sex and age groups, although it appears the RRs for asthma-related or respiratory-related outcomes were higher among women than men, whereas the non-asthma-related and non-respiratory-related RRs were reciprocally lower among women compared with men. The negative association between non-respiratory-related discharges and asthma admissions disappeared in several subgroups but persisted among women and individuals 35–54 years old.

Sensitivity and alternative analyses

Results of the sensitivity and alternative analyses are provided in Figure 3. For the most part the overall direction and significance of the associations remained the same, with one exception: the negative association between non-respiratory-related discharges and asthma-related admissions disappeared in all sensitivity and alternative analyses.

Overall, in 31.6% of case time windows and 29.1% of control time windows a controller medication was dispensed (P < 0.001 for difference). In exposed time windows (time windows with a hospital discharge), this value was 39.9% (43.9% when the discharge was asthma-related and 35.7% when it was non-asthma-related, all P < 0.001 for the difference compared with unexposed time windows). However, in the sensitivity analysis that was adjusted for the use of controller medication, the RR of the exposure only slightly changed compared with the main analysis [RR = 1.38 (95% CI 1.21 - 1.57)].

Discussion

We used population-based administrative health data of an entire geographic region to investigate whether discharge from hospital alters the short-term risk of admission due to asthma. As expected, we found that asthma-related and respiratory-related discharges are significant predictors of asthma-related readmission, but non-asthma-related discharges were not associated with the risk of asthma-related readmissions. Other findings of the study remained the same in several sensitivity analyses. Our overall conclusion is that non-respiratory-related

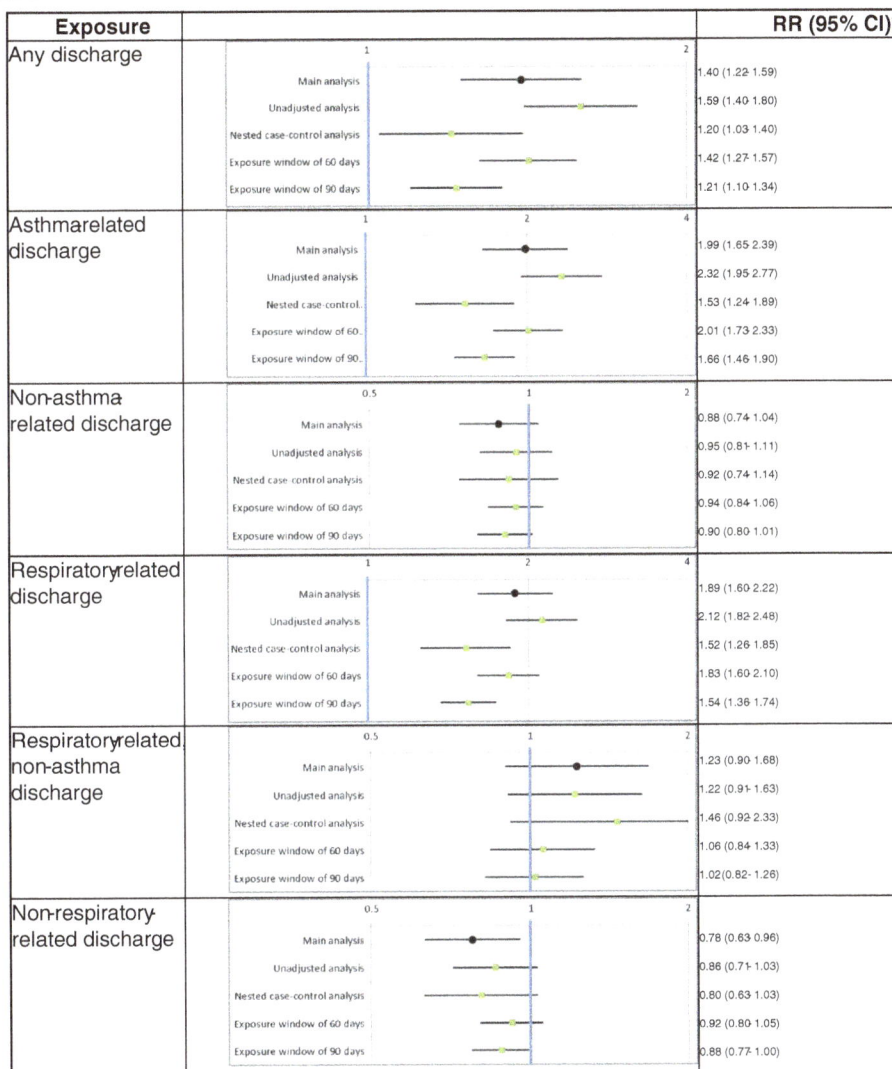

Figure 3 Results of the sensitivity and subgroup analyses. *All RRs, except for the unadjusted case-cross-over, are adjusted for the following variables estimated in the 180 days prior to the start of the time window: number of asthma-related hospital admissions, outpatient services use, medication dispensations, number of dispensations of short-acting beta-agonists, inhaled corticosteroids, and combined inhaled corticosteroids and long-acting beta-agonists, as well as total number of hospital admissions, outpatient services use, medication dispensations, and the Charlson co-morbidity index.

admissions do not appear to alter the short-term risk of severe asthma exacerbation requiring admission, whereas an episode of asthma-related discharge is associated with an elevated rate of readmission. In addition to being a chance finding, a reduced risk of asthma-related admission after an episode of non-asthma-related discharge might indicate that not only the underlying risk of asthma exacerbation is not affected by an episode of inpatient care, but such a discharge might result in a higher threshold for readmitting the patient. In addition, a period of inpatient care independent of asthma might prompt a review of asthma management, thus reducing the risk of asthma exacerbation in the post-discharge period. Evidence for this pattern was observed in our

data, as dispensation of controller medications were more likely to occur in time windows with, compared with those without, a hospital discharge record.

To our knowledge, the association between discharge from hospital and the short-term risk of admission due to asthma has not previously been investigated. Other investigators have assessed the rate of readmission after discharge from a previous asthma-related hospitalization, and factors altering such rates [6,18-21]. But these studies have not attempted to contrast the risk in the post-discharge period with control periods, and thus have not been able to show any change in the risk. In addition, many of such studies have been based on longer-term follow-up periods, and the associations reflect the impact of post-discharge care rather than the short-term effect of previous hospitalization [6,18].

In addition to relying on the data of an entire geographic region that is free from selection bias, the choice of the case-crossover design gives weight to the validity of our findings. Many factors, not necessarily captured in measures of asthma severity and co-morbidity, can alter the risk of hospitalization for an individual (e.g., threshold for hospitalization in the individual's local health setting, availability of hospital beds, to name a few) thus causing a spurious association between the exposure and outcome. As such, we believe the case-crossover design, in which such factor are relatively constant within a patient, is a robust design and the main results are less affected by such biases than the results of the nested case control study (although the overall results were similar).

The limitation of our study should be acknowledged. The identification of asthma was based on resource use records. However, the case definition of asthma, used by several other investigators, in combination with a record of asthma-related hospitalization, must have created a very specific sample of asthma patients. Nonetheless, we acknowledge that the diagnostic accuracy of asthma-related hospitalization in the extreme of age groups might not be optimal. Further, the risk of asthma-related readmissions might well be affected by the cause of the previous hospitalization. We decided not to subdivide the exposure any further than asthma-related and respiratory-related conditions as we were concerned multiple-comparison issues would make the interpretation of the results difficult. Additionally, the risk of asthma-related admission might be a function of events occurring within the prior hospitalization, such as whether appropriate care for asthma was provided at discharge, the discharge medications for asthma, and so on. The observed pattern of medication dispensation indicated that around the time of discharge, whether asthma-related or not, patients were more likely to fill prescriptions for asthma controller medications, but in the sensitivity analysis that adjusted for this pattern, no major changes in the findings were observed. This suggests that dispensation of controller medications did not play a major role in the observed findings. Unfortunately, as in many administrative health databases, medication records during inpatient time were not captured in our data, and in the 30-day time window individuals are most likely taking the medications they received during inpatient time and upon discharge; as such, dispensation records could not have been reliably interrogated for such associations.

While we confirmed the previous findings of an elevated risk of readmission after an asthma-related hospitalization, our study indicates that the risk of an asthma-related hospitalization is not increased after discharge from non-asthma-related admission. This is in line with the general belief that the significance of post-hospital syndrome is primarily related to certain co-morbidities of chronic diseases in the older population, and is not a general period of increased risk affecting an inherently inflammatory condition such as asthma. These findings can be of relevance from a policy and clinical perspectives with regard to the managements and recommendations patients with asthma receive upon discharge from hospital. Lack of association between non-asthma-related admissions with a subsequent risk of an asthma-related hospitalizations means in patients with known asthma who are hospitalized due to non-asthma reasons, care providers need to focus on other health conditions that are known to cause readmission. Future research is required to associate the risk of readmission with such factors as the level of asthma care during admission, outpatient care immediately after discharge, and provision of asthma controller medications in the post-discharge period as potentially relevant and modifiable factors determining the risk of asthma-related readmission.

Competing interests

The authors declare that they have no competing interests.

Authors' contribution

MS proposed the overall research question. MS, JMF, and LL conceived the design of the study and participated in planning the detailed analysis plan. LL helped with the acquisition of the data. MS performed the analyses and wrote the first version. All authors read and approved the final manuscript.

Funding

This study is part of the project "Platform for Outcomes Research and Translation in Asthma and aLlergy (PORTAL)" funded by AllerGen National Center of Excellence. None of the sponsors played a role in the study design, data analysis, interpretation or publication of the results.

Author details

[1]Department of Medicine, Institute for Heart and Lung Health, The University of British Columbia, 7th Floor, 828 West 10th Avenue, Research Pavilion, Vancouver V5Z 1 M9, Vancouver, BC, Canada. [2]Collaboration for Outcomes Research and Evaluation, Faculty of Pharmaceutical Sciences, the University of British Columbia, Vancouver, Canada. [3]Centre for Health Evaluation and Outcome Sciences, the University of British Columbia, Vancouver, Canada.

References

1. Krumholz HM: Post-hospital syndrome–an acquired, transient condition of generalized risk. *N Engl J Med* 2013, **368**(2):100–2.
2. Jencks SF, Williams MV, Coleman EA: Rehospitalizations among patients in the Medicare fee-for-service program. *N Engl J Med* 2009, **360**(14):1418–28.
3. Sandberg S, Paton JY, Ahola S, McCann DC, McGuinness D, Hillary CR, et al: The role of acute and chronic stress in asthma attacks in children. *Lancet* 2000, **356**(9234):982–7.
4. Greene LS: Asthma and oxidant stress: nutritional, environmental, and genetic risk factors. *J Am Coll Nutr* 1995, **14**(4):317–24.

5. Ben-Noun L: Drug-induced respiratory disorders: incidence, prevention and management. *Drug Saf Int J Med Toxicol Drug Exp* 2000, **23**(2):143–64.

6. Minkovitz CS, Andrews JS, Serwint JR: Rehospitalization of children with asthma. *Arch Pediatr Adolesc Med* 1999, **153**(7):727–30.

7. British Columbia Ministry of Health: *Consolidation File (MSP Registration & Premium Billing). V2. [Internet]. Population Data BC*; 2012. http://www.popdata.bc.ca/data.

8. British Columbia Ministry of Health: *Discharge Abstract Database (Hospital Separations). V2. [Internet]. Population Data BC*; 2012. http://www.popdata.bc.ca/data.

9. British Columbia Ministry of Health: *Medical Services Plan (MSP) Payment Information File. V2. Data Extract. [Internet]. Population Data BC*; 2012. http://www.popdata.bc.ca/data.

10. British Columbia Ministry of Health: *PharmaNet. V2. Data Extract. Data Stewardship Committee [Internet]. British Columbia Ministry of Health.* http://www.popdata.bc.ca/data.

11. Ministry of Health: *PharmaNet [Internet]. [cited 2012 Mar 29].* http://www.health.gov.bc.ca/pharmacare/pharmanet/netindex.html.

12. Maclure M: The case-crossover design: a method for studying transient effects on the risk of acute events. *Am J Epidemiol* 1991, **133**(2):144–53.

13. Delaney Chris JA, Suissa S: The case-crossover study design in pharmacoepidemiology. *Stat Methods Med Res* 2009, **18**(1):53–65.

14. Canadian Institute for Health Information: *CIHI Data Quality Study of the 2005–2006 Discharge Abstract Database [Internet].* Ottawa, Ontario; 2009. https://secure.cihi.ca/free_products/DAD_DQ_study_2005_2006_August_2009_e.pdf.

15. Schlesselman JJ, Stolley PD: *Case–control studies: design, conduct, analysis.* Oxford University Press; 1982.

16. Charlson M, Szatrowski TP, Peterson J, Gold J: Validation of a combined comorbidity index. *J Clin Epidemiol* 1994, **47**(11):1245–51.

17. Kelly PJ, Lim LL: Survival analysis for recurrent event data: an application to childhood infectious diseases. *Stat Med* 2000, **19**(1):13–33.

18. Bisgaard H, Møller H: Changes in risk of hospital readmission among asthmatic children in Denmark, 1978–93. *BMJ* 1999, **319**(7204):229–30.

19. Ather S, Chung KD, Gregory P, Demissie K: The association between hospital readmission and insurance provider among adults with asthma. *J Asthma Off J Assoc Care Asthma* 2004, **41**(7):709–13.

20. Reznik M, Hailpern SM, Ozuah PO: Predictors of early hospital readmission for asthma among inner-city children. *J Asthma Off J Assoc Care Asthma* 2006, **43**(1):37–40.

21. McCaul KA, Wakefield MA, Roder DM, Ruffin RE, Heard AR, Alpers JH, *et al*: Trends in hospital readmission for asthma: has the Australian National Asthma Campaign had an effect? *Med J Aust* 2000, **172**(2):62–6.

16

IL-17-producing peripheral blood CD177+ neutrophils increase in allergic asthmatic subjects

Carlos Ramirez-Velazquez[1,2], Elena Cristina Castillo[1], Leopoldo Guido-Bayardo[3] and Vianney Ortiz-Navarrete[1*]

Abstract

Background: A T helper cell (T_H) 17-biased response has been observed in patients with allergic asthma, particularly in those with neutrophil accumulation in the lung. Therefore, we sought to test the hypothesis that neutrophils might be an important source of interleukin (IL)-17 in allergic asthma.

Methods: Whole peripheral blood cells from non-asthmatic control subjects (n = 17) and patients with mild asthma (n = 7), moderate but persistent asthma (n = 4), or acute asthma (n = 6) were analyzed for IL-17A expression in CD177+ neutrophils. IL-17A expression was also analyzed in CD3+CD4+ and CD3+CD8+ lymphocyte populations. Asthmatic patients were classified as allergic to fungi, indoor allergens, or other allergens (*e.g.*, pollen) based on a positive intradermal allergy test reaction.

Results: The percentage of CD177+ neutrophils in whole blood of asthmatic patients was higher than in healthy controls and highest in the moderate asthma group. Furthermore, the percentage of CD177+IL-17+ neutrophils was elevated in patients with mild asthma, whereas the CD4+ IL-17+ lymphocyte population was higher in asthmatic patients and highest in those with moderate but persistent asthma. We also found that the four patients that were allergic to fungi had the highest percentage of CD177+IL17+ neutrophils and CD8+IL17+ lymphocytes.

Conclusion: IL17+CD177+ Neutrophils increase in allergic asthma patients especially when allergic to fungi. This cell population, through release of IL-17, might be contributing during the initial phase asthmatic disease and/or during disease progression but its role has not yet been established.

Keywords: Neutrophils, IL-17, Allergic asthma, Blood

Background

Asthma is a heterogeneous chronic inflammatory respiratory disease characterized by overproduction of mucus and airway-wall remodeling that leads to bronchial hyperactivity and airway obstruction [1]. Allergens and some pathogens have been implicated in the worsening of asthma [2,3], and the disease can be classified as mild, moderate, or severe according to the magnitude of the inflammation [4].

For many years, allergic asthma has been considered a T helper 2 (T_H2)-biased disease, characterized by eosinophil infiltration and the production of the cytokines interleukin (IL)-4, IL-5, and IL-13 [5]. A T_H17-biased response has also been observed in patients that exhibit chronic inflammation [6] and particularly in those with severe asthma who respond poorly to steroids, where inflammatory cellular infiltration in the airway is primarily due to CD4+ T_H17 cells and neutrophils [7-9].

Neutrophils have been associated with the severity of asthma [10,11]. Moreover, studies in humans have demonstrated neutrophil recruitment in response to allergen challenge that coincides with the peak of CD4+ T-cell recruitment. The peak of eosinophil recruitment occurs several days later [12], suggesting the importance of neutrophils in the pathogenesis of the disease. In addition, it has been reported that IL-17 favors neutrophil recruitment and leads to the induction of neutrophilia rather than eosinophilia in rodents [13,14]. The numbers of neutrophils in the sputum [9,10,15], bronchoalveolar lavage [12], bronchial biopsies [16,17], and peripheral blood [18] of allergic asthmatic patients have been shown to increase concomitantly with IL-17 levels [7,19-21].

---

* Correspondence: vortiz@cinvestav.mx
[1]Molecular Biomedicine Department, Centro de Investigación y de Estudios Avanzados (CINVESTAV)-IPN, Av. IPN No. 2508, Colonia San Pedro Zacatenco, México, DF CP. 07360, México
Full list of author information is available at the end of the article

IL-17 is mainly produced by T_H17 cells, but also by $CD8^+$ T cells, $\gamma\delta$ T cells, natural killer cells, and granulocytes [22]. In addition, it has been shown that murine neutrophils release IL-17 [13,23], but no further studies have investigated the expression and release of IL-17A -the most common form of IL-17- from human peripheral blood neutrophils in neither a normal state or during disease (e.g., allergic asthma).

In this study, we demonstrated that in fact human neutrophils are able to express IL-17. We also observed increased numbers of IL-17A + neutrophils in peripheral blood of asthmatic patients particularly in those suffering from fungal allergy-associated asthma.

Methods

Patients and control subjects

We recruited 17 asthmatic patients and all of them tested positive in the allergen skin prick test (Alerquim, Mexico City) to at least one of following: house dust mites, pollens, and fungi. We classified the asthma severity in our patients according to Global strategy for asthma management and prevention: GINA executive summary 2008 [24]. In our study we only included patients who matched the mild (seven patients) or moderate (four patients) categories according to GINA.

We also included acute asthma patients (six patients) defined as those who show exacerbation in symptoms such as wheezing, breathlessness, and chest tightness 48 hours prior to admission to the emergency department and received only rescue medication. These patients were enrolled within 24 hours of admission to the emergency department. Prior to the start of treatment, a blood sample was obtained for this study. However, three out of the six patients with acute asthma had inhaled β2-agonist short acting bronchodilators 48 h before their hospital admission. Patients who had an infection process along with the exacerbation were not included.

All subjects (asthmatic and control) were either non-smokers or former smokers who had quit smoking for at least 12 months. Subjects who had used corticosteroids, long-acting β2-agonists, leukotriene antagonists, or antihistamines in the month preceding the study were excluded, so were subjects with history of respiratory tract infection in the 4 weeks preceding the study. Healthy subjects without history of allergy or bronchial symptoms and who tested negative in the allergen skin prick test (Alerquim) made up the control group. Total serum immunoglobulin E was measured in every subject as well as the forced expiratory volume in 1 second (FEV1). Table 1. Three different independent measurements of FEV1 were performed with a dry spirometer (Medgraphics, Minnesota, USA) and the optimum value was expressed as a percentage of the predicted value. The Ethics Committee of the Fernando Quiroz Hospital approved the study, and each subject gave written informed consent.

Preparation of human mononuclear cells

Whole blood cells were obtained from 17 healthy volunteers and 17 asthmatic patients. Peripheral blood mononuclear cells (PBMCs) were isolated using a differential centrifugation gradient (Ficoll-Paque PLUS, GE Healthcare). The PBMCs were analyzed for viability with trypan blue, washed, and grouped into two, either for the ex-vivo staining or in vitro activation.

Cell activation

Heparinized whole blood (HWB; 500 µL) was stimulated with 2 µg/mL ionomycin (Sigma-Aldrich) and 40 ng/mL phorbol myristate acetate (PMA; Sigma-Aldrich) for 18 h at 37°C. PBMCs were stimulated with 200 ng/mL ionomycin and 2 ng/mL PMA for 18 hours at 37°C. In both cases 10 µg/mL brefeldin A (BFA; Sigma-Aldrich) was added during the last 6 hours of culture activation.

Surface staining and intracellular cytokine detection

Cells from activated and non-activated HWB were stained with fluorescein isothiocyanate (FITC)-conjugated anti-CD177 and phycoerythrin (PE)-conjugated anti-IL-5Rα (R&D) for 20 min at 4°C. Blood erythrocytes were lysed with lysis buffer solution (155 mM NH4C1, 10 mM KHCO3, and 0.1 mM EDTA, pH 7.3) for 15 min at room temperature (RT). Subsequently, cells were permeabilized using FACS Perm2 solution (BD Biosciences, San Jose, CA, USA) for 10 min based on manufacturer recommendations. Then samples were stained with peridinin chlorophyll-A protein (PerCP)/Cy5.5 conjugated anti-IL-17A (BioLegend). Finally cells were fixed with 2% paraformaldehyde (PFA) and analyzed using a CyAn ADP cytometer (Beckman Coulter, Inc. Indianapolis, IN; USA). Activated and non-activated PBMCs were stained with FITC-conjugated anti-CD-3, allophycocyanin

Table 1 Characteristics of study subjects

	Asthmatics	Non-asthmatic controls
Sex (female/male)	6/11	7/10
Age (y) (mean ± SEM)	22.35 ± 3.82	24.12 ± 1.38
Atopy (N°)[1]	17/17	0/17
Serum total IgE levels (IU/mL) (mean ± SEM)	425.2 ± 105.2**	278.89 ± 14.6
FEV1 (% predicted)	48-117	88-111
(mean ± SEM)	(77.65% ± 4.77)**	(96.59% ± 1.61)

[1]Atopy is defined as at least one positive prick test.
**$P < .01$ compared to non-asthmatic controls.
Abbreviations: FEV1 Forced expiratory volume in 1 second, Ig Immunoglobulin, SEM Standard error of the mean.

(APC)-Cy7-conjugated anti-CD4 and PE-conjugated anti-CD8 for 20 min at 4°C and afterwards permeabilized, stained for IL-17A and CD69, and fixed as described above. Cells were washed after fixation and analyzed with a CyAn ADP cytometer (Beckman Coulter). Isotype-control matched mAbs (BioLegend) were used as negative controls for each fluorochrome.

Flow cytometry analysis

Neutrophils were identified according to size (forward scatter, FSC) and complexity (side scatter, SSC) and by the expression of CD177 (BioLegend). Eosinophils IL-5Rα marker was used to distinguish them from neutrophils in HWB to further determine the percentage of $CD177^+IL17^+$ neutrophils. IL-17 expression was also evaluated in $CD3^+CD4^+$ and $CD3^+CD8^+$ lymphocytes from PBMCs previously gated according to FSC and SSC as well. CD69 was used as an activation marker for T cells which were activated with ionomycin-PMA. Data analysis was performed using the FlowJo 5.6.4. software.

Statistical analysis

Distributions of continuous variables are expressed as mean ± standard error (SEM) and median. A nonparametric Mann–Whitney U test was used to compare continuous variables, the Wilcoxon test for 2-group comparisons, and the Kruskal-Wallis test for multiple comparisons. The Friedman post hoc test was used to confirm differences in individual groups. P values less than .05 were interpreted to indicate significance.

Results

Peripheral blood neutrophils express IL-17 and increase in number in allergic asthma patients

The neutrophils population in HWB was analyzed by flow cytometry according to size (forward scatter, FSC) and complexity (side scatter, SSC) as well as the expression of CD177 (Figure 1). The percentage of neutrophils in the whole blood of asthmatic patients was higher than in healthy controls (P = .012; Figure 2A), and was highest in patients with moderate asthma (P = .0001), but no differences were observed between patients with acute

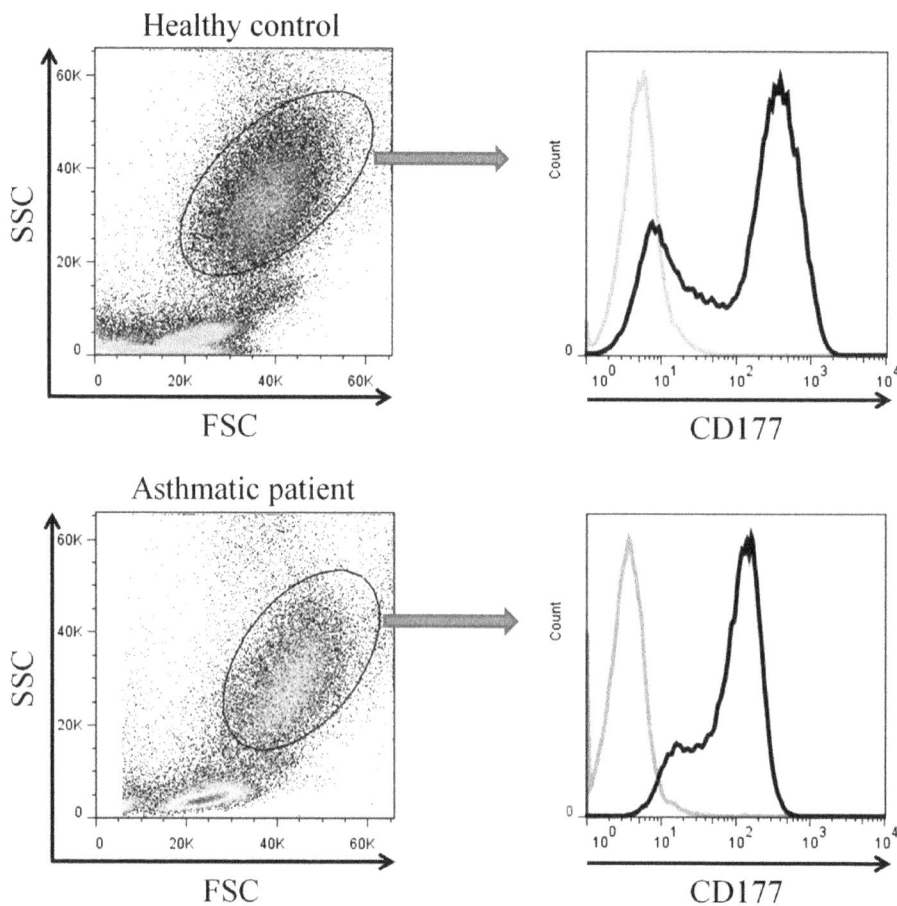

Figure 1 Peripheral blood neutrophils were identified within the granulocytes cells according to size (forward scatter), complexity (side scatter) and CD177 expression. A representative dot plot and histogram is shown from one patient and one healthy control.

asthma and healthy controls (Figure 2B). We observed that the percentage of CD177$^+$IL-17$^+$ neutrophils in allergic asthmatic patients was higher ($P = .003$) when compared to healthy controls (Figure 3A, 3B). No further increase was observed when neutrophils were stimulated with ionomycin/PMA (data not shown). In addition, we found that the percentage of CD177$^+$IL-17$^+$ neutrophils increased in mild ($P = .01$), moderate ($P = .005$) and acute asthma ($P = .041$) in comparison to healthy controls. The CD177$^+$IL-17$^+$ neutrophils percentage was highest in patients diagnosed with mild asthma, as compared to that in those with moderate asthma ($P = .0108$) or acute asthma ($P = .0001$). However, no significant difference was observed between the latter two groups (Figure 3C).

The percentage of IL-17A$^+$ neutrophils in peripheral blood is higher in asthma patients with fungal allergy

We sought to determine if a specific type of allergen preferentially activated the neutrophil response. To address this we analyzed the percentage of CD177$^+$ IL-17A$^+$ neutrophils from asthmatic patients that are allergic to specific groups of allergens based on positive intradermal allergy test reactions. Patients were divided into two groups: asthmatic patients allergic to fungi (*Penicilium, Rhizopus, Candida albicans, Alternaria alternata,* and *Aspergillus fumigatus*) and asthmatic patients allergic to other allergens such as pollens (*Lolium perenne, Fraxinus, Liquidambar, Pinus, Quercus, Olea europeae, Amaranthus palmeri, Prosopis,* and *Chenopodium album*) and indoor allergens (dust mites, dogs, cats, and cockroaches). We found that asthmatic patients that are allergic to fungi (4 out of 17) had a higher percentage of CD177$^+$ IL-17$^+$ neutrophils in their peripheral blood compared to patients with allergic asthma that are reactive to other allergens ($P = .0001$; Table 2). Figure 3D shows that patients with mild asthma who are allergic to fungi (2 out of 6) exhibited the highest percentage of CD177$^+$ IL-17$^+$ neutrophils as compared to those patients with mild asthma who are allergic to other allergens ($P = .029$) and to healthy controls (allergic fungal $P = .0001$, other allergens

& $P = .04$). While analyzing the numbers of neutrophils, we observed an increase in both the percentage of cells that express IL-17 and the number of neutrophils ($P = .006$; Table 2). This data suggests a positive association between neutrophils, fungal allergens, and asthma.

In addition, we analyzed the percentage of IL-17A$^+$ T cells stratified according to the two groups of allergens in the asthmatic patients. We found that the percentage of CD8$^+$ IL-17$^+$ T cells was higher in patients that are allergic to fungi ($P = .006$; Table 2). On the other hand the percentage of CD4$^+$ IL-17A$^+$ T cells remained unchanged ($P = .38$; Table 2) even between patients allergic to pollens and indoor allergens (data not shown).

CD4$^+$ IL-17$^+$ T lymphocytes increase in number according to asthma severity

PBMCs were isolated from peripheral blood of allergic asthma patients and healthy controls in order to identify IL-17+ CD4$^+$ T cells. Analysis was performed using flow cytometry based on the expression of molecular markers by selecting the CD4$^+$ IL17A$^+$ population by gating for lymphocytes. We observed that the percentage of CD4$^+$ IL-17A$^+$ T cells was higher in allergic asthma patients than in healthy controls ($P = .02$; Figure 4A). We found that the percentage of CD4$^+$ T cells was higher in all groups (mild $P = .007$, moderate $P = .0001$, acute $P = .04$) the highest being in moderate asthma patients ($P = .03$). We found no difference between patients with acute asthma and those with moderate asthma (Figure 4B).

Discussion

Multiple lines of evidence show a link between an increase in neutrophil numbers and the exacerbation, progression, severity, and difficulties in the control of asthmatic disease [9,10,15], not just at the bronchial level but also in peripheral blood [18]. Some mediators of these cells such as matrix metalloproteinase-9 [25], lactoferrin [26], reactive oxygen species [27], and IL-8 [28] have been associated with poor clinical evolution of the disease. During this study, even though only a small

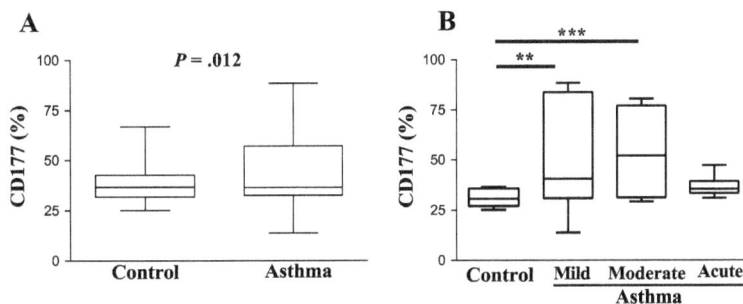

Figure 2 Neutrophils increase in patients with allergic asthma. (A) The percentage of CD177$^+$ neutrophils in allergic asthma and healthy control subjects is shown. **(B)** Percentages of CD177$^+$ neutrophils from patients with mild, moderate, and acute asthma in comparison with control non-asthmatic subjects. The asterisks indicate **$P = .01$, ***$P = .0001$. Error bars indicate SEM.

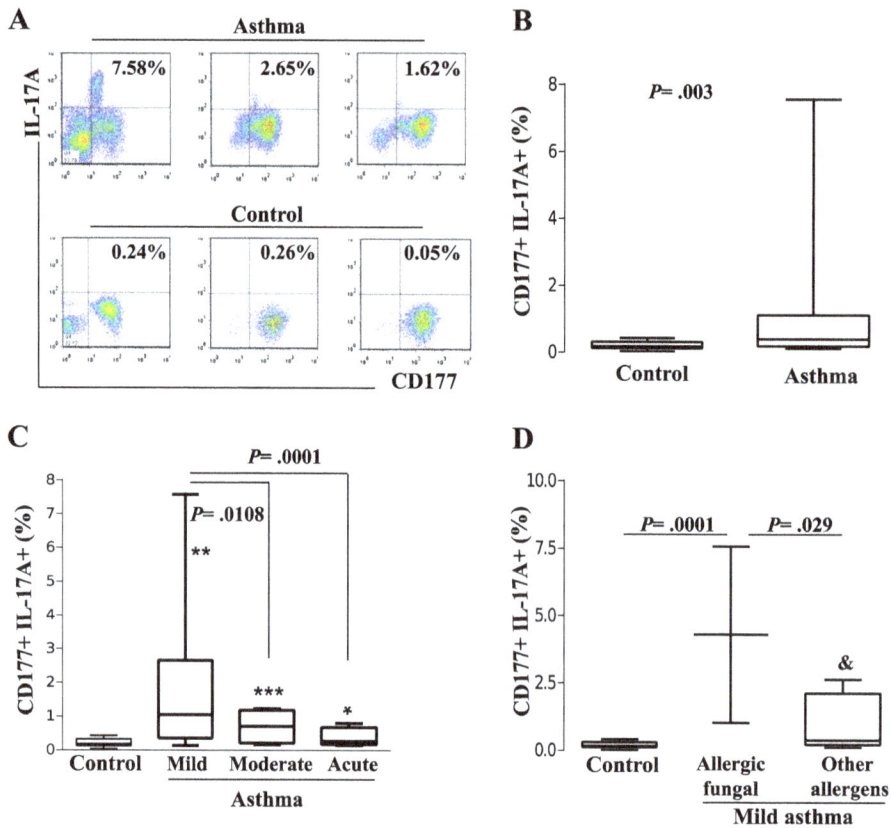

Figure 3 Neutrophils express IL-17A. **(A)** Percentages of CD177[+] IL-17A[+] neutrophils from allergic asthma patients and healthy controls. **(B)** Percentages of CD177[+] cells that are IL-17A[+]. **(C)** Percentage of IL-17A[+] cells stratified by the severity of allergic asthma and **(D)** by responses to allergy tests in mild asthma patients. The symbols indicate *P = .04, **P = .01, ***P = .005, and &P = .001. Error bars indicate SEM., and &P = .001.

number of patients was analyzed, we found an increase in the percentage of neutrophils in peripheral blood from allergic asthmatic patients. In this same group of patients we observed an IL-17[+] neutrophil subpopulation increase. The highest increase in this subpopulation was seen in patients with mild asthma. This result suggests that CD177[+] IL-17A + neutrophils might play a role in the early stages of the response. The difference in the number of IL-17A[+] neutrophils in the three evaluated groups did not change even after cells were

Table 2 Comparisons of biomarkers in patients allergic to fungal allergens and to other allergens

	Fungal allergens (n = 4)	Other allergens (indoor and pollen allergens) (n = 13)	P value*
CD177+ IL-17A + (%)	2.465 ± 1.716	0.6938 ± 0.205	0.0001
IL-17+ TCD4+ (%)	0.405 ± 0.233	0.417 ± 0.165	0.3801
IL-17+ TCD8+ (%)	0.277 ± 0.196	0.148 ± 0.042	0.0065
Neutrophil count (mm³)	7325 ± 1656	3761 ± 356.0	0.0067
Eosinophil count (mm³)	390.8 ± 218.3	693.5 ± 102.7	0.2931
CD4[+] T cells (mm³)	347.8 ± 147.8	507.9 ± 79.41	0.4001
CD8[+] T cells (mm³)	229.9 ± 56.56	363.5 ± 90.93	0.0528
Serum total IgE levels (IU/mL)	496.43 ± 294.0	352.0 ± 81.82	0.0352
FEV1 (% predicted)	83.75 ± 14.21	75.00 ± 4.99	0.1097

Data are shown as mean ± standard errors of the mean.
Abbreviations: *FEV1* Forced expiratory volume in 1 second, *Ig* Immunoglobulin, *IL* Interleukin.

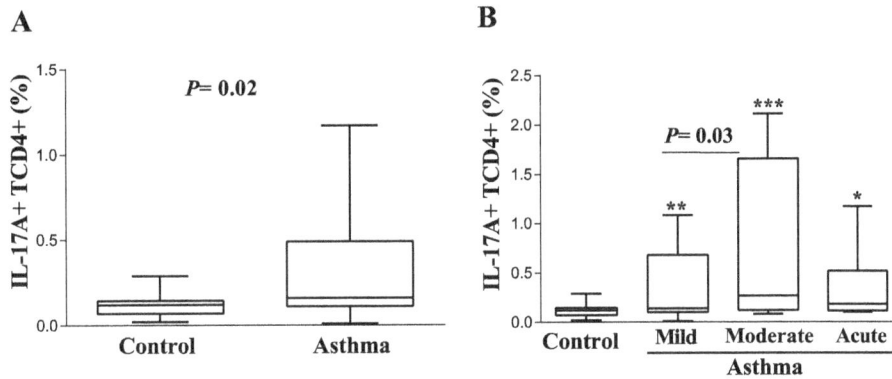

Figure 4 Percentage of CD4⁺ T cells expressing IL-17 (Th17) in asthmatic patients. (A) Comparison of the percentages of Th17 cells from patients and controls. **(B)** Percentage of Th17 cells stratified according to disease severity. Asterisks indicate *$P = .04$, **$P = .007$, *** $P = .0001$. Error bars indicate SEM.

stimulated *in vitro* with ionomycin/PMA (data not shown). This indicates the possible existence of neutrophils that have been polarized to produce IL-17A, as has been described for CD4⁺ IL-17⁺ T cells. However, further studies are required to evaluate whether or not these neutrophils subpopulation express the nuclear hormone receptor RORγt [22]. Recently, Tan Z et al., demonstrated that Gr-1^hi mouse neutrophils express RORγt and these cells express IL-17A mRNA after stimulation with LPS, LPS/IL-1β, or PMA/ionomycin suggesting that these cells have the capacity to produce IL-17A. The RORγt neutrophils appear to amplify inflammation and damage in ischemia-reperfusion (I/R) injury. Taz Z et al. also showed the presence of CD15^hi IL-17⁺ neutrophils population in peripheral blood from seven patients who underwent partial hepatectomy. Remarkably these CD15^hi neutrophils expressing IL-17A increased upon surgical intervention[29]. However, they are yet to prove whether these cells express RORγt. Their results resemble ours in that there is an IL-17A subpopulation of neutrophils in peripheral blood and that those cells might play a role in pathogenesis thought the release of IL-17A. However, whether this CD15^hi IL-17⁺ neutrophil subpopulation is the same as the one described by us is yet to be determined.

We found that patients with fungal allergies (4 of 17) had the highest number of CD177⁺ IL-17⁺ neutrophils. In this regard, Inoue et al. reported that the use of β-glucan from *Candida albicans* in the lungs of mice induces neutrophilic airway inflammation and the expression of different cytokines such as IL-17 [30]. Furthermore, Werner et al. reported that mouse neutrophils produce IL-17 in a dectin-1-dependent manner following infection with *Aspergillus fumigatus* [31]. Thus, we suggest that fungal allergens and their derivatives might activate neutrophils through the dectin-1 receptor, inducing IL-17 production

and contributing to bronchial inflammation during allergic asthma.

Additionally, we observed that the numbers of CD8⁺ T IL-17⁺ cells also increased in patients with fungal allergy asthma. Consistent with this observation, it has been reported that neutrophils regulate the infiltration of CD8⁺ T cells to the inflammation site in an animal model for fungal airway allergy [32]. Neutrophils could also act as antigen-presenting cells to promote IL-17 production by CD4 and CD8⁺ T cells [33-35].

Finally, we observed that the percentage of CD4⁺IL-17⁺ T cells in peripheral blood of patients was associated with the severity of asthma, confirming observations described by other groups [6-9,21,36]. We also observed an increase of CD4⁺IL-17⁺ T cells in acute asthma, reinforcing the importance of IL-17A in the immunopathology of asthma. Furthermore, in contrast to neutrophils, the production of IL-17 by CD4⁺ T cells was independent of the type of allergen. Importantly, Pelletier, M et al., described a chemokine-dependent reciprocal cross-talk between human neutrophils and Th17 cells. They described that activated neutrophils induce chemotaxis of Th17 cells by release of CCL2 and CCL20 chemokines. At the same time, CXCL8 is produced by Th17 to chemoattract neutrophils. They also found that CD15⁺ neutrophils and RORγt⁺ cells colocalize in gut tissue from patients with Crohn disease and synovial fluid from rheumatoid arthritis patients [37]. It is likely that the recruitment of neutrophils and Th17 in response to allergen is mediated by the chemokine cross-talk described above.

As it is now known, Th17 response is important for host defense against extracellular bacteria and fungi by indirectly inducing and activating neutrophils through production of IL-17A and IL-17 F. In this context, our study found higher percentage of IL-17⁺ neutrophils in asthma patients who are allergic to fungi. This suggests that this cell subpopulation might be activated by fungal allergens to release IL-17.

Conclusion

We identified a subpopulation of CD177[+] IL-17A[+] neutrophils in peripheral blood of asthmatic patients and healthy controls. Even though we were able to appreciate differences between asthmatic groups, due to the number of analyzed patients, it is not possible to define the relation between this subpopulation and severity of asthma.

Abbreviations
FEV1: Forced expiratory volume in 1 second; FITC: Fluorescein isothiocyanate; PMA: Phorbol myristate acetate; FACS: Flow cytometry (fluorescence-activated cell sorting); SEM: Standard error of the mean; FSC: Forward scatter; SSC: Side scatter; HWB: Heparinized whole blood; PBMC: Peripheral blood mononuclear cell; IL: Interleukin; T_H: T helper.

Competing interest
The authors declared no conflict of interest.

Authors' contributions
CRV and VON designed the experiments; LGB selected the patients; CRV did the experiments; CRV, ECC and VON analyzed the data and wrote the manuscript. All authors read and approve the final manuscript.

Acknowledgments
The authors are grateful for the support of CONACyT (grant 24312 to VON and scholarship 20700 to CRV) and CINVESTAV-IPN, Zacatenco. We thank María de Los Angeles Hernandez-Cueto for assistance with statistical analysis, and Ismael Carrillo-Martín on the discussion of manuscript.

Author details
[1]Molecular Biomedicine Department, Centro de Investigación y de Estudios Avanzados (CINVESTAV)-IPN, Av. IPN No. 2508, Colonia San Pedro Zacatenco, México, DF CP. 07360, México. [2]Allergy Department, Hospital General Dr. Fernando Quiroz Gutiérrez, ISSSTE, Calle Felipe Angeles y Canario. Colonia Bellavista, Mexico, DF CP 01140, Mexico. [3]Allergy Department, Centro Médico Nacional 20 de Noviembre ISSSTE, Felix Cuevas 540, Colonia del Valle, Mexico, DF CP 03229, Mexico.

References
1. Hammad H, Lambrecht BN: The airway epithelium in asthma. *Nat Med* 2012, 18:684–692.
2. Thumerelle C, Deschildre A, Bouquillon C, *et al*: Role of viruses and atypical bacteria in exacerbations of asthma in hospitalized children: A prospective study in the Nord-Pas de Calais region (France). *Pediatr Pulmonol* 2003, 35:75–82.
3. Murray CS: Study of modifiable risk factors for asthma exacerbations: virus infection and allergen exposure increase the risk of asthma hospital admissions in children. *Thorax* 2006, 61:376–382.
4. Hamid Q, Tulic M: Immunobiology of asthma. *Ann Rev Physiol* 2009, 71:489–507.
5. Woodruff PG, Modrek B, Choy DF, *et al*: T-helper type 2-driven inflammation defines major subphenotypes of asthma. *Am J Resp Crit Care Med* 2009, 180:388–395.
6. Pène J, Chevalier S, Preisser L, *et al*: Chronically inflamed human tissues are infiltrated by highly differentiated Th17 lymphocytes. *J Immunol* 2008, 180:7423–7430.
7. Al-Ramli W, Préfontaine D, Chouiali F, *et al*: TH17-associated cytokines (IL-17A and IL-17F) in severe asthma. *J Allergy Clin Immunol* 2009, 123:1185–1187.
8. McKinley L, Alcorn JF, Peterson A, *et al*: TH17 cells mediate steroid-resistant airway inflammation and airway hyperresponsiveness in mice. *J Immunol* 2008, 181:4089–4097.
9. Green RH, Brightling CE, Woltmann G, *et al*: Analysis of induced sputum in adults with asthma: identification of subgroup with isolated sputum neutrophilia and poor response to inhaled corticosteroids. *Thorax* 2002, 57:875–879.
10. Jatakanon A, Uasuf C, Maziak W, *et al*: Neutrophilic inflammation in severe persistent asthma. *Am J Respir Crit Care Med* 1999, 160:1532–1539.
11. Hastie AT, Moore WC, Meyers DA, *et al*: Analyses of asthma severity phenotypes and inflammatory proteins in subjects stratified by sputum granulocytes. *J Allergy Clin Immunol* 2010, 125:1028–1036.
12. Lommatzsch M, Julius P, Kuepper M, *et al*: The course of allergen-induced leukocyte infiltration in human and experimental asthma. *J Allergy Clin Immunol* 2006, 118:91–97.
13. Ferretti S, Bonneau O, Dubois GR, *et al*: IL-17, produced by lymphocytes and neutrophils, is necessary for lipopolysaccharide-induced airway neutrophilia: IL-15 as a possible trigger. *J Immunol* 2003, 170:2106–2112.
14. Fei M, Bhatia S, Oriss TB, *et al*: TNF-α from inflammatory dendritic cells (DCs) regulates lung IL-17A/IL-5 levels and neutrophilia versus eosinophilia during persistent fungal infection. *PNAS* 2011, 108:5360–5365.
15. Fahy J, Kim K, Boushey H: Prominent neutrophilic inflammation in sputum from subjects with asthma exacerbation. *J Allergy Clin Immunol* 1995, 95:843–852.
16. Foley SC, Hamid Q: Images in allergy and immunology: neutrophils in asthma. *J Allergy Clin Immunol* 2007, 119:1282–1286.
17. Qiu Y, Zhu J, Bandi V, *et al*: Bronchial mucosal inflammation and upregulation of CXC chemoattractants and receptors in severe exacerbations of asthma. *Thorax* 2007, 62:475–482.
18. Asman B, Strand V, Bylin G, *et al*: Peripheral neutrophils after allergic asthmatic reactions. *Int J Clin Lab Res* 1997, 27:185–188.
19. Sun YC, Zhou QT, Yao WZ: Sputum interleukin-17 is increased and associated with airway neutrophilia in patients with severe asthma. *Chin Med J (Engl)* 2005, 118:953–956.
20. Song C, Luo L, Lei Z, *et al*: IL-17-producing alveolar macrophages mediate allergic lung inflammation related to asthma. *J Immunol* 2008, 181:6117–6124.
21. Zhao Y, Yang J, Gao YD, *et al*: Th17 Immunity in patients with allergic asthma. *Int Arch Allergy Immunol* 2010, 151:297–307.
22. Korn T, Bettelli E, Oukka M, *et al*: IL-17 and Th17 Cells. *Ann Rev Immunol* 2009, 27:485–517.
23. Li L, Huang L, Vergis AL, *et al*: IL-17 produced by neutrophils regulates IFN-γ–mediated neutrophil migration in mouse kidney ischemia-reperfusion injury. *J Clin Invest* 2010, 120:331–342.
24. Bateman E, Hurd S, Barnes P, *et al*: Global strategy for asthma management and prevention: GINA executive summary. *Eur Respir J* 2008, 31:143–178.
25. Pinto LA, Depner M, Klopp N, *et al*: MMP-9 gene variants increase the risk for non-atopic asthma in children. *Respir Res* 2010, 11:23.
26. Taylor M, Zweiman B, Moskovitz A, *et al*: Platelet-activating factor- and leukotriene B4-induced release of lactoferrin from blood neutrophils of atopic and nonatopic individuals. *J Allergy Clin Immunol* 1990, 86:740–748.
27. Loukides S, Bouros D, Papatheodorou G, *et al*: The relationships among hydrogen peroxide in expired breath condensate, airway inflammation, and asthma severity. *Chest* 2002, 121:338–346.
28. Gibson PG, Simpson JL, Saltos N: Heterogeneity of airway inflammation in persistent asthma: evidence of neutrophilic inflammation and increased sputum interleukin-8. *Chest* 2001, 119:1329–1336.
29. Tan Z, Jiang R, Wang X, *et al*: RORgt + IL-17+ neutrophils play a critical role in hepatic ischemia–reperfusion injury. *J Mol Cell Biol* 2013, 5:143–146.
30. Inoue K, Takano H, Koike E, *et al*: Candida soluble cell wall beta-glucan facilitates ovalbumin-induced allergic airway inflammation in mice: Possible role of antigen-presenting cells. *Respir Res* 2009, 10:68.
31. Werner JL, Gessner MA, Lilly LM, *et al*: Neutrophils produce interleukin 17A (IL-17A) in a dectin-1- and IL-23-dependent manner during invasive fungal infection. *Infect Immun* 2011, 79:3966–3977.
32. Park S, Wiekowski M, Lira S, Mehrad B: Neutrophils regulate airway responses in a model of fungal allergic airways disease. *J Immunol* 2006, 176:2538–2545.

33. Abi Abdallah DS, Egan CE, Butcher BA, *et al:* Mouse neutrophils are professional antigen-presenting cells programmed to instruct Th1 and Th17 T-cell differentiation. *Int Immunol* 2011, **23:**317–326.
34. Beauvillain C, Delneste Y, Scotet M, *et al:* Neutrophils efficiently cross-prime naive T cells in vivo. *Blood* 2007, **110:**2965–2973.
35. Yang CW, Strong BSI, Miller MJ, *et al:* Neutrophils influence the level of antigen presentation during the immune response to protein antigens in adjuvants. *J Immunol* 2010, **185:**2927–2934.
36. Kudo M, Melton AC, Chen C, *et al:* IL-17A produced by αβ T cells drives airway hyper-responsiveness in mice and enhances mouse and human airway smooth muscle contraction. *Nat Med* 2012, **18:**547–554.
37. Pelletier M, Maggi L, Micheletti A, *et al:* Evidence for a cross-talk between human neutrophils and Th17 cells. *Blood* 2010, **115:**335–343.

Epigenetic regulation of asthma and allergic disease

Philippe Bégin and Kari C Nadeau[*]

Abstract

Epigenetics of asthma and allergic disease is a field that has expanded greatly in the last decade. Previously thought only in terms of cell differentiation, it is now evident the epigenetics regulate many processes. With T cell activation, commitment toward an allergic phenotype is tightly regulated by DNA methylation and histone modifications at the Th2 locus control region. When normal epigenetic control is disturbed, either experimentally or by environmental exposures, Th1/Th2 balance can be affected. Epigenetic marks are not only transferred to daughter cells with cell replication but they can also be inherited through generations. In animal models, with constant environmental pressure, epigenetically determined phenotypes are amplified through generations and can last up to 2 generations after the environment is back to normal. In this review on the epigenetic regulation of asthma and allergic diseases we review basic epigenetic mechanisms and discuss the epigenetic control of Th2 cells. We then cover the transgenerational inheritance model of epigenetic traits and discuss how this could relate the amplification of asthma and allergic disease prevalence and severity through the last decades. Finally, we discuss recent epigenetic association studies for allergic phenotypes and related environmental risk factors as well as potential underlying mechanisms for these associations.

Keywords: Epigenetic, Asthma, Allergy, Atopy, Inheritance, Transgenerational, Methylation, Histone, Th2, Amplification hypothesis

Introduction

The term epigenetics was coined by C.H. Waddington in the 1950's to describe means in addition to genetics to explain cell differentiation [1]. The concept of epigenetics was initially limited to cell differentiation from pluripotent stem cells to unipotent well differentiated cells, but the modern definition of epigenetics has been broaden beyond differentiation to include non-sequence inheritance. Epigenetic mechanisms have been shown to regulate many genes including those involved in inflammation and the immune response and to ensure inheritance of phenotype with cell division [2,3].

The purpose of this review is to provide allergy/immunology professionals and researchers with a broad, yet easy-to-follow, review of the epigenetic regulation of asthma and allergic disease. The main focus will be on DNA methylation and histone modifications, their relevance in the process of allergic sensitization, their impact on disease heritability and association with environmental exposure and allergy phenotype. MicroRNA, which constitute a distinct epigenetic mechanism, are beyond the scope of this review. Their role in allergic disease has been reviewed recently elsewhere [4].

The basics

DNA methylation was the first epigenetic mechanism recognised and the one that is most extensively studied. De novo methylation occurs in response to various cellular stressors and signal by DNA methyltransferases (Dnmt3a and Dmnt3b) which add a methyl group to position 5 of cytosine residues at a CpG site (Figure 1). CpG sites are dinucleotides consisting of a cytosine and guanine (the "p" stands for the phosphodiester bond linking the 2 nucleotides) which occur throughout the genome but may be concentrated in clusters referred to as CpG islands found at important regulatory sites, such as promoter and enhancer regions [5]. CpG islands are defined as a region with 200 base pairs containing an observed-to-expected CpG ratio that is greater than 60

* Correspondence: knadeau@stanford.edu
Allergy, Immunology, and Rheumatology Division, Stanford University, 269 Campus Drive, Stanford, California, USA

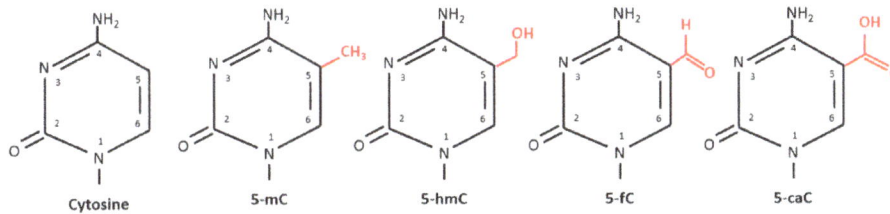

Figure 1 Structure of methylcytosine and its by-products. 5-mC = 5'methylcytosine; 5-hmC = 5'-hydroxymethylcytosine; 5-fC = 5'-formylcytosine; 5-caC = 5'-carboxymethylcytosine.

[6,7]. In terminally differentiated cells up to 90% of genome CpG sites are methylated with most unmethylated CpG islands found in functionally active genes [5].

The palindromic nature of a CpG site is important as it ensures replication of the methylation pattern with each cell division [5]. With DNA replication, both separated strands of DNA will each carry one methylated cytosine to be used as a template for duplication (Figure 2). The resulting daughter DNA duplex strands will thus be hemi-methylated. This hemi-methylated DNA is recognized by a different DNA methyltransferase isoform (Dnmt1) which methylates CpG sites on the new strand using the old one as a template. This maintenance methylation ensures conservation of the methylation pattern during cell division.

Conversely, a CpG site can be demethylated by oxidation of the methyl group. Physiologically, this process is initiated by the enzyme Ten-eleven translocation (TET) dioxygenase which gives rise to 5-hydroxymethylcytosine and then to 5-formylcytosine and 5-carboxylcytosine [8]. These modified nucleic acids can also be generated, although far less efficiently, by radical reactions involving hydroxyl radical and one-electron oxidants. They are then excised by the DNA repair enzyme thymine DNA glycosylase and replaced by a normal cytosine [9].

The mechanism by which DNA methylation is associated with gene silencing is still not fully understood. Earlier studies reported that methylation could directly limit the access to transcription factors (TF) [10]. Although this is true for some TF, it is not an absolute rule as some TF have been shown to have greater specificity for methylated binding motifs [11]. Methylated DNA can also recruit methyl-CpG binding proteins which compete with TF for access to binding sites [12]. Some of these proteins, such as MeCP2, can further recruit histone modifying enzymes to add another level of epigenetic modifications (discussed below) [13]. However, the interaction between DNA methylation and other epigenetic mechanisms is not unidirectional as histone modifications can also affect DNA methylation [14]. In fact, studies in stem cells and thymocytes have shown chromatin inactivation by histone and chromatin modifying enzymes to precede de novo DNA methylation

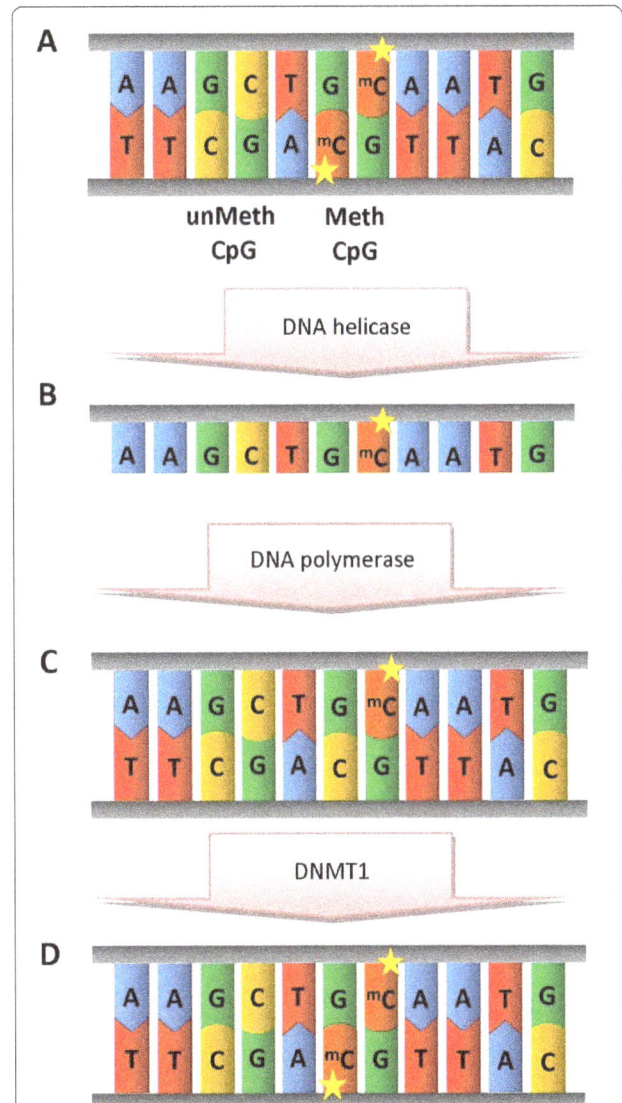

Figure 2 Replication of methylated DNA. The palindromic nature of CpG sites is key to their inheritance **(A)**. With replication, each separated strand carries one methylated cytosine **(B)**. The daughter hemi-methylated DNA **(C)** is recognised by DNMT isoform 1 which methylates CpG sites on the new strand using the old one as a template **(D)**.

during progressive epigenetic silencing [15-17]. Regardless of its underlying mechanism, DNA methylation is important in itself and should not be viewed as an epiphenomenon of other epigenetic mechanism as DNMT mutants display a multitude of defects, including aberrant gene expression, activation of mobile DNA elements and reduced genome stability [18].

Chromatin, the complex of DNA and nucleic proteins in the nucleus, is another central target of epigenetic modifications. Transcriptionally inactive heterochromatin is packed densely whereas active euchromatin is less condensed (Figure 3). The core component of chromatin is the histone octamer which organises DNA in structural units called nucleosomes [18]. The histone octamer consists of 2 dimers of core histones H2A and H2B and 2 dimers of core histones H3 and H4. Chromatin remodelling is a fundamental mechanism for establishing somatic cell memory of gene expression pattern. It is a dynamic process which is regulated by histones and ATP-dependent chromatin remodeling complexes which either move, eject or restructure nucleosomes. The "open" or "closed" state of the chromatin near a particular gene can be revealed by examining DNA sensitivity to the enzyme DNAse I by way of a procedure known as a DNAse sensitivity assay. This technique is based on the fact that DNAse I degrades open DNA more quickly than closed DNA, hence the term DNAse I hypersensitivity site (DHS) [19].

Core histones have long N-terminal tails protruding from the nucleosome which can undergo posttranslational modifications that alter their interaction with DNA and nuclear proteins. The standard way of reporting those modifications is by naming the histone, followed by the amino acid, and the modification. For example, H3K4me1 would denote single methylation (me1) of lysine 4 (k4) on histone 3 (H3). Research has shown a strong relation between covalent histone modifications and gene expression [18]. As a general rule, histone acetylation or phosphorylation are associated with an active state. Histone methylation, on the other hand, appears to have diverse function in the control of gene activity, depending on the amino acid and the number of methyl- groups added. The nature and combination of these changes determine the extent of expression, with those highly expressed genes associated with greater permissive histone modifications and those less frequently transcribed ones associated with repressive changes and more tightly packaged chromatin, although the relationship between gene expression status and histone modification is not absolute [20]. In addition to influencing chromatin structure, recruitment of chromatin-remodelling complexes by covalently modified amino acid on histone tails may also help target gene locus for pre-initiation of transcription gene [21,22]. The addition or removal of the various chemical elements on histones is catalyzed by histone modifying complexes such as histone acetyl transferase (HAT) and histone deactetylase (HDAC) which add and remove acetyl- groups on histone residues, respectively.

Epigenetic control of T cell phenotype
Th2 differentiation
While epigenetic changes have been coined as the hallmark of cell differentiation, their importance in other

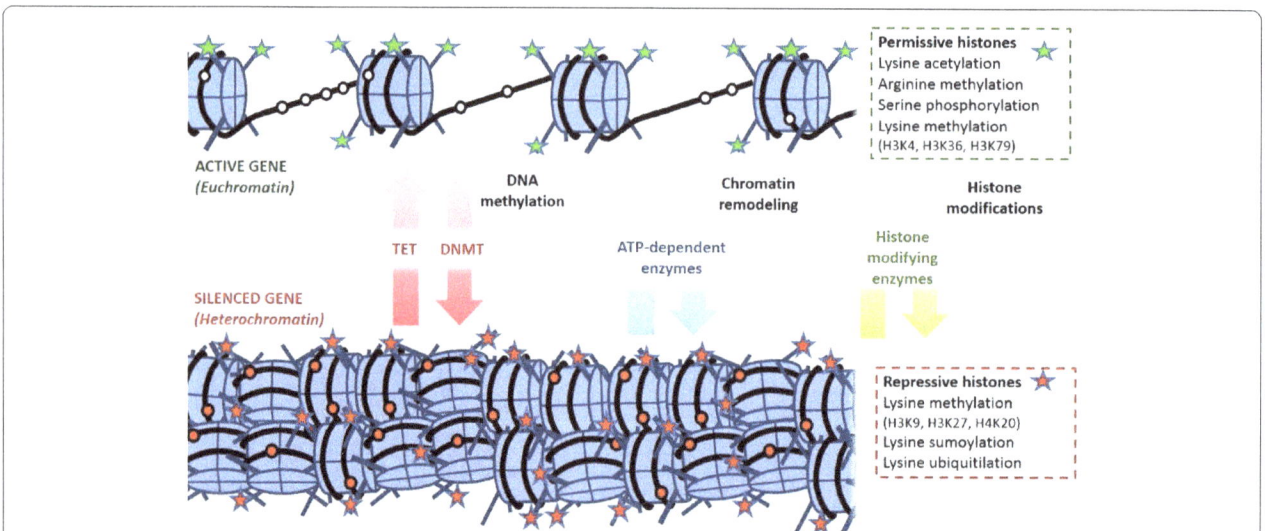

Figure 3 Euchromatin and heterochromatin. Unmethylated CpG islands (blank circles), permissive histone modifications (green stars) and loose chromatin structure promote gene transcription in the euchromatin state. Conversely, DNA methylation (red circles), repressive histone modifications (red stars) and condensed structure prevent transcription in the heterochromatin state. Although governed by distinct enzymes, cooperativity and interaction between the different epigenetic modifications provide a self-reinforcing mechanism for epigenetic regulation. TET=Ten-eleven translocation dioxygenase; DNMT=DNA methyltransferase.

processes is now coming to light. Of note, T cell activation and skewing, which could be viewed as a certain type of cell differentiation, is governed in great parts by epigenetic changes which insure that the clone of a T cell will retain its phenotype (Th2, Th1 or otherwise) [23].

Th2 skewing is triggered by simultaneous TCR and IL4 receptor activation, which leads to the phosphorylation of STAT6 and expression of Th2 master regulator GATA-3 and Th2 signature cytokines, including IL-4. Th1 differentiation is similarly triggered by simultaneous TCR and IL-12 receptor activation, phosphorylation of STAT4 and expression of Th1 master regulator TBET and Th1 signature cytokine INF-γ, with silencing of Th2 cytokines.

In resting CD4 T cells, both IL-4 and IFN-g genes are methylated [24]. Upon allergenic sensitization, the IL-4 promoter in allergen-specific T cells is demethylated, the extent of which correlates with IL-4 expression [24]. The IL-4 locus of Th2 cells is also marked with permissive histone modifications H3K4me which are absent in Th1 or naïve T cells [25]. Similar modifications are found at the IFN-γ locus in Th1 cells or the IL-17 locus in Th17 cells.

The main Th2 genes are positioned in the Th2 locus control region (LCR) on chromosome 5 which forms a chromatin hub that interacts with GATA-3 (Figure 4) [23]. GATA-3 then interacts with HAT enzyme p300 and with chromatin remodeling complex component Chd to induce permissive histone and chromatin changes at the Th2 LCR [26]. The GATA-3/Chd complex also binds HDAC to repress the tbx21 locus encoding TBET, the master regulator of Th1 differentiation which activates Th1 genes and suppresses Th2 genes [26], and recruits the H3k27m3 methyltransferase EZH2 to the IFN-g locus, causing its inhibition [27]. Further suppression of Th1 cytokines is achieved by the increase of their DNA methylation from naïve state [28]. In Th1 cells, STAT4 and TBET have been shown to exert similar but inverse influence on IFN-g and Th2 genes epigenetics to promote Th1 skewing [29].

The exact mechanism of DNA demethylation of Th2 genes is still incompletely understood, possibly due to the only recent discovery of the TET enzymes which are responsible for physiological DNA demethylation. In a mouse study, GATA-3 was insufficient to induce DNA demethylation of the RAD50 DHS site 7 in the Th2 LCR, although the process was shown to be dependent on STAT6 [30]. Interestingly, knocking-out RAD50 DHS site 6 prevented DNA methylation of IL-4, IL-5 and IL-13, suggesting an interdependence between those genes and an important role for the chromatin hub structure of the Th2 LCR (Figure 4) [31].

Interestingly, the GATA-3 promoter has been shown to keep its repressive histone modification despite TH2 activation and present a bivalent state with both repressive and activating histone modification [25]. This suggests an important role for positive feedback to additionally insure its stable expression, with GATA-3 positive binding to its regulatory elements. It is also worth noting that the main anti-Th1 effect of GATA-3 is exerted through direct inhibition of the IL-12/STAT4 and RUNX pathways [23].

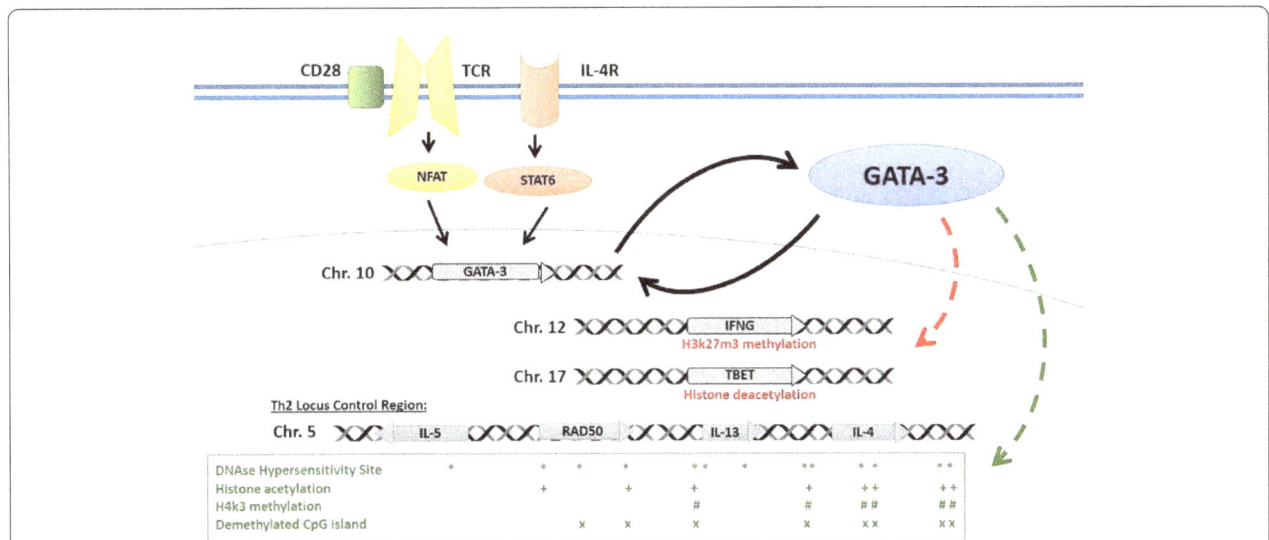

Figure 4 Epigenetic control of the Th2 locus. Master regulator GATA-3 is induced by TCR and IL-4 receptor activation and maintains its own expression with a positive feedback mechanism. GATA-3 induces repressive histone modifications at Th1 loci (TBET, IFNG). It interacts with HAT enzyme p300 with chromatin remodeling complex component Chd to induce permissive histone and chromatin changes at the Th2 LCR. Distribution of main epigenetic marks at the Th2 LCR [23] are presented in the lower box.

Establishment of T regulatory phenotype

T regulatory cells are a subset of T cells which suppress the inflammatory response and thus play an important role in immune tolerance to self and exogenous antigens. Their function and number in tissue has been shown to inversely correlate with allergic phenotypes and their importance in allergic disease has been well described [32].

FOXP3 is the master regulator for regulatory T cells (Treg) [33] which can be divided in two subsets based on their origin: Tregs of thymic origin (tTreg), which were previously referred to as natural Tregs and peripherally-derived Treg (pTregs). FOXP3 expression is controlled by proximal promoter and intronic regulatory elements designated as conserved non coding sequences (CNS1-3) which are highly conserved between species.

In the thymus, tTregs are induced by TCR engagement with self-peptide major histocompatibility complex with specific strength and duration. The subsequent NF-κB signaling induces permissive histone modification (H3K4me1) at the CNS3 and potentially initiates chromatin remodeling in the FOXP3 locus through the c-Rel subunit [34]. In parallel, cAMP response element-binding protein (CREB) binds to the CNS2 element, which inversely correlates with the methylation status of CpG islands [35]. DNA demethylation of the CNS2, also called the Treg-specific demethylated region (TSDR) is a major event in tTreg differentiation and carries an important function in FOXP3 stabilizing FOXP3 expression [36]. CNS2 is the site at which FOXP3 binds to its own gene to maintain expression in a positive feedback mechanism allowing for a persistent phenotype and suppressive function. FOXP3 induces the expression of IL-2 receptor CD25, which activation phosphorylates STAT5 which binds the promoter and CNS2 independently of methylation status providing an additional positive feedback mechanism [37].

Besides Tregs, activated T cells also express FOXP3 upon TCR engagement [38]. However, this expression is only transient as the CNS2 remains methylated. In fact, when comparing tTregs to FOXP3+ activated effector T cells there are hundreds of loci throughout the genome which show demethylation and correspond to binding sites for FOXP3 [39]. These methylation changes are not induced by FOXP3 but rather allow FOXP3 to access its targets and exert its function. The lack of demethylation of these loci could explain the difference in function despite the expression of FOXP3 in activated T cells.

In contrast to thymic-derived Tregs, generation of Tregs from peripheral naïve T cells is favored by suboptimal TCR stimulation in the presence of TGF-β [40]. TGF-β promotes FOXP3 transcription in peripheral CD4 T cells through binding of SMAD3 at CNS1 [41]. A FOXP3-CNS1-deficient mice mouse has shown that CNS1 is critical for FOXP3 induction in peripheral CD4 T cells but not in thymocytes. Interestingly, those mice lacked the self-reactive auto-immune manifestations observed in FOXP3 deficient *scrufy* mice, but had maternal-fetal conflict and inflammatory disease at the mucosal interface, suggesting a specific role for pTregs in acquired tolerance to exogenous antigens [42]. The generation of TGF-β-induced Tregs can be augmented by the addition of retinoic acid, which has been shown to induce histone acetylation at the CNS1 region [43]. While in vitro differentiated Treg cells appear to lack TSDR demethylation, in vivo pTregs gradually demethylate the TSDR which could contribute to phenotype stability [44].

Inheritance of epigenetic traits

Development of allergy and asthma is determined by interplay between environmental and inherited factors, the later accounting for over half of the risk [45]. Interestingly, this is in high contrast with the low fraction of variance in asthma prevalence (4%) that can be accounted for by genetic loci in a large-scale genome wide association study [46,47]. This missing heritability could be due in part to the difficulty of accounting for rare polymorphisms with a high penetrance in some families (private mutations) but it also raises the possibility of non-genetic means of inheritance [46].

Genetics also fail to explain the sudden rise in allergies and asthma as even with significant selection pressure, any change in population genetics would necessitate multiple generations to occur. Epigenetic changes on the other hand can be induced much more rapidly with various environmental exposures and, like with genetics, these changes can be passed down from parents to offspring. There are several ways in which epigenetics can influence phenotype inheritance, including gene imprinting, in utero modifications and transgenerational inheritance.

Parental imprinting and maternal influence

Asthma and atopy are complex genetic traits meaning that the phenotype is the result of the interaction of multiple genes each with their own Mendelian pattern of inheritance. The expected result is that no clear pattern of inheritance would be discernable, with risk from both parents being very similar overall. In reality, the risk for allergy and asthma inherited from the mother is up to 5 fold greater than the paternal risk [48-51].

The discrepancy in parental risk could be explained in part by parental imprinting. Parental imprinting is a process by which some genes are epigenetically silenced during gametogenesis in a parent-of-origin-specific manner, which results in only one allele being expressed for the imprinted loci. The best example probably consists of polymorphisms of FcεR1-β which are only associated with atopy when the risk allele is inherited from the mother in multiple cohorts [49,52,53].

A more recent study showed that maternal but not paternal atopy predicted the expression profile of 18 cytokines and chemokine in the airway mucosal fluid of newborns [54]. However, it is unclear whether this is the result of true genomic imprinting or from a direct modification of the foetal immune system by the mother's atopic phenotype in utero. Animal studies have shown that challenging previously sensitized mice to ovalbumin during pregnancy resulted in an increased allergic phenotype in offsprings [55]. Transferring T cells from sensitized to naïve pregnant mice had the same effect, suggesting this in utero influence was mediated at least in part by the maternal immune system after conception [56]. In humans, one groups has evaluated the methylome of over 300 pregnant women using a high throughput DNA methylation analysis and found that a score of differentially methylated regions better predicted atopic disease in children than clinical data [57]. The same group is currently looking at the correlation of DNA methylation in the neonates cord blood to better understand the mechanisms involved.

Transgenerational inheritance

It has been well described that through development, with the shift from pluripotent stem cells to well differentiated specialized cell types, chromatin becomes increasingly repressed by histone modifications and less activated by permissive histones [58]. However, while it was originally thought that epigenetic marks were completely erased from germline upon conception, this concept has been disproved over a decade ago [59,60]. It is now evident that epigenetic changes induced by environmental exposure may alter the epigenome of the germline and persist through generations.

In their canonical experiment with the agouti mouse model, Morgan et al., fed mice with a methyl-donor rich diet that favored the methylation of the agouti gene, which codes for signalling peptide in mice, which affects coat colour pigmentation. Not only did this influence their immediate offspring's fur color, but throughout five generations with the exact same diet, the fur coat would get darker and darker showing transgenerational transmission of the phenotype, which is not only inherited but augmented [60]. The experiment was repeated recently by Cropley and colleagues who studied the effect of stopping the methyl donor rich diet after 5 generations [61]. Interestingly they found that the following generation (F_6), which was not exposed to the diet, actually exhibited a further increase in fur pigmentation, with normal color returning only with the second generation off therapy (F_7). Mice from the fifth generation had been weaned and put on normal control diet before mating, showing the effect of the diet did not take place in utero. Rather, it suggests that germ cells exposed to excess methyl donors within

the developing F_5 females retained a memory of the methyl donor effect, manifested in F_6 mice [61].

In utero diet supplementation with methyl donors has similarly been shown to increase allergic disease in a mouse model [62]. The F1 progeny exposed to an in utero diet supplemented with methyl donors demonstrated enhanced cardinal features of allergic airway disease, including airway hyperreactivity, lung lavage eosinophilia and IL-13, higher concentrations of serum IgE as well as change in splenocyte phenotype compared to controls on normal diet. More importantly, these traits were passed down transgenerationally, although somewhat less robustly, in F2 "grand-children" mice which did not have in utero supplementation. In human, transgenerational inheritance is exemplified by the effects of tobacco, which may last for 2 generations. Li et al. compared 338 children diagnosed with asthma in their first 5 years of life to 570 countermatched controls and found that a child whose maternal grandmother smoked during pregnancy had double the chance of developing asthma [63]. This risk was even greater if the mother also smoked during pregnancy (OR = 2.6, compared to 1.8 if she did not) supporting the epigenetic transgenerational model in which persistent exposure leads to inheritance and augmentation of the phenotype. However, this association was only replicated for paternal grandmother smoking (which had not been investigated in the former report) in a recent study [64]. The reason for these discordant results is unclear. It could relate to differences in study populations. The first study included children from a southern California cohort [65] (66% white, relatively high levels of air pollution) with slightly earlier diagnosis of asthma (before 5 years) while the second one, from Avon, UK (96% white), included subjects with diagnosis before 7 years of age.

Transgenerational inheritance of epigenetic traits is extremely interesting from an epidemiologic point of view as it provides a new hypothesis for the persistently increasing prevalence of allergy and related disorders. If the recent increase had been due to a change in environment, prevalence should have increased at once and remained stable as long as this environment remained the same. However, if the new environment induces epigenetic changes, a transgenerational amplification of the atopic phenotype would be expected even with stable exposure (Figure 5). Furthermore, according to this hypothesis, it would be expected that the benefit of some interventions to prevent allergies (such as pro- and prebiotics) could take a full generation before reaching their full effect, hence possibly the somewhat disappointing results so far [66].

Association studies in asthma and allergy

At this stage, most of the epigenetic literature on asthma and allergy consists of association studies [67-88]. As with genetic association studies, both candidate gene and

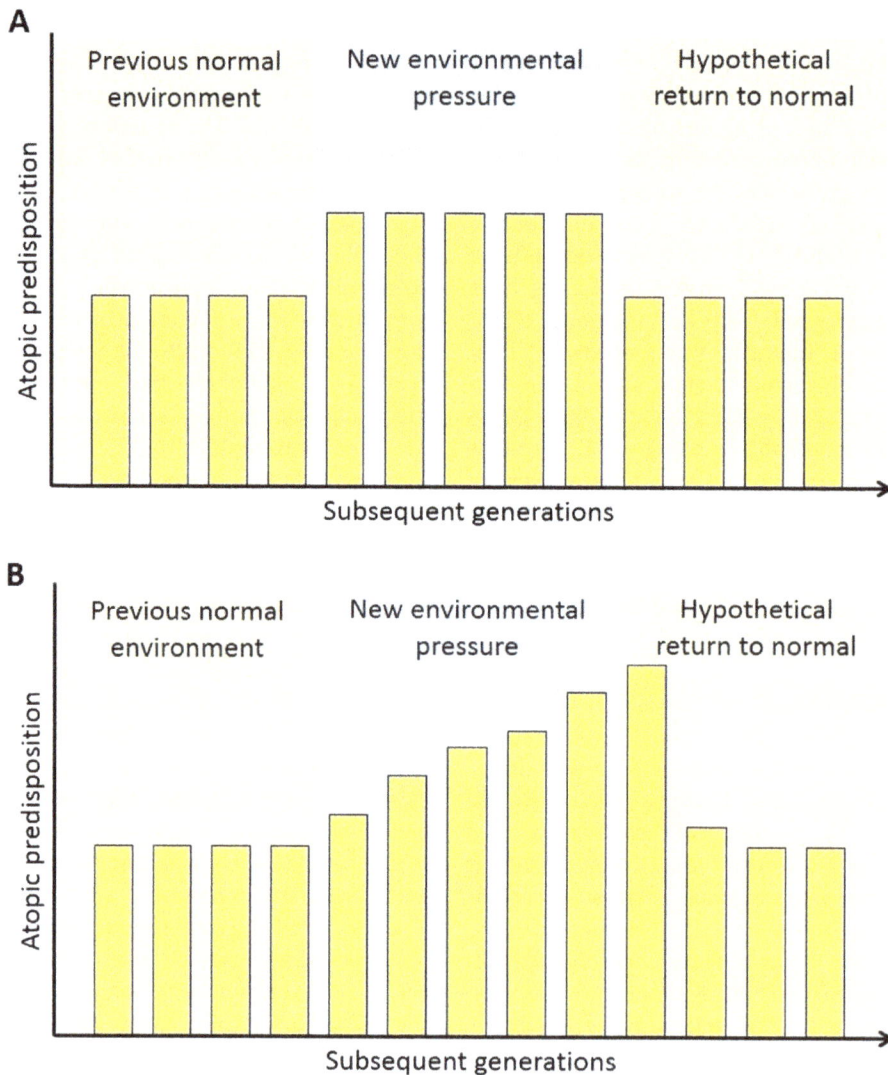

Figure 5 Transgenerational amplification hypothesis. Panel **A** depicts a purely environmental model for the rise of atopic disease, in which a change in environment increases baseline genetic risk for the disease. Panel **B** depicts an epigenetic transgenerational inheritance model, in which a persistent change in environment does not only increase baseline risk but induces transmittable epigenetic changes leading to amplification of the phenotype with every subsequent generation. Return to a normal environment, will lead to resolution of the phenotype but only after 2 generations.

genome-wide approaches are used. Candidate gene approach has the benefit of allowing the specific study of a certain number of particularly relevant genes. Its main disadvantage is the fact that it relies on the investigators hypothesis as to which gene(s) to study. Genome-wide approaches do not have this limitation. However, the amount of analysed data is so great that some relevant but weakly associated loci may be lost after statistical corrections.

Figure 6 provides a list of selected loci that have been reported to be associated with allergic phenotypes and/or environmental risk factors. Association studies are extremely helpful to provide a description of the epigenetic landscape of a given phenotype, which can lead to the identification of potential biomarkers or targets for

therapy. However, they are not sufficient to conclude causality, especially when dealing with a mixed cell population (biopsy or whole PBMCs). Since different differentiated cell types exhibit a different methylation pattern (i.e. Th2 vs Th1 vs Treg cells), changes in the proportion of these subsets will directly affect the methylation pattern of the overall population. Thus, finding more demethylation of the Th2 LCR genes (IL-4, IL-13) in PBMCs from atopic individuals may be only a reflection of the larger proportion of Th2 cells in those individuals, and not the cause of it.

An exciting aspect of epigenetics is that it sheds a new light on previous genetic association studies. Since epigenetic marks have the potential to silence a gene, it is to be expected that it can modulate the effect of an

Associations with phenotype
Asthma
Immune response: *FOXP3(67), INF-g(67), STAT5A(68), CRIP1(68),* IL-4R(69)
NO synthesis: *ARG2(70)*
Lipid pathway: *ALOX12(71), ASCL3(72)*
Pharmacologic receptor: *ADRB2(73)*
Atopy
Immune response: *TLSP(74)*
Lipid pathway: *PTGDR(75)*
Xenobiotics: *CYP26A1(76)*
Various: *58 genes (77)*
Associations with environmental exposure
Tobacco smoke
Immune response: *TGFB3(78)*
Xenobiotic metabolism: *AHRR(79), CYP1A1(79)*
Signaling: *NPSR1(80), GFI1(79), PTPRO(78)*
Oncogenes: *SPDEF(78), SNCG(78), AXL(78), MET(78), NBL1(78), KLK11(78)*
Farming
Immune response: *STAT6(82), RAD50(82), IL13(82), IL4(82), CD14(81)*
Sphyngolipid synthesis: *ORMDL1(82)*
Pollution
Immune response: *FOXP3(83), IFN-g(83), CTLA-4(84), IL-10(84), IL1-R2(84), IFN-g(85)*
NO synthesis: *NOS2A(86), NOS3(86), iNOS(87)*
Lipid Pathway: *ASCL3(72)*
Xenobiotics metabolism: *CYPBRD1(84)*
Signaling:*CLK2(84), MAP3K7(84), PIK3CG(84)*
DNA-binding: *ZNF445(84), PHF20L1(84), TRPS1(84)*
Pet keeping
Immune response: *CD14(88)*

Figure 6 Loci identified from previous DNA methylation association studies for asthma, atopy and related exposures.

underlying polymorphism on disease risk. For example, IL-4R single-nucleotide polymorphism (SNP) rs3024685, which is not associated with asthma on its own, carries a significant risk for the disease when controlled for IL4-R methylation [69].

Similarly, the 17q12-21 which carries 2 polymorphisms associated with maternally inherited risk for asthma was found to be highly methylated in adult males [89]. In fact, epigenetic changes can alter the effect of gene polymorphisms over time. The decreasing effect of CD14 polymorphism on soluble CD14 levels has been shown to be paralleled by small but significant increases in CD14 methylation from 2 to 10 years of age [90].

Genetic polymorphisms can also in turn affect epigenetics regulation of gene expression at a given locus [71,75]. Morales and colleagues showed that hypomethylation of CpG site in the arachidonate 12-lipoxygenase (ALOX12) gene correlated with wheezing in two Spanish cohorts. In both cohorts, they found that the extent of hypomethylation correlated with the genotype for haplotype-tagging single nucleotide polymorphism (SNP) rs312466. In the Menorca cohort for example, subjects with G/G genotype had a 25% genome methylation at CpG site E85, compared to 15% and 7% methylation for genotypes G/A and A/A, respectively) [71]. Recently, North and colleagues found that DNA methylation of the Ephrin-B3 gene (EFNB3), a transmembrane ligand for receptor tyrosine kinases involved in bidirectional signaling, correlated with total symptom scores recorded after exposure to grass for two days in an Environmental Exposure Unit [91]. They also identified two SNPs which influenced on methylation status. One of those, rs3744262 changes a cytosine for a thymine on a CpG site (CpG-SNP) and therefore directly impacted on its methylation. These studies show how polymorphisms and epigenetic regulations are interrelated and how future studies should be structured to examine these interactions.

Potential underlying mechanisms

Although our understanding is still superficial, there is an increasing amount of literature looking into the mechanisms by which allergic phenotypes and environmental exposures could be associated with specific epigenetic changes.

In lung biopsies, the HDAC: HAT ratio has been shown to be lower in asthmatic samples and to correct with treatment [92-96]. This is significant as endogenous HDAC activity may play a crucial role in maintaining the balance of pre-established Th1-like and Th2-like responses. When their endogenous HDAC activity is inhibited, ex vivo memory T cells show an increase in Th2-associated recall response (IL-13, IL-5) and reduction in Th1- (IFN-γ, CXCL10) or Tr1-associated (IL-10) recall response, shifting the Th1:Th2 ratios by 3-fold to 8-fold [97]. However, the relation between HDAC/HAT activity and allergic inflammation is not that simple. Inhibition HDAC may also increase the suppressive function of FOXP3+ Tregs ex vivo [98] and the induction of pTregs by the metabolites of commensal bacterias has been shown to relate to their HDAC inhibitory property which decreases proinflammatory cytokine expression in dendritic cell [99]. The transmaternal asthma protection provided by the farm-derived gram-negative bacterium Acinetobacter lwoffii F78 was associated with an increase in permissive H4 acetylation of the INF-γ locus and this protection was abolished when mice were treated with an HAT inhibitor [100]. It is important to point out that histones are not the only targets of acetylation. Multiple cellular proteins with important functions are also regulated by acetylation and will be affected by changes of HDAC/HAT activities. This includes signal transducers and nuclear factors that are relevant to the immune response such as GATA-3 and FOXP3 [101]. More specifically, mice studies have shown that optimal Treg function requires acetylation of several lysines in the forkhead domain of Foxp3 which enhance binding to the Il2 promoter and suppress endogenous IL-2 production [102,103]. In the end, the question remains as to what causes this change in HDAC/HAT activity in the first place in atopic subjects.

Environmental tobacco smoke supresses the expression and activity of HDAC2 and HDAC3 [104,105]. Exposure to tobacco smoke has also been shown to alter the expression of dnmt1 and dnmt3b [106]. Both tobacco smoke and pollution induce oxidative stress which are thought to favour the demethylation process, as well as to cause lesions to DNA which prevent binding of Dnmt, resulting in a non-specific decrease in methylation across the genome [107-109]. This non-specific interference with the epigenetic process could potentially have a major impact on a concomitant immune response to an allergen given the complex epigenetic control involved in mounting such a response.

Although a diet rich in methyl-donor nutrients has been shown to promote DNA methylation and to induce an allergic phenotype in mice, the same has yet to be shown for humans [62]. Maternal intake of folic acid (a methyl donor) during pregnancy does not influence risk for atopy [110], asthma [111] or food allergy [112]. Whether the previously reported protective effect of antioxidant supplement can be related to an effect on DNA demethylation is still undetermined [113-116].

Conclusion

Epigenetics is an exciting new field in allergy and asthma research that has strongly evolved in the last decade. Recent studies shed a new light on the pathogenesis of this complex group of disease, not only with regards to gene-environment interaction but also with regards to the model of inheritance and its epidemiological implications. The field is still at its infancy stage and more work needs to be done to dissect the epigenome of asthma and allergy and to better understand its underlying mechanisms.

Abbreviations
DNMT: DNA methyltransferase; HAT: Histone acetyltransferase; HDAC: Histone deacetylase; TET: Ten-eleven translocation; DHS: DNAse I Hypersensitivity site; TSDR: Treg-specific demethylated region; LCR: Locus control Region; TCR: T cell receptor; SNP: Single nucleotide polymorphism.

Competing interests
The authors declare that they have no competing interests.

Authors' contributions
PB performed litterature review and wrote the manuscript. NK reviewed the manuscript. Both authors read and approved the manuscript.

Acknowledgment
The authors would like to aknowledge Dr Sharon Chinthrajah for careful proof reading of the manuscript. Philippe Bégin MD, FRCPC is supported by AllerGen NCE Inc. (the Allergy, Gene and Environment Network), a member of the Networks of Centre of Excellence Canada program.

References
1. Baedke J: The epigenetic landscape in the course of time: Conrad Hal Waddington's methodological impact on the life sciences. *Stud Hist Phil Biol Biomed Sci* 2013, **44**(4):756–773. PubMed PMID: 23932231.
2. Barnes PJ: Targeting the epigenome in the treatment of asthma and chronic obstructive pulmonary disease. *Proc Am Thorac Soc* 2009, **6**(8):693–696. PubMed PMID: 20008877.
3. Suarez-Alvarez B, Baragano Raneros A, Ortega F, Lopez-Larrea C: Epigenetic modulation of the immune function: a potential target for tolerance. *Epigenetics* 2013, **8**(7):694–702. PubMed PMID: 23803720. Pubmed Central PMCID: 3781188.
4. Lu TX, Rothenberg ME: Diagnostic, functional, and therapeutic roles of microRNA in allergic diseases. *J Allergy* 2013, **132**(1):3–13. quiz 4. PubMed PMID: 23735656. Pubmed Central PMCID: 3737592.
5. Wu SC, Zhang Y: Active DNA demethylation: many roads lead to Rome. *Nat Rev Mol Cell Biol* 2010, **11**(9):607–620. PubMed PMID: 20683471. Pubmed Central PMCID: 3711520.
6. Gardiner-Garden M, Frommer M: CpG islands in vertebrate genomes. *J Mol Biol* 1987, **196**(2):261–282. PubMed PMID: 3656447.
7. Saxonov S, Berg P, Brutlag DL: A genome-wide analysis of CpG dinucleotides in the human genome distinguishes two distinct classes of promoters. *Proc Natl Acad Sci U S A* 2006, **103**(5):1412–1417. PubMed PMID: 16432200. Pubmed Central PMCID: 1345710.
8. Cadet J, Wagner JR: TET enzymatic oxidation of 5-methylcytosine, 5-hydroxymethylcytosine and 5-formylcytosine. *Mutat Res* 2013, **764-765**:18–35. PubMed PMID: 24045206.
9. Hashimoto H, Hong S, Bhagwat AS, Zhang X, Cheng X: Excision of 5-hydroxymethyluracil and 5-carboxylcytosine by the thymine DNA glycosylase domain: its structural basis and implications for active DNA demethylation. *Nucleic Acids Res* 2012, **40**(20):10203–10214. PubMed PMID: 22962365. Pubmed Central PMCID: 3488261.
10. Adams RL: DNA methylation. The effect of minor bases on DNA-protein interactions. *Biochem J* 1990, **265**(2):309–320. PubMed PMID: 2405840. Pubmed Central PMCID: 1136889.
11. Hu S, Wan J, Su Y, Song Q, Zeng Y, Nguyen HN, Shin J, Cox E, Rho HS, Woodard C, Xia S, Liu S, Lyu H, Ming GL, Wade H, Song H, Qian J, Zhu H: DNA methylation presents distinct binding sites for human transcription factors. *eLife* 2013, **2**:e00726. PubMed PMID: 24015356. Pubmed Central PMCID: 3762332.
12. Boyes J, Bird A: DNA methylation inhibits transcription indirectly via a methyl-CpG binding protein. *Cell* 1991, **64**(6):1123–1134. PubMed PMID: 2004419.
13. Nan X, Ng HH, Johnson CA, Laherty CD, Turner BM, Eisenman RN, Bird A: Transcriptional repression by the methyl-CpG-binding protein MeCP2 involves a histone deacetylase complex. *Nature* 1998, **393**(6683):386–389. PubMed PMID: 9620804.
14. Murr R: Interplay between different epigenetic modifications and mechanisms. *Adv Genet* 2010, **70**:101–141. PubMed PMID: 20920747.

15. Su RC, Brown KE, Saaber S, Fisher AG, Merkenschlager M, Smale ST: Dynamic assembly of silent chromatin during thymocyte maturation. *Nat Genet* 2004, **36**(5):502–506. PubMed PMID: 15098035.

16. Su RC, Sridharan R, Smale ST: Assembly of silent chromatin during thymocyte development. *Semin Immunol* 2005, **17**(2):129–140. PubMed PMID: 15737574.

17. Cedar H, Bergman Y: Linking DNA methylation and histone modification: patterns and paradigms. *Nat Rev Genet* 2009, **10**(5):295–304. PubMed PMID: 19308066.

18. Weissmann F, Lyko F: Cooperative interactions between epigenetic modifications and their function in the regulation of chromosome architecture. *BioEssays* 2003, **25**(8):792–797. PubMed PMID: 12879449.

19. Gregory RI, Khosla S, Feil R: Probing chromatin structure with nuclease sensitivity assays. *Methods Mol Biol* 2001, **181**:269–284. PubMed PMID: 12843457.

20. Wang Z, Zang C, Rosenfeld JA, Schones DE, Barski A, Cuddapah S, Cui K, Roh TY, Peng W, Zhang MQ, Zhao K: Combinatorial patterns of histone acetylations and methylations in the human genome. *Nat Genet* 2008, **40**(7):897–903. PubMed PMID: 18552846. Pubmed Central PMCID: 2769248.

21. Dey A, Chitsaz F, Abbasi A, Misteli T, Ozato K: The double bromodomain protein Brd4 binds to acetylated chromatin during interphase and mitosis. *Proc Natl Acad Sci U S A* 2003, **100**(15):8758–8763. PubMed PMID: 12840145. Pubmed Central PMCID: 166386.

22. Zeng L, Zhang Q, Li S, Plotnikov AN, Walsh MJ, Zhou MM: Mechanism and regulation of acetylated histone binding by the tandem PHD finger of DPF3b. *Nature* 2010, **466**(7303):258–262. PubMed PMID: 20613843. Pubmed Central PMCID: 2901902.

23. Zeng WP: 'All things considered': transcriptional regulation of T helper type 2 cell differentiation from precursor to effector activation. *Immunology* 2013, **140**(1):31–38. PubMed PMID: 23668241. Pubmed Central PMCID: 3809703.

24. Kwon NH, Kim JS, Lee JY, Oh MJ, Choi DC: DNA methylation and the expression of IL-4 and IFN-gamma promoter genes in patients with bronchial asthma. *J Clin Immunol* 2008, **28**(2):139–146. PubMed PMID: 18004650.

25. Wei G, Wei L, Zhu J, Zang C, Hu-Li J, Yao Z, Cui K, Kanno Y, Roh TY, Watford WT, Schones DE, Peng W, Sun HW, Paul WE, O'Shea JJ, Zhao K: Global mapping of H3K4me3 and H3K27me3 reveals specificity and plasticity in lineage fate determination of differentiating CD4+ T cells. *Immunity* 2009, **30**(1):155–167. PubMed PMID: 19144320. Pubmed Central PMCID: 2722509.

26. Hosokawa H, Tanaka T, Kato M, Shinoda K, Tohyama H, Hanazawa A, Tamaki Y, Hirahara K, Yagi R, Sakikawa I, Morita A, Nagira M, Poyurovsky MV, Suzuki Y, Motohashi S, Nakayama T: Gata3/Ruvbl2 complex regulates T helper 2 cell proliferation via repression of Cdkn2c expression. *Proc Natl Acad Sci U S A* 2013, **110**(46):18626–18631. PubMed PMID: 24167278. Pubmed Central PMCID: 3832009.

27. Chang S, Aune TM: Dynamic changes in histone-methylation 'marks' across the locus encoding interferon-gamma during the differentiation of T helper type 2 cells. *Nat Immunol* 2007, **8**(7):723–731. PubMed PMID: 17546034.

28. Brand S, Kesper DA, Teich R, Kilic-Niebergall E, Pinkenburg O, Bothur E, Lohoff M, Garn H, Pfefferle PI, Renz H: DNA methylation of TH1/TH2 cytokine genes affects sensitization and progress of experimental asthma. *J Allergy Clin Immunol* 2012, **129**(6):1602–10 e6. PubMed PMID: 22277202.

29. Williams CL, Schilling MM, Cho SH, Lee K, Wei M, Aditi, Boothby M: STAT4 and T-bet are required for the plasticity of IFN-gamma expression across Th2 ontogeny and influence changes in Ifng promoter DNA methylation. *J Immunol* 2013, **191**(2):678–687.

30. Kim ST, Fields PE, Flavell RA: Demethylation of a specific hypersensitive site in the Th2 locus control region. *Proc Natl Acad Sci U S A* 2007, **104**(43):17052–17057. PubMed PMID: 17940027. Pubmed Central PMCID: 2040439.

31. Williams A, Lee GR, Spilianakis CG, Hwang SS, Eisenbarth SC, Flavell RA: Hypersensitive site 6 of the Th2 locus control region is essential for Th2 cytokine expression. *Proc Natl Acad Sci U S A* 2013, **110**(17):6955–6960. PubMed PMID: 23569250. Pubmed Central PMCID: 3637752.

32. Pellerin L, Jenks JA, Begin P, Bacchetta R, Nadeau KC: Regulatory T cells and their roles in immune dysregulation and allergy. *Immunol Res* 2014, **58**(2-3):358–368. PubMed PMID: 24781194.

33. Passerini L, de Sio FR S, Roncarolo MG, Bacchetta R: Forkhead box P3: The Peacekeeper of the Immune System. *Int Rev Immunol* 2013, **33**(2):129–145. PubMed PMID: 24354325.

34. Zheng Y, Josefowicz S, Chaudhry A, Peng XP, Forbush K, Rudensky AY: Role of conserved non-coding DNA elements in the Foxp3 gene in regulatory T-cell fate. *Nature* 2010, **463**(7282):808–812. PubMed PMID: 20072126. Pubmed Central PMCID: 2884187.

35. Kim HP, Leonard WJ: CREB/ATF-dependent T cell receptor-induced FoxP3 gene expression: a role for DNA methylation. *J Exp Med* 2007, **204**(7):1543–1551. PubMed PMID: 17591856. Pubmed Central PMCID: 2118651.

36. Polansky JK, Kretschmer K, Freyer J, Floess S, Garbe A, Baron U, Olek S, Hamann A, von Boehmer H, Huehn J: DNA methylation controls Foxp3 gene expression. *Eur J Immunol* 2008, **38**(6):1654–1663. PubMed PMID: 18493985.

37. Haiqi H, Yong Z, Yi L: Transcriptional regulation of Foxp3 in regulatory T cells. *Immunobiology* 2011, **216**(6):678–685. PubMed PMID: 21122941.

38. Ohkura N, Kitagawa Y, Sakaguchi S: Development and maintenance of regulatory T cells. *Immunity* 2013, **38**(3):414–423. PubMed PMID: 23521883.

39. Zhang Y, Maksimovic J, Naselli G, Qian J, Chopin M, Blewitt ME, Oshlack A, Harrison LC: Genome-wide DNA methylation analysis identifies hypomethylated genes regulated by FOXP3 in human regulatory T cells. *Blood* 2013, **122**(16):2823–2836. PubMed PMID: 23974203. Pubmed Central PMCID: 3798997.

40. Shevach EM, Thornton AM: tTregs, pTregs, and iTregs: similarities and differences. *Immunol Rev* 2014, **259**(1):88–102. PubMed PMID: 24712461. Pubmed Central PMCID: 3982187.

41. Schlenner SM, Weigmann B, Ruan Q, Chen Y, von Boehmer H: Smad3 binding to the foxp3 enhancer is dispensable for the development of regulatory T cells with the exception of the gut. *J Exp Med* 2012, **209**(9):1529–1535. PubMed PMID: 22908322. Pubmed Central PMCID: 3428940.

42. Samstein RM, Josefowicz SZ, Arvey A, Treuting PM, Rudensky AY: Extrathymic generation of regulatory T cells in placental mammals mitigates maternal-fetal conflict. *Cell* 2012, **150**(1):29–38. PubMed PMID: 22770213. Pubmed Central PMCID: 3422629.

43. Lu L, Ma J, Li Z, Lan Q, Chen M, Liu Y, Xia Z, Wang J, Han Y, Shi W, Quesniaux V, Ryffel B, Brand D, Li B, Liu Z, Zheng SG: All-trans retinoic acid promotes TGF-beta-induced Tregs via histone modification but not DNA demethylation on Foxp3 gene locus. *PLoS One* 2011, **6**(9):e24590. PubMed PMID: 21931768. Pubmed Central PMCID: 3172235.

44. Ohkura N, Hamaguchi M, Morikawa H, Sugimura K, Tanaka A, Ito Y, Osaki M, Tanaka Y, Yamashita R, Nakano N, Huehn J, Fehling HJ, Sparwasser T, Nakai K, Sakaguchi S: T cell receptor stimulation-induced epigenetic changes and Foxp3 expression are independent and complementary events required for Treg cell development. *Immunity* 2012, **37**(5):785–799. PubMed PMID: 23123060.

45. Palmer LJ, Burton PR, Faux JA, James AL, Musk AW, Cookson WO: Independent inheritance of serum immunoglobulin E concentrations and airway responsiveness. *Am J Respir Crit Care Med* 2000, **161**(6):1836–1843. PubMed PMID: 10852754.

46. Cookson W, Moffatt M, Strachan DP: Genetic risks and childhood-onset asthma. *J Allergy Clin Immunol* 2011, **128**(2):266–270. quiz 71–2. PubMed PMID: 21807248.

47. Moffatt MF, Gut IG, Demenais F, Strachan DP, Bouzigon E, Heath S, von Mutius E, Farrall M, Lathrop M, Cookson WO, GABRIEL Consortium: A large-scale, consortium-based genomewide association study of asthma. *N Engl J Med* 2010, **363**(13):1211–1221. PubMed PMID: 20860503.

48. Litonjua AA, Carey VJ, Burge HA, Weiss ST, Gold DR: Parental history and the risk for childhood asthma. Does mother confer more risk than father? *Am J Respir Crit Care Med* 1998, **158**(1):176–181. PubMed PMID: 9655726.

49. Cookson WO, Young RP, Sandford AJ, Moffatt MF, Shirakawa T, Sharp PA, Faux JA, Julier C, Nakumuura Y: Maternal inheritance of atopic IgE responsiveness on chromosome 11q. *Lancet* 1992, **340**(8816):381–384. PubMed PMID: 1353553.

50. Ruiz RG, Kemeny DM, Price JF: Higher risk of infantile atopic dermatitis from maternal atopy than from paternal atopy. *Clin Exp Allergy* 1992, **22**(8):762–766. PubMed PMID: 1525695.

51. Barrett EG: Maternal influence in the transmission of asthma susceptibility. *Pulm Pharmacol Ther* 2008, **21**(3):474–484. PubMed PMID: 17693106. Pubmed Central PMCID: 2478516.

52. Rigoli L, Salpietro DC, Lavalle R, Cafiero G, Zuccarello D, Barberi I: **Allelic association of gene markers on chromosome 11q in Italian families with atopy.** *Acta Paediatr* 2000, **89**(9):1056–1061. PubMed PMID: 11071084.

53. Hill MR, James AL, Faux JA, Ryan G, Hopkin JM, le Souef P, Musk AW, Cookson WO: **Fc epsilon RI-beta polymorphism and risk of atopy in a general population sample.** *BMJ* 1995, **311**(7008):776–779. PubMed PMID: 7580438. Pubmed Central PMCID: 2550787.

54. Folsgaard NV, Chawes BL, Rasmussen MA, Bischoff AL, Carson CG, Stokholm J, Pedersen L, Hansel TT, Bønnelykke K, Brix S, Bisgaard H: **Neonatal cytokine profile in the airway mucosal lining fluid is skewed by maternal atopy.** *Am J Respir Crit Care Med* 2012, **185**(3):275–280. PubMed PMID: 22077068.

55. Hamada K, Suzaki Y, Goldman A, Ning YY, Goldsmith C, Palecanda A, Coull B, Hubeau C, Kobzik L: **Allergen-independent maternal transmission of asthma susceptibility.** *J Immunol* 2003, **170**(4):1683–1689. PubMed PMID: 12574331.

56. Hubeau C, Apostolou I, Kobzik L: **Adoptively transferred allergen-specific T cells cause maternal transmission of asthma risk.** *Am J Pathol* 2006, **168**(6):1931–1939. PubMed PMID: 16723708. Pubmed Central PMCID: 1606611.

57. Hauk PJ, Forssen A, Pedersen B, Strand M, Munoz L, Schedel M, Lynch A, Winn V, Schwartz DA, Gelfand EW: **Differential DNA Methylation In Mothers Increases The Prevalence Of Atopic Dermatitis In Their Offspring.** *J Allergy Clin Immunol* 2014, **133**(22):AB149.

58. Zhu J, Adli M, Zou JY, Verstappen G, Coyne M, Zhang X, Durham T, Miri M, Deshpande V, De Jager PL, Bennett DA, Houmard JA, Muoio DM, Onder TT, Camahort R, Cowan CA, Meissner A, Epstein CB, Shoresh N, Bernstein BE: **Genome-wide chromatin state transitions associated with developmental and environmental cues.** *Cell* 2013, **152**(3):642–654. PubMed PMID: 23333102. Pubmed Central PMCID: 3563935.

59. Waterland RA, Jirtle RL: **Transposable elements: targets for early nutritional effects on epigenetic gene regulation.** *Mol Cell Biol* 2003, **23**(15):5293–5300. PubMed PMID: 12861015. Pubmed Central PMCID: 165709.

60. Morgan HD, Sutherland HG, Martin DI, Whitelaw E: **Epigenetic inheritance at the agouti locus in the mouse.** *Nat Genet* 1999, **23**(3):314–318. PubMed PMID: 10545949.

61. Cropley JE, Dang TH, Martin DI, Suter CM: **The penetrance of an epigenetic trait in mice is progressively yet reversibly increased by selection and environment.** *Proceedings Biological sciences/The Royal Society* 2012, **279**(1737):2347–2353. PubMed PMID: 22319121. Pubmed Central PMCID: 3350677.

62. Hollingsworth JW, Maruoka S, Boon K, Garantziotis S, Li Z, Tomfohr J, Bailey N, Potts EN, Whitehead G, Brass DM, Schwartz DA: **In utero supplementation with methyl donors enhances allergic airway disease in mice.** *J Clin Invest* 2008, **118**(10):3462–3469. PubMed PMID: 18802477. Pubmed Central PMCID: 2542847.

63. Li YF, Langholz B, Salam MT, Gilliland FD: **Maternal and grandmaternal smoking patterns are associated with early childhood asthma.** *Chest* 2005, **127**(4):1232–1241. PubMed PMID: 15821200.

64. Miller LL, Henderson J, Northstone K, Pembrey M, Golding J: **Do grandmaternal smoking patterns influence the aetiology of childhood asthma?** *Chest* 2013, Published online Oct 24 2013, PubMed PMID: 24158349.

65. Peters JM, Avol E, Navidi W, London SJ, Gauderman WJ, Lurmann F, Linn WS, Margolis H, Rappaport E, Gong H, Thomas DC: **A study of twelve Southern California communities with differing levels and types of air pollution. I Prevalence of respiratory morbidity.** *Am J Respir Crit Care Med* 1999, **159**(3):760–767. PubMed PMID: 10051248.

66. Elazab N, Mendy A, Gasana J, Vieira ER, Quizon A, Forno E: **Probiotic administration in early life, atopy, and asthma: a meta-analysis of clinical trials.** *Pediatrics* 2013, **132**(3):e666–e676. PubMed PMID: 23958764.

67. Runyon RS, Cachola LM, Rajeshuni N, Hunter T, Garcia M, Ahn R, Lurmann F, Krasnow R, Jack LM, Miller RL, Swan GE, Kohli A, Jacobson AC, Nadeau KC: **Asthma discordance in twins is linked to epigenetic modifications of T cells.** *PLoS One* 2012, **7**(11):e48796. PubMed PMID: 23226205. Pubmed Central PMCID: 3511472.

68. Stefanowicz D, Hackett TL, Garmaroudi FS, Gunther OP, Neumann S, Sutanto EN, Ling KM, Kobor MS, Kicic A, Stick SM, Paré PD, Knight DA: **DNA methylation profiles of airway epithelial cells and PBMCs from healthy, atopic and asthmatic children.** *PLoS One* 2012, **7**(9):e44213. PubMed PMID: 22970180. Pubmed Central PMCID: 3435400.

69. Soto-Ramirez N, Arshad SH, Holloway JW, Zhang H, Schauberger E, Ewart S, Patil V, Karmaus W: **The interaction of genetic variants and DNA methylation of the interleukin-4 receptor gene increase the risk of asthma at age 18 years.** *Clinical epigenetics* 2013, **5**(1):1. PubMed PMID: 23286427. Pubmed Central PMCID: 3544634.

70. Breton CV, Byun HM, Wang X, Salam MT, Siegmund K, Gilliland FD: **DNA methylation in the arginase-nitric oxide synthase pathway is associated with exhaled nitric oxide in children with asthma.** *Am J Respir Crit Care Med* 2011, **184**(2):191–197. PubMed PMID: 21512169. Pubmed Central PMCID: 3172885.

71. Morales E, Bustamante M, Vilahur N, Escaramis G, Montfort M, de Cid R, Garcia-Esteban R, Torrent M, Estivill X, Grimalt JO, Sunyer J: **DNA hypomethylation at ALOX12 is associated with persistent wheezing in childhood.** *Am J Respir Crit Care Med* 2012, **185**(9):937–943. PubMed PMID: 22323304.

72. Perera F, Tang WY, Herbstman J, Tang D, Levin L, Miller R, Ho SM: **Relation of DNA methylation of 5'-CpG island of ACSL3 to transplacental exposure to airborne polycyclic aromatic hydrocarbons and childhood asthma.** *PLoS One* 2009, **4**(2):e4488. PubMed PMID: 19221603. Pubmed Central PMCID: 2637989.

73. Fu A, Leaderer BP, Gent JF, Leaderer D, Zhu Y: **An environmental epigenetic study of ADRB2 5'-UTR methylation and childhood asthma severity.** *Clin Exp Allergy* 2012, **42**(11):1575–1581. PubMed PMID: 22862293. Pubmed Central PMCID: 3673701.

74. Luo Y, Zhou B, Zhao M, Tang J, Lu Q: **Promoter demethylation contributes to TSLP overexpression in skin lesions of patients with atopic dermatitis.** *Clin Exp Dermatol* 2014, **39**(1):48–53. PubMed PMID: 24341479.

75. Isidoro-Garcia M, Sanz C, Garcia-Solaesa V, Pascual M, Pescador DB, Lorente F, Dávila I: **PTGDR gene in asthma: a functional, genetic, and epigenetic study.** *Allergy* 2011, **66**(12):1553–1562. PubMed PMID: 21883277.

76. Pascual M, Suzuki M, Isidoro-Garcia M, Padron J, Turner T, Lorente F, Dávila I, Greally JM: **Epigenetic changes in B lymphocytes associated with house dust mite allergic asthma.** *Epigenetics* 2011, **6**(9):1131–1137. PubMed PMID: 21975512.

77. Kim YJ, Park SW, Kim TH, Park JS, Cheong HS, Shin HD, Park CS: **Genome-wide methylation profiling of the bronchial mucosa of asthmatics: relationship to atopy.** *BMC medical genetics* 2013, **14**:39. PubMed PMID: 23521807. Pubmed Central PMCID: 3616917.

78. Breton CV, Byun HM, Wenten M, Pan F, Yang A, Gilliland FD: **Prenatal tobacco smoke exposure affects global and gene-specific DNA methylation.** *Am J Respir Crit Care Med* 2009, **180**(5):462–467. PubMed PMID: 19498054. Pubmed Central PMCID: 2742762.

79. Joubert BR, Haberg SE, Nilsen RM, Wang X, Vollset SE, Murphy SK, Huang Z, Hoyo C, Midttun Ø, Cupul-Uicab LA, Ueland PM, Wu MC, Nystad W, Bell DA, Peddada SD, London SJ: **450 K epigenome-wide scan identifies differential DNA methylation in newborns related to maternal smoking during pregnancy.** *Environ Health Perspect* 2012, **120**(10):1425–1431. PubMed PMID: 22851337. Pubmed Central PMCID: 3491949.

80. Reinius LE, Gref A, Saaf A, Acevedo N, Joerink M, Kupczyk M, D'Amato M, Bergström A, Melén E, Scheynius A, Dahlén SE, Pershagen G, Söderhäll C, Kere J, BIOAIR Study Group: **DNA methylation in the Neuropeptide S Receptor 1 (NPSR1) promoter in relation to asthma and environmental factors.** *PLoS One* 2013, **8**(1):e53877. PubMed PMID: 23372674. Pubmed Central PMCID: 3553086.

81. Slaats GG, Reinius LE, Alm J, Kere J, Scheynius A, Joerink M: **DNA methylation levels within the CD14 promoter region are lower in placentas of mothers living on a farm.** *Allergy* 2012, **67**(7):895–903. PubMed PMID: 22564189.

82. Michel S, Busato F, Genuneit J, Pekkanen J, Dalphin JC, Riedler J, Mazaleyrat N, Weber J, Karvonen AM, Hirvonen MR, Braun-Fahrländer C, Lauener R, von Mutius E, Kabesch M, Tost J, PASTURE study group: **Farm exposure and time trends in early childhood may influence DNA methylation in genes related to asthma and allergy.** *Allergy* 2013, **68**(3):355–364. PubMed PMID: 23346934.

83. Kohli A, Garcia MA, Miller RL, Maher C, Humblet O, Hammond SK, Nadeau K: **Secondhand smoke in combination with ambient air pollution exposure is associated with increasedx CpG methylation and decreased expression of IFN-gamma in T effector cells and Foxp3 in T regulatory cells in children.** *Clinical epigenetics* 2012, **4**(1):17. PubMed PMID: 23009259. Pubmed Central PMCID: 3483214.

84. Rossnerova A, Tulupova E, Tabashidze N, Schmuczerova J, Dostal M, Rossner P Jr, Gmuender H, Sram RJ: Factors affecting the 27K DNA methylation pattern in asthmatic and healthy children from locations with various environments. *Mutat Res* 2013, 741–742:18–26. PubMed PMID: 23458556.

85. Tang WY, Levin L, Talaska G, Cheung YY, Herbstman J, Tang D, Miller RL, Perera F, Ho SM: Maternal exposure to polycyclic aromatic hydrocarbons and 5'-CpG methylation of interferon-gamma in cord white blood cells. *Environ Health Perspect* 2012, 120(8):1195–1200. PubMed PMID: 22562770. Pubmed Central PMCID: 3440069.

86. Breton CV, Salam MT, Wang X, Byun HM, Siegmund KD, Gilliland FD: Particulate matter, DNA methylation in nitric oxide synthase, and childhood respiratory disease. *Environ Health Perspect* 2012, 120(9):1320–1326. PubMed PMID: 22591701. Pubmed Central PMCID: 3440108.

87. Tarantini L, Bonzini M, Apostoli P, Pegoraro V, Bollati V, Marinelli B, Cantone L, Rizzo G, Hou L, Schwartz J, Bertazzi PA, Baccarelli A: Effects of particulate matter on genomic DNA methylation content and iNOS promoter methylation. *Environ Health Perspect* 2009, 117(2):217–222. PubMed PMID: 19270791. Pubmed Central PMCID: 2649223.

88. Munthe-Kaas MC, Bertelsen RJ, Torjussen TM, Hjorthaug HS, Undlien DE, Lyle R, Gervin K, Granum B, Mowinckel P, Carlsen KH, Carlsen KC: Pet keeping and tobacco exposure influence CD14 methylation in childhood. *Pediatr Allergy Immunol* 2012, 23(8):747–754. PubMed PMID: 23194293.

89. Naumova AK, Al Tuwaijri A, Morin A, Vaillancourt VT, Madore AM, Berlivet S, Kohan-Ghadr HR, Moussette S, Laprise C: Sex- and age-dependent DNA methylation at the 17q12-q21 locus associated with childhood asthma. *Hum Genet* 2013, 132(7):811–822. PubMed PMID: 23546690.

90. Munthe-Kaas MC, Torjussen TM, Gervin K, Lodrup Carlsen KC, Carlsen KH, Granum B, Hjorthaug HS, Undlien D, Lyle R: CD14 polymorphisms and serum CD14 levels through childhood: a role for gene methylation? *J Allergy Clin Immunol* 2010, 125(6):1361–1368. PubMed PMID: 20398919.

91. North M, Mah S, Day AG, Kobor M, Ellis AK: Effects Of rs3744262 On DNA Methylation and Symptoms In Participants With Allergic Rhinitis During Grass Pollen Exposure In The Environmental Exposure Unit (EEU). *J Allergy Clin Immunol* 2014, 133(2):AB89.

92. Ito K, Caramori G, Lim S, Oates T, Chung KF, Barnes PJ, Adcock IM: Expression and activity of histone deacetylases in human asthmatic airways. *Am J Respir Crit Care Med* 2002, 166(3):392–396. PubMed PMID: 12153977.

93. Cosio BG, Mann B, Ito K, Jazrawi E, Barnes PJ, Chung KF, Adcock IM: Histone acetylase and deacetylase activity in alveolar macrophages and blood mononocytes in asthma. *Am J Respir Crit Care Med* 2004, 170(2):141–147. PubMed PMID: 15087294.

94. Su RC, Becker AB, Kozyrskyj AL, Hayglass KT: Altered epigenetic regulation and increasing severity of bronchial hyperresponsiveness in atopic asthmatic children. *J Allergy Clin Immunol* 2009, 124(5):1116–1118. PubMed PMID: 19895998.

95. Gunawardhana LP, Gibson PG, Simpson JL, Powell H, Baines KJ: Activity and expression of histone acetylases and deacetylases in inflammatory phenotypes of asthma. *Clin Exp Allergy* 2014, 44(1):47–57. PubMed PMID: 24355018.

96. Cosio BG, Tsaprouni L, Ito K, Jazrawi E, Adcock IM, Barnes PJ: Theophylline restores histone deacetylase activity and steroid responses in COPD macrophages. *J Exp Med* 2004, 200(5):689–695. PubMed PMID: 15337792. Pubmed Central PMCID: 2212744.

97. Su RC, Becker AB, Kozyrskyj AL, Hayglass KT: Epigenetic regulation of established human type 1 versus type 2 cytokine responses. *J Allergy Clin Immunol* 2008, 121(1):57–63 e3. PubMed PMID: 17980413.

98. Akimova T, Ge G, Golovina T, Mikheeva T, Wang L, Riley JL, Hancock WW: Histone/protein deacetylase inhibitors increase suppressive functions of human FOXP3+ Tregs. *Clin Immunol* 2010, 136(3):348–363. PubMed PMID: 20478744. Pubmed Central PMCID: 2917523.

99. Arpaia N, Campbell C, Fan X, Dikiy S, van der Veeken J, deRoos P, Liu H, Cross JR, Pfeffer K, Coffer PJ, Rudensky AY: Metabolites produced by commensal bacteria promote peripheral regulatory T-cell generation. *Nature* 2013, 504(7480):451–455. PubMed PMID: 24226773. Pubmed Central PMCID: 3869884.

100. Brand S, Teich R, Dicke T, Harb H, Yildirim AO, Tost J, Schneider-Stock R, Waterland RA, Bauer UM, von Mutius E, Garn H, Pfefferle PI, Renz H: Epigenetic regulation in murine offspring as a novel mechanism for transmaternal asthma protection induced by microbes. *J Allergy Clin Immunol* 2011, 128(3):618–25 e1-7. PubMed PMID: 21680015.

101. Glozak MA, Sengupta N, Zhang X, Seto E: Acetylation and deacetylation of non-histone proteins. *Gene* 2005, 363:15–23. PubMed PMID: 16289629.

102. Tao R, de Zoeten EF, Ozkaynak E, Chen C, Wang L, Porrett PM, Li B, Turka LA, Olson EN, Greene MI, Wells AD, Hancock WW: Deacetylase inhibition promotes the generation and function of regulatory T cells. *Nat Med* 2007, 13(11):1299–1307. PubMed PMID: 17922010.

103. Beier UH, Akimova T, Liu Y, Wang L, Hancock WW: Histone/protein deacetylases control Foxp3 expression and the heat shock response of T-regulatory cells. *Curr Opin Immunol* 2011, 23(5):670–678. PubMed PMID: 21798734. Pubmed Central PMCID: 3190028.

104. Kobayashi Y, Bossley C, Gupta A, Akashi K, Tsartsali L, Mercado N, Barnes PJ, Bush A, Ito K: Passive smoking impairs histone deacetylase-2 in children with severe asthma. *Chest* 2013, 145(2):305–312. PubMed PMID: 24030221.

105. Winkler AR, Nocka KN, Williams CM: Smoke exposure of human macrophages reduces HDAC3 activity, resulting in enhanced inflammatory cytokine production. *Pulm Pharmacol Ther* 2012, 25(4):286–292. PubMed PMID: 22613758.

106. Liu F, Killian JK, Yang M, Walker RL, Hong JA, Zhang M, Davis S, Zhang Y, Hussain M, Xi S, Rao M, Meltzer PA, Schrump DS: Epigenomic alterations and gene expression profiles in respiratory epithelia exposed to cigarette smoke condensate. *Oncogene* 2010, 29(25):3650–3664. PubMed PMID: 20440268.

107. Franco R, Schoneveld O, Georgakilas AG, Panayiotidis MI: Oxidative stress, DNA methylation and carcinogenesis. *Cancer Lett* 2008, 266(1):6–11. PubMed PMID: 18372104.

108. Baccarelli A, Wright RO, Bollati V, Tarantini L, Litonjua AA, Suh HH, Zanobetti A, Sparrow D, Vokonas PS, Schwartz J: Rapid DNA methylation changes after exposure to traffic particles. *Am J Respir Crit Care Med* 2009, 179 (7):572–578. PubMed PMID: 19136372. Pubmed Central PMCID: 2720123.

109. Bollati V, Baccarelli A, Hou L, Bonzini M, Fustinoni S, Cavallo D, Byun HM, Jiang J, Marinelli B, Pesatori AC, Bertazzi PA, Yang AS: Changes in DNA methylation patterns in subjects exposed to low-dose benzene. *Cancer Res* 2007, 67(3):876–880. PubMed PMID: 17283117.

110. Bekkers MB, Elstgeest LE, Scholtens S, Haveman-Nies A, de Jongste JC, Kerkhof M, Koppelman GH, Gehring U, Smit HA, Wijga AH: Maternal use of folic acid supplements during pregnancy, and childhood respiratory health and atopy. *Eur Respir J* 2012, 39(6):1468–1474. PubMed PMID: 22034647.

111. Martinussen MP, Risnes KR, Jacobsen GW, Bracken MB: Folic acid supplementation in early pregnancy and asthma in children aged 6 years. *Am J Obstet Gynecol* 2012, 206(1):72 e1-7. PubMed PMID: 21982024. Pubmed Central PMCID: 3246127.

112. Binkley KE, Leaver C, Ray JG: Antenatal risk factors for peanut allergy in children. Allergy, asthma, and clinical immunology : official journal of the Canadian Society of Allergy and. *Clin Immunol* 2011, 7:17.

113. Li-Weber M, Giaisi M, Treiber MK, Krammer PH: Vitamin E inhibits IL-4 gene expression in peripheral blood T cells. *Eur J Immunol* 2002, 32(9):2401–2408. PubMed PMID: 12207324.

114. McKeever TM, Lewis SA, Smit H, Burney P, Britton J, Cassano PA: Serum nutrient markers and skin prick testing using data from the Third National Health and Nutrition Examination Survey. *J Allergy Clin Immunol* 2004, 114(6):1398–1402. PubMed PMID: 15577844.

115. Sato Y, Akiyama H, Suganuma H, Watanabe T, Nagaoka MH, Inakuma T, Goda Y, Maitani T: The feeding of beta-carotene down-regulates serum IgE levels and inhibits the type I allergic response in mice. *Biol Pharm Bull* 2004, 27(7):978–984. PubMed PMID: 15256726.

116. Hoppu U, Rinne M, Salo-Vaananen P, Lampi AM, Piironen V, Isolauri E: Vitamin C in breast milk may reduce the risk of atopy in the infant. *Eur J Clin Nutr* 2005, 59(1):123–128. PubMed PMID: 15340369.

18

A retrospective study of the clinical benefit from acetylsalicylic acid desensitization in patients with nasal polyposis and asthma

Christine Ibrahim[1]*, Kulraj Singh[1], Gina Tsai[1,2], David Huang[1,2], Jorge Mazza[1,2], Brian Rotenberg[1,3], Harold Kim[1,2] and David William Moote[1,2]*

Abstract

Background: Aspirin-exacerbated respiratory disease (AERD), also known as Samter's triad, is a clinical syndrome which consists of aspirin (ASA) intolerance, chronic rhinosinusitis with nasal polyposis, and intrinsic bronchial asthma (Press Med 119:48-51, 1922). ASA challenge is the gold standard for diagnosing AERD (Curr Allergy Asthma 9:155-163, 2009). The practice of ASA challenge and desensitization in Canada is infrequently utilized, which may explain its omission as a viable therapeutic option in the latest Canadian clinical practice guidelines for acute and chronic rhinosinusitis (AACI 7:1-38, 2011).

Methods: This retrospective study assessed 111 patients who underwent ASA desensitization in the Allergy and Immunology clinic at St. Joseph's Healthcare (SJHC) in London, Ontario. The mean age was 50.7 years, and 52.5% (n = 58) were male. Sixty-one percent (n = 68) claimed prior, significant reactions to ASA, and all patients had features of AERD.

Results: Seventy-three percent (n = 81) claimed symptom improvement after achieving maintenance dosing on the desensitization protocol. Of this population, 21.6% (n = 24) improved in all 3 areas of interest (sense of taste or smell, upper respiratory symptoms and lower respiratory symptoms). Twenty-six percent (n = 29) had adverse effects, mostly in the way of gastrointestinal upset, but no severe adverse events were seen.

Conclusions: ASA desensitization helps improve symptoms in patients with AERD. Further, it allows patients to tolerate additional ASA and other non-steroidal anti-inflammatories (NSAIDs) when needed for supplemental analgesia or for cardio-protection. This is of particular benefit in those who require these medications for improved quality of life, and for reduced morbidity and mortality, such as those with cardiovascular disease or chronic pain. There should be further studies conducted in Canada as well as consideration for ASA desensitization to be included in the next clinical practice guidelines.

Keywords: Aspirin desensitization, Nasal polyposis, Rhinosinusitis, Asthma, Aspirin-exacerbated respiratory disease

Background

Aspirin-exacerbated respiratory disease (AERD) is a clinical syndrome which consists of aspirin intolerance, chronic rhinosinusitis with nasal polyposis and intrinsic bronchial asthma as first described by Widal in 1922 [1]. Max Samter, an American immunologist, revisited the association and proposed the possible pathogenesis in the 1960s. His name is often associated with the syndrome—Samter's triad [2]. AERD affects 0.3-0.9% of the general population, but its prevalence rises to 10-20% in asthmatics, and up to 30-40% in asthmatics with nasal polyposis [3,4]. Clinical features include onset of nasal congestion with anosmia, with progression to chronic pansinusitis and nasal polyposis. The nasal polyps often re-grow rapidly after repeated surgeries [5]. Asthma may precede the upper airway disease or develop later.

ASA challenge is the gold standard for diagnosing AERD [5]. Zeiss and Lockey were the first authors to

* Correspondence: cibrahim@uwo.ca; dmoote@uwo.ca
[1]Schulich School of Medicine and Dentistry, London, Ontario, Canada
[2]Department of Allergy and Immunology, London, Ontario, Canada
Full list of author information is available at the end of the article

describe a 72-hour refractory period after oral ASA challenge in ASA-sensitive patients in 1976 [6]. Since then, multiple studies have shown that desensitization and daily treatment with aspirin can not only allow the medication to be tolerated, but can significantly improve overall symptoms and quality of life, decrease formation of nasal polyps and sinus infections, reduce the need for oral corticosteroids and sinus surgery, and improve nasal and asthma scores in patient with AERD. The effects are noticeable as early as 4 weeks following desensitization [7], and persist at least up to 5 years in to follow-up [8]. Much of what we know about ASA challenge and desensitization derives from studies of over 1400 patients who have undergone the procedure at Scripps Clinic in San Diego, CA, USA. ASA challenge and desensitization has received little attention in Canada, which may explain its omission as a viable therapeutic option in the latest Canadian clinical practice guidelines for acute and chronic rhinosinusitis [9].

Since the use of aspirin desensitization was first described in 1984, and shown to clinically improve the underlying inflammatory airway disease [10], much research has been done to further optimize this procedure. Premedication with leukotriene receptor antagonists, alone or in combination with inhaled corticosteroids and long-acting β2-agonists, was able to reduce lower respiratory tract reactions during aspirin challenge in some patients, but did not change the overall rate of positive aspirin challenge and desensitization [11,12].

The aim of this study was two-fold. First, to assess patient-specific improvement scores and address questions surrounding patient discontinuation. Second, to assess the severity of adverse effects from high-dose ASA maintenance therapy.

Methods
Study population
This retrospective study of 111 patients took place at the Allergy and Immunology clinic at St. Joseph's Healthcare (SJHC) in London, Ontario, from 2007–2011.

Inclusion criteria involved patients seen in consultation at the Allergy and Immunology clinic, an adult (≥ age of 17), who had nasal polyposis, asthma, and a history of ASA or non-steroidal anti-inflammatory (NSAIDs) sensitivity, and had a stable clinical course. They must have then completed a trial of ASA desensitization and attended follow-up for at least one year after. Baseline medical illness and therapies were assessed (Table 1). The use of steroids and antibiotics related to AERD were determined (Table 2).

Subjects were excluded if they had significant concomitant disease, history of life-threatening ASA or NSAID reactions, or other chronic conditions or treatments that may have confounded the interpretation of the study results.

Table 1 Baseline characteristics of patients

Age-year, mean (range)	50.7 (17–75)	
Male, n (%)	58 (52.2)	
Female, n (%)	53 (47.8%)	
Length of upper respiratory disease (%)		
<5 years	22.2	
5-10 years	28.3	
10-15 years	15.2	
>15 years	34.3	
Length of lower respiratory disease (%)		
<5 years	33.7	
5-10 years	25.3	
10-15 years	10.8	
>15 years	30.2	
Baseline FEV1 (n)		Post ASA FEV1 (n)
Mild (≥80)	25	32
Moderate (<80 × ≥50)	36	36
Severe (<50)	2	2
Unknown	48	41

Ethics approval was received from Western University in London, Ontario. Informed consent was obtained, and clinical records were reviewed, looking specifically for ASA desensitization over a two-day protocol. This previously validated protocol is from the Scripps Clinic, with an initial dose of 40 mg titrated up to 162 mg on day one, and then 325 mg on day two [3,7,8]. From past literature, maintenance dose is kept at 325 mg or 650 mg twice daily [3,8,13].

Patient characteristics
Patient characteristics prior to ASA challenge and desensitization were obtained, including age, duration of

Table 2 Indications of disease severity

Prednisone use in past 12 months (%)	63.80%
Antibiotic use in past 12 months (%)	22.90%
Number of endoscopic sinus surgeries (%)	
None	11.4
1 to 3	65.7
4 to 6	19.1
7 to 10	1.9
>10	1.9
Lund-MacKay CT Score (%, from n = 72)	
0-6	2.6
7-12	13.2
13-18	35.5
19-24	48.7

upper and/or lower respiratory disease, and baseline percent predicted FEV1 (Table 1). Further severity of disease was assessed based on number of prednisone bursts and antibiotic treatment in the preceding 12 months to desensitization, current asthma and rhinitis controller medications, number of endoscopic sinus operations, and severity of disease on imaging (Tables 2 and 3).

Types of reactions during desensitization were recorded and classified based on the data available (Table 4), as was medication used prior to and during desensitization (Table 5). Any adverse reactions to continued ASA use, and reasons for discontinuation of therapy were also assessed, and analyzed, as provided through chart review.

Outcomes assessment

A priori rules were used regarding clinical benefit of ASA desensitization through patient statements, clinical notes, and imaging. Although ideal to compare imaging pre- and post- desensitization, the time interval and completeness of each patient was variable, and/or confounded by repeated surgical intervention or patient withdrawal. These data will be collected for a future, prospective study. Initial CT imaging was scored via the validated Lund-MacKay CT score (Table 2).

Assessment of safety

Given the potential for significant reactions in a patient with known sensitivity to ASA and/or NSAIDs, the desensitization process was done in a controlled setting in hospital, with medications, including epinephrine close at hand. It was carried out using a validated protocol [3], conducted in a step-wise approach, with safety as a priority. Subjects were monitored closely by the physicians and nurses. Vital signs and physical examinations

Table 4 ASA data

History of ASA reaction (n, %)	64 (61)
Type of reaction (%)	
Mixed symptoms*	2.1
Significant reaction**	14.9
Unknown	83.0

*Mixed (flushing, worsening nasal congestion, swelling).
**Significant reaction (anaphylactoid).

were taken, at a minimum, before and after each interval dose. Subjects were monitored for at least 1 hour after last dose of the day.

Statistical analysis

Statistical analysis was performed using SAS 9.3 (SAS Institute, Cary, NC) and through Microsoft Excel™, including assessment of patient demographics and percentage calculations.

Results

Patient characteristics

The median age was 50.7 (17–75), and the population was split between males at 52.2% (n = 58) and females at 47.8% (n = 53). Most of the population had upper respiratory

Table 5 ASA Desensitization

Total desensitized (n = 111)	
Treatment during desensitization (n, %)	
Yes	39 (35.1)
No	66 (59.5)
Unknown	6 (5.4)
Treatment medication (n)	
Nasal Steroid	2
Oral Steroid	21
Puffer (SABA, ICS, combination)	13
Epinephrine	1
Patient improvement on ASA (n, %)	
Yes	81 (73.0)
No	23 (20.7)
Unknown	7 (6.3)
Patient improvement score (out of 3)	
Change in taste or smell (1 pt)	34/111
Change in upper respiratory symptoms (1 pt)	78/111
Change in lower respiratory symptoms (1 pt)	67/111
0 out of 3	17 (15.3)
1 out of 3	20 (18.1)
2 out of 3	45 (40.5)
3 out of 3	24 (21.6)
Unknown	5 (4.5)

Table 3 Asthma and rhinitis medications

Skin test positivity (%)		63.8	
Baseline asthma therapy (%)		*Post-ASA asthma therapy (%)*	
SABA	1.9	SABA	2.7
ICS	2.9	ICS	3.6
LABA	0.0	LABA	0.0
Leukotriene	1.9	Leukotriene	4.5
Combination	80.0	Combination	60.4
Unknown	13.3	Unknown	28.8
Baseline rhinitis therapy (%)		*Post ASA rhinitis therapy (%)*	
Nasal washes	3.8	Nasal washes	2.7
Nasal steroids	46.7	Nasal steroids	46.8
Antihistamines	2.9	Antihistamines	0.9
Combination	28.6	Combination	19.0
Unknown	18.0	Unknown	30.6

disease (77.8%, n = 86) and lower respiratory disease (66.3%, n = 74) for over 5 years. Based on limited retrospective data, it was difficult to assess baseline FEV1 severity and to assess for significant change during ASA desensitization.

In regards to baseline therapy, 80.8% (n = 90) were on a combination therapy for asthma, and 46.7% (n = 52) were on nasal steroids for rhinitis symptoms. After desensitization, there were comments in the patients record about being on less therapy, and the data trended towards decreased upper and lower respiratory therapy once on maintenance ASA therapy, but this did not reach statistical significance. As per the validated protocol [3], patients were started on 40 mg and titrated up to 162 mg on day one. On the second day, they were titrated up to 325 mg. From there the maintenance dose was 325 mg or 650 mg twice daily (Table 6).

In terms of AERD features, overall this population trended towards having more moderate-severe disease. Sixty-four percent (n = 71) required oral steroid therapy within the 12 months prior to desensitization therapy and 22.9% (n = 25) required antibiotics. The majority of the population, as seen in Table 2, had undergone more than one endoscopic sinus surgery, and most showed severe sinus of disease on imaging. This was confirmed by the severity in the Lund-MacKay score prior to desensitization with 97.4% (n = 108) scored $\geq$13 points.

Outcomes assessment

Sixty-one percent (n = 68) had recorded previous reactions to ASA and/or NSAIDs exposure (Table 4).

Of those desensitized, 35.1% (n = 39) received pretreatment or required treatment during desensitization, most commonly the use of an oral steroid (21/39 persons). One patient required epinephrine during the procedure, but was able to continue with the planned day two protocol and was successful in achieving desensitization and eventual improvement in symptoms.

Of those who achieved maintenance therapy, 73% (n = 81) stated improvement in symptoms of AERD. We created a patient improvement score with 1 point for improvement in taste or smell, 1 point for improvement in upper respiratory symptoms, and 1 point for improvement in lower respiratory symptoms for a total out of 3. Fifteen percent (n = 17) had no benefit, 18.1% (n = 20) had improvement in only one area, 40.5% (n = 45) had improvement in two areas, and 21.6% (n = 24) had improvement in all three.

Safety assessment

In other published studies, known adverse effects occurred during the desensitization process (chest symptoms, worsened nasal congestion, rhinorrhea, facial flushing). In our study, one patient developed an anaphylactic reaction requiring epinephrine and prednisone. However, when rechallenged the patient on day 2 and they tolerated the dose of ASA, and did not require further rescue therapy. There has been anecdotal evidence that the more significant the adverse reaction, the more likely the subject is to have clinically significant improvement with desensitization, however, no study has specifically assessed this.

Of those who initially tolerated ASA maintenance therapy, 26.1% (n = 29) eventually developed adverse reactions (Table 7). Most common was gastrointestinal upset (n = 23). Of this group, 8 patients had a history of gastrointestinal reflux, on a proton-pump inhibitor, and 3 patients required the addition of a proton-pump inhibitor. Three patients had issues with easy bruising.

Twelve months after desensitization, 27.9% (n = 31) had discontinued therapy. The most common reasons cited included lack of patient-perceived benefit, lack of compliance and thus subsequent need for repeat desensitization, worsened respiratory symptoms, or intolerable side-effects related to high-dose ASA.

Discussion

This retrospective analysis looked at 111 patients who underwent ASA desensitization for AERD, who were followed for a maintenance period of approximately 12 months.

In regards to the first objective, of those who achieved maintenance therapy, 73% (n = 81) claimed symptom improvement. There was improvement noted in the chart review of overall symptoms, quality of life, and reduced need for rescue therapy for upper and lower respiratory symptoms. Patients were particularly impressed with any return of their sense of smell and/or taste. Using a score out of 3, relating to improved AERD symptoms, 15.3% (n = 17) identified no benefit, however, the remaining 94 patients had some form of improvement, with 21.6% (n =

Table 6 ASA Maintenance therapy, need for resensitization, and sinus surgery during therapy

ASA maintenance	Dose (mg)*	BID (n, %)	TID (n, %)
	325	37/80 (46.3%)	6/80 (7.5%)
	650	37/80 (46.3.)	0/80 (0.0%)
Patients resensitized (n, %)**		30/111 (27.0%)	
Sinus surgery during desensitization	1st year (n, %)	2nd year (n, %)	3rd year (n, %)
	15/111 (13.5%)	5/80 (6.3%)	6/80 (7.5%)

Note:
- N = 80 includes all those who achieved desensitization up to 1 year, with 10 lost to follow up, but kept as 'intention to treat'.
- N = 111, includes all those who initially achieved desensitization.
*Reasons for ASA dose variations included: adverse effects, up- or down-titrated to symptoms or lack thereof, and/or interruption for surgery or illness.
**Reasons for resensitization included: restart post infection, sinus surgery, other surgery, and/or compliance.

Table 7 Adverse reactions and discontinuation of ASA

Adverse reactions (n, %)	
Yes	29 (26.1)
No	71 (64.0)
Unknown	11 (9.9)
Reactions (n)	
Tinnitus	1
Gout	1
Gastrointestinal upset	23
Hypertension	1
Bruising	3
Discontinuation of ASA therapy	
Yes*	31 (27.9)
No	70 (63.1)
Unknown	10 (9.0)

*Most common reasons for discontinuation: patient belief not working, compliance, worsening symptoms, infection, surgery, and/or adverse effects.

24) having had an improvement in all 3 areas of sense of taste/smell, upper, and lower respiratory symptoms.

These values are similar to those seen in the literature. A retrospective study by Berges-Gimeno et al. [8] of 172 patients found a statistically significant improvement in the number of sinus infections, ability to smell, and upper and lower respiratory symptoms after one year of maintenance ASA therapy. There were also fewer hospitalizations for asthma, and a reduction in the use of nasal, inhaled and oral corticosteroids. Overall, 87% were said to have responded to ASA therapy.

A randomized, double blind study by Swierczynska-Krepa M et al. [14] found improved smell, peak nasal inspiratory flow, and quality of life amongst aspirin-intolerant asthma patients on ASA maintenance.

A randomized controlled trial by Lee et al. [13], took 137 patients randomized to receive ASA 325 mg or 625 mg twice daily. Then after 1 month the group either increased or decreased their dosage based on symptoms. There was a statistically significant improvement in sinus infections and operations, hospitalizations for asthma, and upper and lower respiratory symptoms. After one year, there was a statistically significant reduction in intranasal and oral corticosteroid use.

In our study, patients were mostly on ASA 325 mg or 650 mg twice daily (Table 6). Overall, 46.3% were on 325 mg twice daily, and 46.3% were taking 650 mg twice daily. Six patients (7.5%) were on 325 mg three times daily, as they were in-between dosage adjustments. Dosage adjustments varied based on a multitude of factors such as adequate or inadequate symptom control, adverse effects, compliance, and interruptions for surgery or illness.

It is difficult to say that the ideal dose is, and the literature has shown benefit for both regimens [3,5,13]. As such, it becomes an area of individualized therapy based on patient response.

Overall this study had a patient population with severe AERD, and many with a history of multiple nasal surgeries (Table 2). The literature has shown that ASA desensitization has resulted in improved nasal polyposis and less nasal surgeries [5,15]. A recent study by Cho et al. [16] demonstrated a sustained improvement in endoscopic and symptomatic nasal polyposis symptoms of those on ASA maintenance therapy.

In our study, fifteen patients (13.5%) underwent nasal surgery within the first year of desensitization. Then 6.3% and 7.5% underwent nasal surgery within the second and third years of desensitization, respectively (Table 6).

In our study, at the end of 12 months, 27.9%, (n = 31) had discontinued therapy. Two of those patients were asked to discontinue therapy for upcoming surgery. Another two stopped due to infection, with the inability to maintain therapy. Otherwise, the rest who discontinued therapy claimed lack of perceived benefit, issues with compliance of high-dose ASA twice a day, worsened AERD symptoms, or adverse effects related to ASA therapy.

Among those who tolerated ASA therapy, 26.1% (n = 29) had adverse events that were likely due to the ASA. Most commonly this was gastrointestinal upset, and a few patients needed to be started on proton-pump-inhibitor therapy. Three patients had issues with easy bruising, 1 with tinnitus, 1 patient developed gout, and 1 patient had worsened hypertension. There were no life-threatening adverse reactions during the 12-month follow up. This is a similar to past literature where 10-50% of patients discontinue, and 20-30% complain about gastritis and reflux symptoms [3,6,8].

The retrospective study by Berges-Gimeno et al. [8] showed that 13% discontinued, with 67% of that group having gastrointestinal symptoms. Of the 172 patients, 11% failed to respond to therapy.

From the randomized study by Lee et al. [13], 23.4% discontinued due to adverse effects, with 37.5% of that group having dyspepsia.

Limitations in this study include those associated with any retrospective study and analysis, particularly lack of data points, such as pre- and post- FEV1 percent-predicted values. A randomized controlled trial would have been the preferred method. Additionally, not all patients were initially challenged to prove ASA sensitivity, rather the focus was on clinical history. Dosing was carried out by different physicians and not controlled for. In assessing response to ASA maintenance therapy, there was no objective and validated scoring system used. Lastly, follow-up was only 12 months, and it would have been worthwhile following up this population longitudinally to assess benefit-risk ratios for clinical outcomes versus adverse effects. Pre- and post- CT sinus imaging may have provided a better diagnostic assessment of the effectiveness of desensitization therapy, however post-therapy imaging is not the current standard of care, nor is there sufficient data to correlate the association between symptoms and imaging on post-therapy images.

With respect to future directions, a prospective, randomized controlled study, would be beneficial to gather key clinical data points, as well, to assess baselines characteristics, prove ASA sensitivity, and determine if there are certain clinical predictors that indicate which patients would be better candidates for ASA desensitization. In previous studies, those who were able to maintain a high-dose ASA regimen successfully were more likely to be: less than 40 years old, a poor sense of smell, multiple prior respiratory reactions, or to have had severe prior asthmatic reactions associated with aspirin and NSAIDs [15]. However, to our knowledge, there is no published literature on validated and reproducible patient predictors of clinical benefit from ASA desensitization.

Conclusion
This study assessing 111 patients who underwent ASA desensitization for AERD showed overall effectiveness, with 81/111 patients claiming improvement in symptoms and 31/111 discontinuing maintenance ASA therapy. This is the first Canadian study assessing ASA desensitization and maintenance therapy in the AERD population. A validated protocol is in place, and many centres outside of Canada have significant reproducible data showing benefit to ASA desensitization in this population.

The ability to desensitize the patient to ASA not only aids in symptom improvement and a gain in quality of life in this population, but it also allows the use of ASA and NSAIDs in patient populations who require these medications for other reasons. We believe ASA desensitization should be considered and performed more frequently in the appropriate clinical situations in Canada.

Competing interests
The authors declare that they have no competing interests.

Authors' contributions
All authors contributed equally to this study. All authors read and approved the final manuscript.

Author details
[1]Schulich School of Medicine and Dentistry, London, Ontario, Canada.
[2]Department of Allergy and Immunology, London, Ontario, Canada.
[3]Department of Otolaryngology, London, Ontario, Canada.

References
1. Widal MF: Anaphylaxie et idiosyncraise. *Press Med* 1922, 119:48–51.
2. Samter M, Beers RF: Intolerance to aspirin: clinical studies and consideration of its pathogenesis. *Ann Intern Med* 1968, 68:975–983.
3. Lee RU, Stevenson DD: Aspirin-exacerbated respiratory disease: evaluation and management. *Allergy Asthma Immunol Res* 2011, 1:3–10.
4. Fokkens WJ, Lund VJ, Mullol J, Bachert C, Cohen N, Cobo R, Desrosiers M, Hellings P, Holmstrom M, Hytönen M, Jones N, Kalogjera L, Kennedy D, Klossek JM, Kowalski M, Meltzer E, Naclerio B, Passali D, Price D, Riechelmann H, Scadding G, Stammberger H, Thomas M, Voegels R, Wang DY: European position paper on nasal polyps. *Rhinology* 2007, 45(Suppl 20):1–139.
5. Stevenson DD: Aspirin sensitivity and desensitization for asthma and sinusitis. *Curr Allergy Asthma Rep* 2009, 9:155–163.
6. Pfaar O, Klimek L: Aspirin desensitization in aspirin intolerance: update on current standards and recent improvements. *Curr Opin Allergy Clin Immunol* 2006, 6:161–166.
7. Berges-Gimeno MP, Simon RA, Stevenson DD: Early effects of aspirin desensitization treatment in asthmatic patients with aspirin-exacerbated respiratory disease. *Ann Allergy Asthma Immunol* 2003, 3:338–341.
8. Berges-Gimeno MP, Simon RA, Stevenson DD: Long-term treatment with aspirin desensitization in asthmatic patients with aspirin-exacerbated respiratory disease. *J Allergy Clin Immunol* 2003, 1:180–186.
9. Desrosiers M, Evans GA, Keith PK, Wright ED, Kaplan A, Bouchard J, Ciavarella A, Doyle PW, Javer AR, Leith ES, Mukherji A, Schellenberg RR, Small P, Witterick IJ: Canadian clinical practice guidelines for acute and chronic rhinosinusitis. *Allergy Asthma Clin Immunol* 2011, 7:1–38.
10. Stevenson DD, Pleskow WW, Simon RA, Mathison DA, Lumry WR, Schatz M, Zeiger RS: Aspirin sensitive rhinosinusitis-asthma: a double-blind crossover study of treatment with aspirin. *J Allergy Clin Immunol* 1984, 73:500–507.
11. White A, Ludington E, Mehra P, Stevenson DD, Simon RA: Effect of leukotriene modifier drugs on the safety of oral aspirin challenges. *Ann Allergy Asthma Immunol* 2006, 5:688–693.
12. White AA, Stevenson DD, Simon RA: The blocking effect of essential controller medications during aspirin challenges in patients with aspirin-exacerbated respiratory disease. *Ann Allergy Asthma Immunol* 2005, 4:330–335.
13. Lee JY, Simon RA, Stevenson DD: Selection of aspirin dosages for aspirin desensitization treatment in patients with aspirin-exacerbated respiratory disease. *J Allergy Clin Immunol* 2007, 119:157–164.
14. Swierczynska-Krepa M, Sanak M, Bochenek G, Strek P, Cmiel A, Gielicz A, Plutecka H, Szczeklik A, Nizankowska-Mogilnicka E: Aspirin desensitization in patients with aspirin-induced and aspirin-tolerant asthma: a double blind study. *J Allergy Clin Immunol* 2014, 134:883–890.
15. Dursun AB, Woessner KA, Simon RA, Karasoy D, Stevenson DD: Predicting outcomes of oral aspirin challenges in patients with asthma, nasal polyps, and chronic sinusitis. *Ann Allergy Asthma Immunol* 2008, 5:420–425.
16. Cho KS, Soudry E, Psaltis AJ, Nadeau KC, McGhee SA, Nayak JV, Hwang PH: Long-term sinonasal outcomes of aspirin desensitization in aspirin exacerbated respiratory disease. *Otolaryngol Head Neck Surg* 2014, 151:575–581.

19

Th17/Treg ratio derived using DNA methylation analysis is associated with the late phase asthmatic response

Amrit Singh[1,2,3†], Masatsugu Yamamoto[1,2,4,5†], Jian Ruan[1,2,3], Jung Young Choi[1,2], Gail M Gauvreau[6], Sven Olek[7], Ulrich Hoffmueller[7], Christopher Carlsten[1,2,4,5], J Mark FitzGerald[2,4,5], Louis-Philippe Boulet[8], Paul M O'Byrne[6] and Scott J Tebbutt[1,2,3,5*]

Abstract

Background: The imbalance between Th17 and Treg cells has been studied in various diseases including allergic asthma but their roles have not been fully understood in the development of the late phase asthmatic response.

Objectives: To determine changes in Th17 and Treg cell numbers between isolated early responders (ERs) and dual responders (DRs) undergoing allergen inhalation challenge. To identify gene expression profiles associated with Th17 and Treg cells.

Methods: 14 participants (8 ERs and 6 DRs) with mild allergic asthma underwent allergen inhalation challenge. Peripheral blood was collected prior to and 2 hours post allergen challenge. DNA methylation analysis was used to quantifiy the relative frequencies of Th17, Tregs, total B cells, and total T cells. Gene expression from whole blood was measured using microarrays. Technical replication of selected genes was performed using nanoString nCounter Elements.

Results: The Th17/Treg ratio significantly increased in DRs compared to ERs post allergen challenge compared to pre-challenge. Genes significantly correlated to Th17 and Treg cell counts were inversely correlated with each other. Genes significantly correlated with Th17/Treg ratio included the cluster of genes of the leukocyte receptor complex located on chromosome 19q 13.4.

Conclusions: Th17/Treg imbalance post-challenge may contribute to the development of the late phase inflammatory phenotype.

Keywords: Allergen inhalation challenge, Asthma, Asthmatic response, DNA methylation, Epigenetic cell counting, Peripheral blood, Th17/Treg ratio, nCounter Elements

Introduction

The imbalance between a proinflammatory T helper 17 (Th17) and a regulatory T (Treg) cell phenotype may play a crucial role in allergic airway inflammation [1]. Experimental models have shown that Th17 cells typically promote neutrophilic inflammation, and also play important roles in airway hyperresponsiveness in concert with Th2

cells [2]. In peripheral blood, Th17 cell counts have been shown to be higher in subjects with allergic asthma compared to healthy controls [3,4]. The percentage of Th17 cells and IL-17 levels in peripheral blood have been shown to be significantly elevated 24 hours after allergen challenge in dual responders compared to early responders or healthy controls [5]. On the other hand, Treg cells maintain immune homeostasis and regulate immune responses to allergens by preventing excessive inflammatory responses [6]. Treg cells were originally identified as CD4$^+$CD25$^+$ T cells with a function to suppress immune responses [7]. In order to identify Treg cells, *FOXP3* expression as a specific marker has been used, however, it is also

---

* Correspondence: Scott.Tebbutt@hli.ubc.ca
†Equal contributors
[1]James Hogg Research Centre for Heart Lung Innovation, St. Paul's Hospital, University of British Columbia, Vancouver, BC, Canada
[2]Institute for HEART + LUNG Health, Vancouver, BC, Canada
Full list of author information is available at the end of the article

expressed in activated non-suppressor T cells [8,9]. Low levels of the IL-7 receptor (CD127) in combination with high expression of CD4 and CD25 can be used to isolate highly purified suppressive Tregs [10]. Recently, DNA methylation analysis of the Treg specific demethylation region (TSDR) within the *FOXP3* locus has been used to enumerate Treg cells, [11] which have been shown to significantly correlate with $CD4^+CD25^+CD127^{lo}$ and $CD4^+CD25^+CD127^{lo}FOXP3^+$ cells [12].

We have previously demonstrated that peripheral blood is a useful biological material with which to study changes in the blood transcriptome, proteome and metabolome of individuals with mild atopic asthma undergoing allergen inhalation challenge [13-16]. In the present study, we have used qPCR based DNA methylation analysis to estimate the number of Th17 cells, Treg cells, T cells and B cells in peripheral blood of mild atopic asthmatics undergoing allergen inhalation challenge. In the same individuals, we also analysed gene expression profiles in whole blood using microarrays to identify genes correlated with each cell type. We hypothesized that changes in specific immune cell counts in peripheral blood would be associated with the allergen-induced late phase asthmatic response.

Methods
Study participants and allergen inhalation challenge
The Institutional Review Boards of the participating institutions, University of British Columbia, McMaster University and Université Laval, approved this study. Fourteen individuals were recruited as part of the AllerGen NCE Clinical Investigator Collaborative (Canada) and provided written informed consent to undergo an allergen inhalation challenge. All participants were non-smokers, free of other lung diseases, and not pregnant. Diagnosis of asthma was based on the Global Initiative for Asthma criteria. Participants were diagnosed with mild allergic asthma, and only used intermittent short-acting bronchodilators for treatment of their asthma. Participants had a baseline $FEV_1 \geq 70\%$ of predicted, and the PC_{20}, provocative concentration of methacholine required to produce a 20% decrease in FEV_1, was ≤ 16 mg/mL.

Skin prick tests were used to determine allergies to cat, and the dose of cat allergen extract for inhalation. Methacholine and allergen challenges were conducted as triad visits. On the first and third day, participants underwent methacholine inhalation tests for assessments of airway hyperresponsiveness (AHR) as described previously [17,18]. The allergen-induced shift (post/pre in PC_{20}) was evaluated as the change in AHR. On the second day participants underwent allergen inhalation challenge with extracts of cat pelt or hair in doubling doses until a drop in FEV_1 of at least of 20% was achieved, then FEV_1 was measured at regular intervals up to 7 hours post-challenge as

described previously [19]. All participants developed an early response which resolved within 1–3 hours after challenge. Participants that demonstrated a maximum drop in FEV_1 of greater than 15% between 3 to 7 hours after allergen inhalation were classified as dual responders (DRs). Participants having an FEV_1 drop of 10% that was still falling at the end of the 7 hour observation period were categorized as DRs if they also demonstrated a drop in PC_{20} (post compared to pre methacholine challenge). Participants who showed neither a drop in $FEV_1 > 15\%$ between 3 to 7 hours after challenge nor a decreased PC_{20} were classified as isolated early responders (ERs).

Blood collection and isolation of RNA and DNA
Peripheral blood was obtained immediately before and 2 hours post-challenge in PAXgene Blood RNA tubes (PreAnalytiX, Qiagen/BD, Valencia, CA, USA) for RNA and in K2 EDTA Vacutainer tubes (BD, Franklin Lakes, NJ, USA) for buffy coat and complete blood count (CBC) measurements. Cellular RNA was purified from 2.5 mL of whole blood in PAXgene tubes according to the manufacturer's protocols using the RNeasy Mini Kit (Qiagen, Chatsworth, CA, USA). Total DNA was isolated from whole blood or buffy coat from EDTA tubes using QIAamp DNA Blood Mini Kit (Qiagen) according to the manufacturer's protocol.

Epigenetic cell counting of lymphocyte subsets using DNA methylation analysis
Cell counting of lymphocyte subsets was performed by Epiontis (Berlin, Germany) using quantitative real-time PCR (qPCR) based DNA methylation analysis [20,21]. Briefly, bisulphite conversion [22] of genomic DNA resulting in either CpG-variants (if DNA is methylated) or TpG-variants (if DNA is unmethylated) was performed. Each qPCR assay is specific for either the demethylated *FOXP3* TSDR (for Tregs) or the demethylated *CD3D/G* (for T cells) or the demethylated *IL17A* (for Th17 cells) or the B cell specific demethylated gene region (for B cells) templates, since the demethylated version of these regions have been shown to be exclusively present in Treg, T cells, Th17 cells and B cells respectively. The other qPCR assay is specific for a control region within the *GAPDH* gene, a target that is demethylated in all cells. The *GAPDH* PCR assay serves as a "load control" as it estimates the number of "total cells" in a given sample. The percentage of Treg cells, T cells, Th17 cells and B cells in a sample is calculated as:

Percentage of a particular cell-type = [Copy Equivalents as determined with the PCR assay targeting the cell-specific DNA target region (e.g. TpG^{TSDR})]/[Copy Equivalents as determined with the *GAPDH* qPCR assay (TpG^{GAPDH})] × [100] × [2[a]].

In the equation above, the "Copy Equivalents" as determined by the cell-specific PCR assay corresponds to "Treg cells", or "T cells" or "Th17 cells" or "B cells" copies, respectively. The "Copy Equivalents" as determined with the *GAPDH* PCR assay corresponds to the "total cell" copies, respectively. A factor of "100" is used to translate the result into percentage of cells.

a) Only for Tregs a factor of "2" is applied in the equation to correct for the fact that each cell has two copies of the (demethylated) *GAPDH* gene but each Treg has just one copy of the demethylated *FOXP3* gene. As *FOXP3* is X-chromosomally located, each Treg holds exactly one copy of the demethylated *FOXP3* gene. Tregs from male subjects hold one X chromosome on which the *FOXP3* gene is demethylated. In contrast, each Treg from a female subject has two X chromosomes (and thus two copies of the *FOXP3* gene) but one X chromosome is inactivated (i.e. fully methylated) and it exists as a Barr body in the cell.

Microarray gene expression assay
Genome-wide expression profiling, labelling and array hybridization were performed using Affymetrix Human Gene 1.0 ST arrays (Affymetrix, Santa Clara, CA, USA). All microarray data has previously [16] been deposited into the Gene Expression Omnibus (GSE40240). All 'CEL' files were normalized using the Robust Multiarray Average (RMA).

nCounter Elements
Technical replication of selected genes was performed using a new digital technology, nCounter Elements (NanoString, Seattle, USA). nCounter Elements allows users to combine nCounter Elements General Purpose Reagents (GPRs) with unlabelled probes that target specific genes of interest (www.nanostring.com/elements/). 100 ng of each RNA sample is added to the TagSet in hybridization buffer and incubated at 65°C for 16 hours. The TagSet consists of a reporter tag and capture tag that hybridize to the user designed gene-specific probe A and probe B complex. Automated processing per cartridge on the PrepStation (high sensitivity protocol) occurs for 3 hours. After a 2.5 hour scan per cartridge, counts are acquired from the GEN2 Digital Analyzer. Details regarding data normalization can be found in the supplementary material.

Statistical and bioinformatics analysis
Linear models were used to test the association between immune cell frequencies and cell-specific gene expression profiles. Cell counts and all combinations of cell ratios (T, B, Treg and Th17) were compared using linear regression models. All microarray data were analysed using the linear models for microarrays (limma) R-library [23]. The

Benjamini-Hochberg false discovery rate (FDR) was used to correct for multiple testing. Partial least squares (PLS), from the mixOmics R-library [24] was used to identify the relationship between cell-specific gene lists. Statistical analyses were performed in the statistical computing program R version 3.0.1 [25].

To test for the enrichment of gene lists, GeneGo network analysis was performed using MetaCore from Thomson Reuters. Network analyses were performed on gene lists created by ranking genes by the scores which rank the subnetworks to saturation with the objects from the initial gene list.

Results
Participant characteristics
The 14 participants were classified into eight isolated early responders (ERs) and six dual responders (DRs), as shown in Table 1. The mean drop in FEV_1 during the late phase in DRs (21.3 ± 3.2) was 4 times greater ($p < 0.05$) compared to ERs (5.1 ± 1.4). Table 1 also shows that all participants exhibited an immediate drop in FEV_1 of greater than 20%.

Correlation between immune cell frequency and cell-specific gene expression
Sum of the T cell and B cell frequencies obtained using the methylation assays strongly correlate (Spearman r = 0.95) with the lymphocyte frequency obtained using a hematolyzer (Additional file 1: Figure S1). T cell, B cell and Th17 cell counts were significantly positively correlated with the genes targeted in epigenetic cell counting in both the microarray (Figure 1; top row) and nanoString (Figure 1; bottom row) platforms. Treg cell counts were not correlated with *FOXP3* gene expression measured using microarrays but was significantly correlated using nanoString, suggesting greater sensitivity of the platform (Figure 1, red points).

Th17 to Treg ratio discriminates early from dual responders after challenge
Allergen inhalation did not significantly change T cell, B cell, Treg cell and Th17 cell counts in either ERs or DRs. In addition, comparing the change in cell counts in ERs with the change in cell counts in DRs (ΔER vs. ΔDR) no significant cell-types were identified (Table 2A). Next, the ratios between different cell-types were analyzed (Table 2B). Table 2B shows that the Th17/Treg ratio significantly (p = 0.03) increased in DRs compared to ERs, from pre to post challenge. Figure 2 shows that the Th17/Treg ratio did not change from pre to post challenge in ERs (net change = 0.006 ± 0.09), whereas the Th17/Treg ratio increased in DRs (net change = 0.28 ± 0.03).

Table 1 Participant demographics

Participant ID	Age (year)	Sex (M:F)	Allergen	Pre [PC$_{20}$] (mg/mL)	Post [PC$_{20}$] (mg/mL)	Allergen-induced shift[b]	% fall in FEV1	
							Early	Late
ER								
1	28	F	Cat Pelt	12.8	ND	ND	20.3	4.8
2	34	F	Cat Pelt	2.8	6.1	2.3	21	1.5
3	27	M	Cat Pelt	4.5	1.8	0.39	34.4	0
4	42	F	Cat Hair	5.3	8.6	1.6	42.1	11.1
5	29	F	Cat Pelt	0.4	ND	ND	44.3	0
6	31	M	Cat Pelt	11.8	16	1.4	24.2	7.5
7	28	F	Cat Hair	9.4	16	1.7	27.1	7.1
8	42	M	Cat	0.1	ND	ND	23	9
Mean ± SE	32.6 ± 2.2	3:5		2.8[a]	7.5[a]	1.5 ± 0.3	29.6 ± 3.2	5.1 ± 1.4
DR								
9	23	F	Cat Hair	0.3	0.2	0.60	38.9	31.8
10	26	F	Cat Hair	5.1	1.5	0.30	31.4	14.9
11	49	F	Cat Hair	3.6	1.0	0.27	25.3	12.6
12	26	M	Cat Hair	0.9	1.0	1.1	31.5	15.6
13	27	F	Cat Pelt	0.6	0.1	0.19	48.3	25.8
14	52	F	Cat	ND	ND	ND	33	27
Mean ± SE	33.8 ± 3.3	1:5		1.3[a]	0.5[a]	0.5 ± 0.1	34.7 ± 3.2	21.3 ± 3.2[c]

ND - Not determined; all participants were challenged with cat allergen.
[a]geometric mean (PC$_{20}$ values are measured on a log scale).
[b][PC$_{20}$]$_{post}$/[PC$_{20}$]$_{pre}$.
[c]$p < 0.05$ versus ER group.

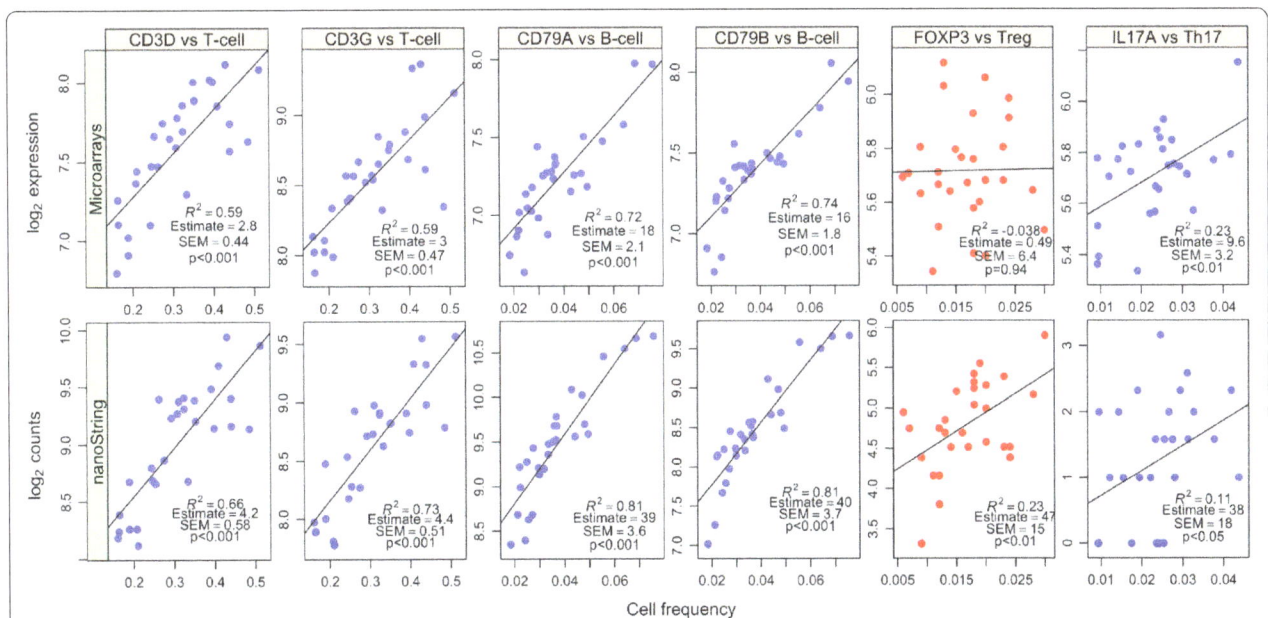

Figure 1 Scatter plots of immune cells quantified using DNA methylation analysis with the corresponding cell-specific gene expressions profiles. x-axis: relative cell-type frequencies of T, B, Treg and Th17 cells in whole blood; y-axis: a) top row: gene (*CD3D, CD3G, CD79A, CD79A, FOXP3,* and *IL17A*) expression intensities measured using microarrays and b) bottom row: gene expression counts measured using nCounter Elements from nanoString.

Table 2 Comparing immune cell-frequencies and cell/cell ratios between early and dual responders after allergen challenge

A. Comparing immune cell-frequencies between ERs and DRs after allergen challenge

	Fold-change (post-pre) in early responders	Fold-change (post-pre) in dual responders	ΔER vs. ΔDR
	Mean ± SEM	Mean ± SEM	p-value
T cell	−2.20 ± 1.40	−4.26 ± 2.39	0.45
B cell	−0.20 ± 0.17	−0.11 ± 0.26	0.77
Th17 cell	−0.22 ± 0.21	0.14 ± 0.16	0.22
Treg cell	−0.12 ± 0.06	−0.42 ± 0.17	0.10

B. Comparing immune cell/cell ratios between ERs and DRs after allergen challenge

	Fold-change (post-pre) in early responders	Fold-change (post-pre) in dual responders	ΔER vs. ΔDR
	Mean ± SEM	Mean ± SEM	p-value
T/B	−0.59 ± 0.70	−0.74 ± 0.43	0.87
Th17/T	0.002 ± 0.006	0.009 ± 0.002	0.31
Treg/T	−0.0008 ± 0.005	−0.006 ± 0.002	0.38
B/Th17	−0.009 ± 0.10	−0.37 ± 0.21	0.13
B/Treg	−0.002 ± 0.22	0.42 ± 0.18	0.18
Th17/Treg	0.006 ± 0.09	0.28 ± 0.03	0.03

Genes associated with Th17 and Treg cells

A multiple linear regression model (limma) was used to identify genes whose expression levels correlated with the frequencies of specific cell-types independent of changes in the frequencies of other cell-types (gene expression ~ Th17 + Treg + B-cells + other T-cells, where other T-cells = overall T-cells minus Th17 and Treg). 10 (99) genes were positively correlated with Th17 (Treg) cells at an FDR of 10%, with no overlapping genes

between the two lists. Th17 genes included *KIR2DS2*, *TAGLN*, *C14orf37*, *KRTAP13-3*, *SAP30*, *KIR2DS4*, *LAIR2*, *FLJ30679*, *RORC* and *KIR2DL2*. The 99 Treg genes were enriched (FDR = 5%) for 27 pathways including many relevant regulatory pathways such as IL-2 regulation of translation, Regulation of telomere length and cellular immortalization, Regulation of T cell function by CTLA-4 (Additional file 1: Figure S2). Partial Least Squares (PLS) was used to determine the correlation between the set of

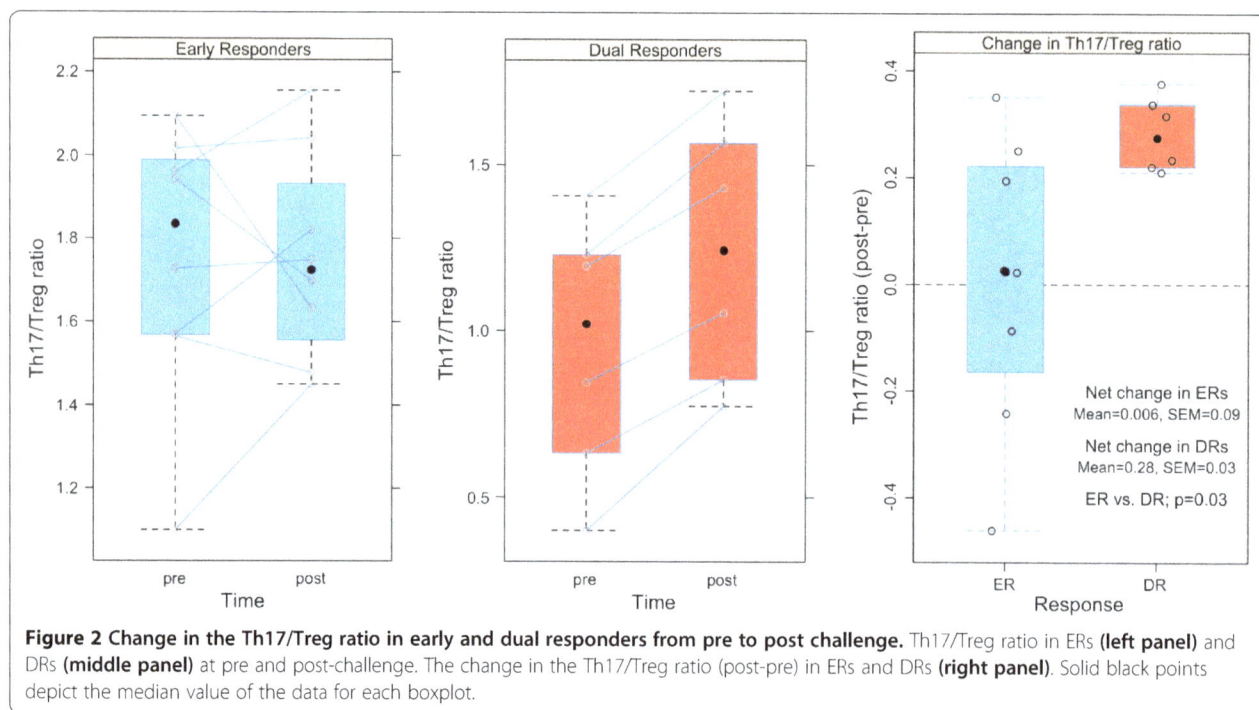

Figure 2 Change in the Th17/Treg ratio in early and dual responders from pre to post challenge. Th17/Treg ratio in ERs **(left panel)** and DRs **(middle panel)** at pre and post-challenge. The change in the Th17/Treg ratio (post-pre) in ERs and DRs **(right panel)**. Solid black points depict the median value of the data for each boxplot.

10 Th17 genes and the set of 99 Treg genes. Figure 3 depicts the results of PLS using a correlation circle (see Gonzalez et al. [26] for complete details on graphical outputs of PLS). Vectors drawn from the origin to each of the points (genes) allows one to determine the relationship between genes: 1) if the angle between two vectors is less than 90°, there exists a positive correlation between the two genes, 2) if the angle between two vectors is greater than 90°, there exists a negative correlation between the two genes, and 3) if the angle between two vectors is equal to 90°, the correlation between the two genes is zero. Figure 3 shows that the Th17 genes were inversely correlated with Treg genes (angle greater than 90°).

Genes significantly correlated with the Th17/Treg ratio
To investigate the relationship of Th17/Treg ratio and gene expression profiles, we identified correlated genes in the entire sample set. We identified 13 genes significantly correlated with Th17/Treg ratio using limma (FDR = 5%, Table 3). Interestingly, 7 genes (KIR3DL1, LAIR2, KIR2DS2, KIR2DL2, CD226, KIR2DS4, KIR2DS1) belong to the leukocyte receptor complex (LRC) located on chromosome 19q13.4, and were shown to be positively correlated except CD226. However, of the four genes profiled

Table 3 Genes significantly correlated to Th17/Treg ratio in Pearson tests (FDR <0.05)

Gene	r	p value	FDR
TAGLN	0.78	7.59E-07	0.02
C14orf37	0.77	3.16E-06	0.02
KIR3DL1*	0.75	3.82E-06	0.02
LAIR2*	0.75	4.80E-06	0.02
CDCP1	0.74	5.77E-06	0.02
KIR2DS2*	0.74	6.19E-06	0.02
SAP30	0.74	7.09E-06	0.02
KIR2DL2*	0.73	8.51E-06	0.02
CD226*	−0.73	9.83E-06	0.02
ZNF286B	−0.73	9.27E-06	0.02
KRTAP13-3	0.72	1.57E-05	0.03
KIR2DS4*	0.71	2.38E-05	0.043
KIR2DS1*	0.70	2.86E-05	0.048

*genes belonging to leukocyte receptor complex (LRC).

using nanoString, only CD226 and KIR2DS4 successfully replicated (Figure 4). The top-listed transcriptional network in GeneGo network analysis for the 13 significant genes included regulatory functions in immune responses (Additional file 1: Table S1).

Significantly different genes between ERs and DRs in Th17 or Treg
In a secondary analysis, we also analysed gene-cell correlations that significantly differed between early and dual responders, irrespective of allergen exposure, using limma. In GeneGo network analysis, genes differentially associated with Th17 (165 genes differentially associated with Th17 between ERs and DRs, p < 0.01) were enriched for immunological processes including immunoglobulin mediated immune response and adaptive immune response. Genes differentially associated with Treg between ER and DR (554 genes, p < 0.01) were enriched for immune processes. Although the genes differentially associated with Th17 cells between ERs and DRs did not achieve a stringent threshold of FDR, the top three genes, S100B, MILR1 and CHI3L1 (p-value < 0.001, FDR = 0.79, Additional file 1: Figure S3), have previously been reported to be involved in allergy or asthma [27-29]. Additional file 1: Figure S3 shows that all three genes were differentially correlated with Th17 cell counts with respect to the response class using both the microarray and nanoString platforms.

Discussion
Although Th17 and Treg cells arise from a common precursor cell [30] they have opposing inflammatory roles which has been demonstrated in the context of autoimmune disease [31], infection [32], and recently allergic airway inflammation [1]. In the present study

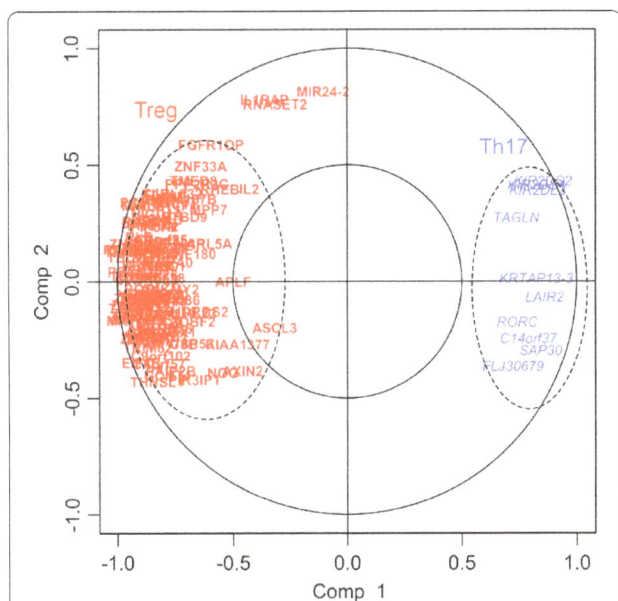

Figure 3 Correlation circle depicting the strength of correlation between Treg genes (red) and Th17 genes (blue) with their respective latent variables (Comp 1 and Comp 2). The Treg genes (red) show a strong negative correlation with the Th17 genes (blue). Vectors drawn from the origin to each of the points (genes) allows one to determine the relationship between genes: 1) if the angle between two vectors is less than 90°, there exists a positive correlation between the two genes, 2) if the angle between two vectors is greater than 90°, there exists a negative correlation between the two genes, and 3) if the angle between two vectors is equal to 90°, the correlation between the two genes is zero.

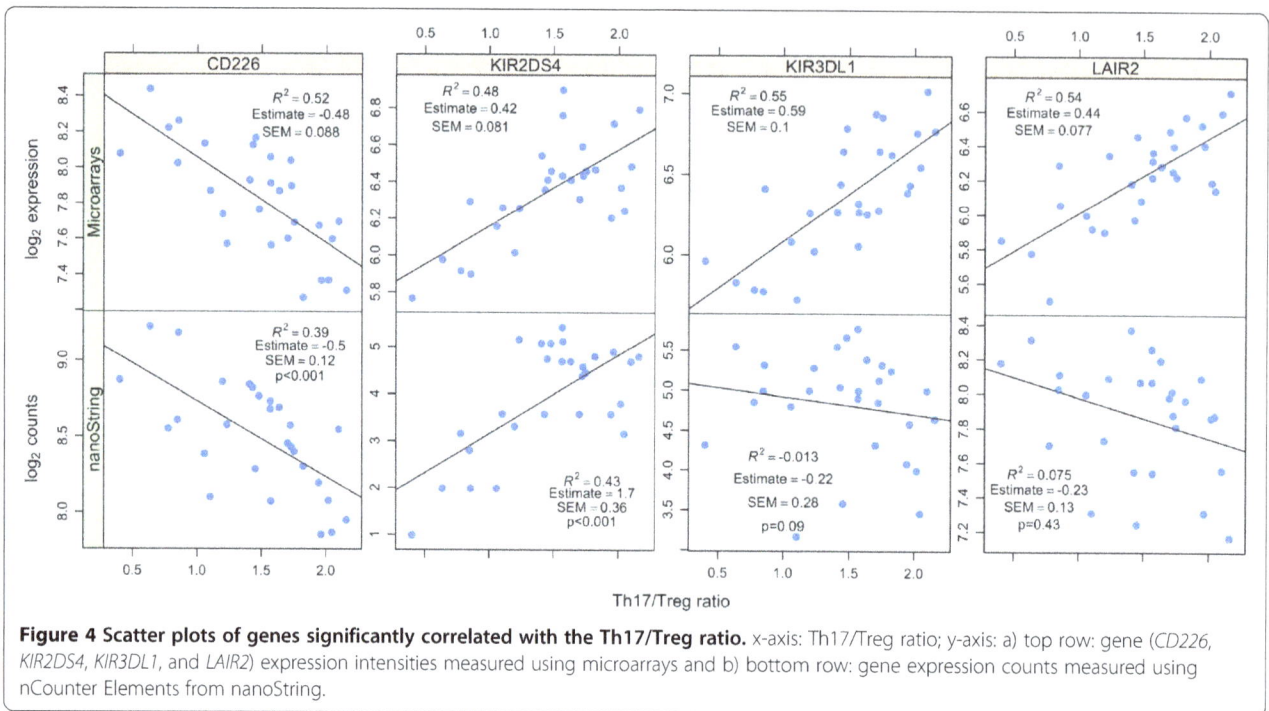

Figure 4 Scatter plots of genes significantly correlated with the Th17/Treg ratio. x-axis: Th17/Treg ratio; y-axis: a) top row: gene (*CD226*, *KIR2DS4*, *KIR3DL1*, and *LAIR2*) expression intensities measured using microarrays and b) bottom row: gene expression counts measured using nCounter Elements from nanoString.

we demonstrate a potential Th17/Treg homeostatic imbalance using peripheral blood of isolated early and dual asthmatic responders (ERs and DRs) undergoing allergen inhalation challenge.

DNA methylation analysis used to enumerate various immune cells revealed good correlation with the cell-specific gene expression profiles as measured using microarrays. Technical replication using nCounter Elements from nanoString, a more sensitive platform indicated that *FOXP3* expression was indeed correlated with Treg cell counts. As a marker for human Tregs, however, *FOXP3* expression is of doubtful value, due to its transient expression in activated non-regulatory effector T cells [21]. In addition, other cell-surface markers such as CD127 or CD45RA have been used to isolate FOXP3$^+$ Treg cell populations with high efficiency [33,34]. Epigenetic enumeration of Treg cells in the present study has been shown to positively correlate with CD4$^+$CD25$^+$CD127^{lo}, and CD4$^+$ CD25$^+$CD127^{lo}FOXP3$^+$ [12] and thus are truly representative of suppressive Tregs.

The percentage of Treg cells did not significantly change in either ERs (−0.12 ± 0.06; p = 0.11) or DRs (−0.42 ± 0.17; p = 0.054), two hours post-challenge. Previous studies have also not shown significant changes in Treg cells in peripheral blood in DRs undergoing allergen inhalation challenge [35,36]. This may be due to many factors such as the time of the post-challenge blood draw, the cell-surface markers used to isolate the Treg cells as well as the small sample sizes (n = 6-11) used in these studies. Similarly, the percentage of Th17 cells also did not significantly change in ERs (−0.22 ± 0.21; p = 0.30) or DRs (0.14 ± 0.16; p = 0.44),

after allergen challenge. Th17 cells have been shown to be increased 7 and 24 hours post-challenge in both ERs and DRs and the increase in DRs was greater than in ERs 24 hours post challenge [5]. Th17 cells as well as the concentrations of IL-17 and IL-22, have also been shown to be increased with the severity of allergic asthma [37]. Genes significantly positively correlated with Th17 cells included *RORC*, the transcription factor involved in Th17 differentiation, whereas genes significantly positively correlated with Treg genes was enriched for regulatory functions. Furthermore, Th17 and Treg cell associated genes were inversely correlated with each other, further implicating the phenotypic roles of these cell-types in allergic asthma.

Although neither cell-type significantly changed pre to post challenge, the change in the Th17/Treg ratio from pre to post challenge significantly (p = 0.03) differed between ERs and DRs. The Th17/Treg ratio increased in DRs whereas little change occurs in ERs after challenge. The increase in the Th17/Treg ratio in DRs is driven by an increase in the number of Th17 cells (0.14 ± 0.16) and a decrease in the number of Treg cells (−0.42 ± 0.17) due to allergen exposure. A possible mechanism of Th17/Treg imbalance was suggested by the genes that were correlated with Th17/Treg ratio. LRC on chromosome 19q13.4 encodes immunoglobulin super family receptors including killer immunoglobulin like receptors (KIRs) expressed on hematopoietic cells. Almost all LRC significant genes were positively correlated to Th17/Treg, whilst *CD226* is the only LRC gene negatively correlated. A previous study on differential expression of LRC genes revealed that KIRs and inhibitory receptor ILT2/LIR1 were expressed in activated T cells and that KIR levels in T cells are associated with resistance to activation-induced cell death [38]. These may suggest a new hypothesis that LRC gene expression patterns might be related to Th17/ Treg ratio and involved in immune responses to inhaled allergen in asthmatics.

The statistical interaction analyses suggested differences in gene expression profiles in Th17 or Tregs between ERs and DRs. Interestingly, top-listed differentially expressed Th17-associated genes *S100B*, *MILR1* and *CHI3L1* have been reported to play roles in allergy and asthma. S100B$^+$ lymphocytes in blood have been reported to consist of two subtypes; a cytotoxic T cell and a NK subtype [27]. In connection with the significant correlations between Th17 and KIR family, Th17 measured by epigenetic cell counting for *IL17A* might be related to other types of immune cells. This is supported by reports showing that IL-17 genes are expressed in non-CD4$^+$ T cells such as γδ T cells, NK cells and Type 3 innate lymphoid cells, suggesting that innate immunity might be responsible for initiating this type of inflammation commonly associated with Th17 immunity [39,40]. Further studies are needed to clarify the disparity between true Th17 and IL17A-demethylated cells. *MILR1* is the gene for allergin-1 protein, which was recently identified to play an inhibitory role in mast cell functions [28]. Polymorphisms in *CHI3L1* as well as the concentration of its corresponding protein YKL-40 in serum has been associated with asthma and pulmonary function [29]. Our findings suggest that Th17 cell gene expression profiles are divergent between asthmatic responses and that these profiles might be related to immune mechanisms.

A limitation of this study is its small sample size, which reduces the statistical power in identifying true positives. Therefore we deemed a technical validation using a highly sensitive platform appropriate for this study. Independent replication will be important as part of future studies with larger sample sizes. Another limitation of the present study is that only a limited number of cell-types were studied using DNA methylation analysis, whereas quantification of a wide array of cell-types such as Th1, Th2, and Th9 cells would provide deeper biological insights into the mechanisms of allergic asthmatic responses. DNA methylation based qPCR assays for these cell-types will allow for tissue samples to remain unperturbed, and additional sources of variability, such as those observed in fluorescence activated cell sorting to be avoided.

The careful phenotyping of our participants, together with innovative epigenetic- and gene expression-based methodologies, have nevertheless revealed interesting directions for further investigations using large sample sizes and different allergens.

Abbreviations
Th17: T helper 17; Treg: Regulatory T; FOXP3: Forkhead box protein 3; TSDR: Treg specific demethylation region; ER: Isolated early responder; DR: Dual responder; Limma: Linear models for microarrays; PLS: Partial least squares; LRC: Leukocyte receptor complex.

Competing interests
The authors declare that they have no competing interests.

Authors' contributions
AS and MY contributed equally to this work. GMG, PMO, CC, JMF, LPB, SJT participated in research design and provision of samples. MY, JR, SJT participated in the sample processing and following experiments. SO and UH performed the epigenetic cell counting assay. AS, MY, JYC, SJT conducted data analyses. AS, MY, CC, SJT participated in the writing of the paper. All authors read and approved the final manuscript.

Acknowledgements
We thank the research participants for taking part in these studies, as well as Johane Lepage, Philippe Prince, Joanne Milot, Mylène Bertrand, Richard Watson, George Obminski, Heather Campbell, Abbey Torek, Tara Strinich and Karen Howie for their expertise and assistance with participant recruitment, allergen challenge and sample collection, as part of the AllerGen NCE Clinical Investigator Collaborative. We also thank Peter Paré for technical advice. This research was supported by funding from AllerGen NCE Inc. (Allergy, Genes and Environment Network) and the Canadian Institutes of Health Research. We are grateful for additional funding support from the Peter Wall Institute for Advanced Studies. AS is the recipient of the CIHR Doctoral Award – Frederick Banting and Charles Best Canada Graduate Scholarship. MY was supported in part by the fellowship grants of a Canadian Institutes of Health Research (CIHR) Integrated and Mentored Pulmonary and Cardiovascular Training Program (IMPACT), the Sumitomo Life Social Welfare Services Foundation and the Mochida Memorial Foundation for Medical and Pharmaceutical Research.

Author details
[1]James Hogg Research Centre for Heart Lung Innovation, St. Paul's Hospital, University of British Columbia, Vancouver, BC, Canada. [2]Institute for HEART + LUNG Health, Vancouver, BC, Canada. [3]Prevention of Organ Failure (PROOF) Centre of Excellence, Vancouver, BC, Canada. [4]Vancouver Coastal Health Research Institute, Vancouver General Hospital, Vancouver, BC, Canada. [5]Department of Medicine, Division of Respiratory Medicine, UBC, Vancouver, BC, Canada. [6]Department of Medicine, McMaster University, Hamilton, ON, Canada. [7]Epiontis GmbH, Berlin, Germany. [8]Quebec Heart and Lung Institute, Laval University, Québec City, QC, Canada.

References
1. Zhao J, Lloyd CM, Noble A: **Th17 responses in chronic allergic airway inflammation abrogate regulatory T-cell-mediated tolerance and contribute to airway remodeling.** *Mucosal Immunol* 2013, **6**(2):335–346.
2. Cosmi L, Liotta F, Maggi E, Romagnani S, Annunziato F: **Th17 cells: New players in asthma pathogenesis.** *Allergy* 2011, **66**(8):989–998.
3. Wong CK, Lun SW, Ko FW, Wong PT, Hu SQ, Chan IH, Hui DS, Lam CW: **Activation of peripheral Th17 lymphocytes in patients with asthma.** *Immunol Invest* 2009, **38**(7):652–664.

4. Kerzel S, Dehne J, Rogosch T, Schaub B, Maier RF, Zemlin M: Th17 cell frequency in peripheral blood from children with allergic asthma correlates with the level of asthma control. *J Pediatr* 2012, **161**(6):1172–1174.
5. Bajoriuniene I, Malakauskas K, Lavinskiene S, Jeroch J, Gasiuniene E, Vitkauskiene A, Sakalauskas R: Peripheral blood Th17 cells and neutrophils in dermatophagoides pteronyssinus-induced early- and late-phase asthmatic response. *Medicina (Kaunas)* 2012, **48**(9):442–451.
6. Langier S, Sade K, Kivity S: Regulatory T cells in allergic asthma. *Isr Med Assoc J* 2012, **14**(3):180–183.
7. Takahashi T, Kuniyasu Y, Toda M, Sakaguchi N, Itoh M, Iwata M, Shimizu J, Sakaguchi S: Immunologic self-tolerance maintained by CD25 + CD4+ naturally anergic and suppressive T cells: Induction of autoimmune disease by breaking their anergic/suppressive state. *Int Immunol* 1998, **10**(12):1969–1980.
8. Tran DQ, Ramsey H, Shevach EM: Induction of FOXP3 expression in naive human CD4 + FOXP3 T cells by T-cell receptor stimulation is transforming growth factor-beta dependent but does not confer a regulatory phenotype. *Blood* 2007, **110**(8):2983–2990.
9. d'Hennezel E, Piccirillo CA: Analysis of human FOXP3+ treg cells phenotype and function. *Methods Mol Biol* 2011, **707**:199–218.
10. Liu W, Putnam AL, Xu-Yu Z, Szot GL, Lee MR, Zhu S, Gottlieb PA, Kapranov P, Gingeras TR, Fazekas de St Groth B, Clayberger C, Soper DM, Ziegler SF, Bluestone JA: CD127 expression inversely correlates with FoxP3 and suppressive function of human CD4+ T reg cells. *J Exp Med* 2006, **203**(7):1701–1711.
11. Baron U, Floess S, Wieczorek G, Baumann K, Grutzkau A, Dong J, Thiel A, Boeld TJ, Hoffmann P, Edinger M, Turbachova I, Hamann A, Olek S, Huehn J: DNA demethylation in the human FOXP3 locus discriminates regulatory T cells from activated FOXP3(+) conventional T cells. *Eur J Immunol* 2007, **37**(9):2378–2389.
12. Nettenstrom L, Alderson K, Raschke EE, Evans MD, Sondel PM, Olek S, Seroogy CM: An optimized multi-parameter flow cytometry protocol for human T regulatory cell analysis on fresh and viably frozen cells, correlation with epigenetic analysis, and comparison of cord and adult blood. *J Immunol Methods* 2013, **387**(1–2):81–88.
13. Kam SH, Singh A, He JQ, Ruan J, Gauvreau GM, O'Byrne PM, Fitzgerald JM, Tebbutt SJ: Peripheral blood gene expression changes during allergen inhalation challenge in atopic asthmatic individuals. *J Asthma* 2012, **49**(3):219–226.
14. Yamamoto M, Singh A, Ruan J, Gauvreau GM, O'Byrne PM, Carlsten CR, Fitzgerald JM, Boulet LP, Tebbutt SJ: Decreased miR-192 expression in peripheral blood of asthmatic individuals undergoing an allergen inhalation challenge. *BMC Genomics* 2012, **13**:655. 2164-13-655.
15. Singh A, Freue GV, Oosthuizen JL, Kam SH, Ruan J, Takhar MK, Gauvreau GM, O'Byrne PM, Fitzgerald JM, Boulet LP, Borchers CH, Tebbutt SJ: Plasma proteomics can discriminate isolated early from dual responses in asthmatic individuals undergoing an allergen inhalation challenge. *Proteomics Clin Appl* 2012, **6**(9-10):476–485.
16. Singh A, Yamamoto M, Kam SH, Ruan J, Gauvreau GM, O'Byrne PM, Fitzgerald JM, Schellenberg R, Boulet LP, Wojewodka G, Kanagaratham C, De Sanctis JB, Radzioch D, Tebbutt SJ: Gene-metabolite expression in blood can discriminate allergen-induced isolated early from dual asthmatic responses. *PLoS One* 2013, **8**(7):e67907.
17. Crapo RO, Casaburi R, Coates AL, Enright PL, Hankinson JL, Irvin CG, MacIntyre NR, McKay RT, Wanger JS, Anderson SD, Cockcroft DW, Fish JE, Sterk PJ: Guidelines for methacholine and exercise challenge testing-1999. this official statement of the american thoracic society was adopted by the ATS board of directors, July 1999. *Am J Respir Crit Care Med* 2000, **161**(1):309–329.
18. Cockcroft DW, Murdock KY: Changes in bronchial responsiveness to histamine at intervals after allergen challenge. *Thorax* 1987, **42**(4):302–308.
19. O'Byrne PM, Dolovich J, Hargreave FE: Late asthmatic responses. *Am Rev Respir Dis* 1987, **136**(3):740–751.
20. Sehouli J, Loddenkemper C, Cornu T, Schwachula T, Hoffmuller U, Grutzkau A, Lohneis P, Dickhaus T, Grone J, Kruschewski M, Mustea A, Turbachova I, Baron U, Olek S: Epigenetic quantification of tumor-infiltrating T-lymphocytes. *Epigenetics* 2011, **6**(2):236–246.
21. Wieczorek G, Asemissen A, Model F, Turbachova I, Floess S, Liebenberg V, Baron U, Stauch D, Kotsch K, Pratschke J, Hamann A, Loddenkemper C, Stein H, Volk HD, Hoffmuller U, Grutzkau A, Mustea A, Huehn J, Scheibenbogen C, Olek S: Quantitative DNA methylation analysis of FOXP3 as a new method for counting regulatory T cells in peripheral blood and solid tissue. *Cancer Res* 2009, **69**(2):599–608.
22. Olek A, Oswald J, Walter J: A modified and improved method for bisulphite based cytosine methylation analysis. *Nucleic Acids Res* 1996, **1524**(24):5064–5066.
23. Symth GK: Linear models and empirical bayes methods for assessing differential expression in microarrays experiments. *Stat Appl Genet Mol Biol* 2004, **3**:Article3.
24. Le Cao KA, Gonzalez I, Dejean S: integrOmics: An R package to unravel relationships between two omics datasets. *Bioinformatics* 2009, **25**(21):2855–2856.
25. R Development Core Team: *R: A language and environment for statistical computing*. Vienna, Austria: R Foundation for Statistical Computing; 2011.
26. Gonzalez I, Cao KA, Davis MJ, Dejean S: Visualising associations between paired 'omics' data sets. *BioData Min* 2012, **5**(1):19. 0381-5-19.
27. Miki Y, Gion Y, Mukae Y, Hayashi A, Sato H, Yoshino T, Takahashi K: Morphologic, flow cytometric, functional, and molecular analyses of S100B positive lymphocytes, unique cytotoxic lymphocytes containing S100B protein. *Eur J Haematol* 2013, **90**(2):99–110.
28. Hitomi K, Tahara-Hanaoka S, Someya S, Fujiki A, Tada H, Sugiyama T, Shibayama S, Shibuya K, Shibuya A: An immunoglobulin-like receptor, allergin-1, inhibits immunoglobulin E-mediated immediate hypersensitivity reactions. *Nat Immunol* 2010, **11**(7):601–607.
29. Ober C, Tan Z, Sun Y, Possick JD, Pan L, Nicolae R, Radford S, Parry RR, Heinzmann A, Deichmann KA, Lester LA, Gern JE, Lemanske RF Jr, Nicolae DL, Elias JA, Chupp GL: Effect of variation in CHI3L1 on serum YKL-40 level, risk of asthma, and lung function. *N Engl J Med* 2008, **358**(16):1682–1691.
30. Bettelli E, Carrier Y, Gao W, Korn T, Strom TB, Oukka M, Weiner HL, Kuchroo VK: Reciprocal developmental pathways for the generation of pathogenic effector TH17 and regulatory T cells. *Nature* 2006, **441**(7090):235–238.
31. Yang J, Chu Y, Yang X, Gao D, Zhu L, Yang X, Wan L, Li M: Th17 and natural treg cell population dynamics in systemic lupus erythematosus. *Arthritis Rheum* 2009, **60**(5):1472–1483.
32. Cua DJ, Kastelein RA: TGF-beta, a 'double agent' in the immune pathology war. *Nat Immunol* 2006, **7**(6):557–559.
33. Brusko T, Bluestone J: Clinical application of regulatory T cells for treatment of type 1 diabetes and transplantation. *Eur J Immunol* 2008, **38**(4):931–934.
34. Hoffmann P, Eder R, Boeld TJ, Doser K, Piseshka B, Andreesen R, Edinger M: Only the CD45RA + subpopulation of CD4 + CD25high T cells gives rise to homogeneous regulatory T-cell lines upon in vitro expansion. *Blood* 2006, **108**(13):4260–4267.
35. Moniuszko M, Kowal K, Zukowski S, Dabrowska M, Bodzenta-Lukaszyk A: Frequencies of circulating CD4 + CD25 + CD127low cells in atopics are altered by bronchial allergen challenge. *Eur J Clin Invest* 2008, **38**(3):201–204.
36. Kinoshita T, Baatjes A, Smith SG, Dua B, Watson R, Kawayama T, Larche M, Gauvreau GM, O'Byrne PM: Natural regulatory T cells in isolated early responders compared with dual responders with allergic asthma. *J Allergy Clin Immunol* 2013, **133**(3):696–703.
37. Zhao Y, Yang J, Gao YD, Guo W: Th17 immunity in patients with allergic asthma. *Int Arch Allergy Immunol* 2010, **151**(4):297–307.
38. Young NT, Uhrberg M, Phillips JH, Lanier LL, Parham P: Differential expression of leukocyte receptor complex-encoded ig-like receptors correlates with the transition from effector to memory CTL. *J Immunol* 2001, **166**(6):3933–3941.
39. Scanlon ST, McKenzie AN: Type 2 innate lymphoid cells: New players in asthma and allergy. *Curr Opin Immunol* 2012, **24**(6):707–712.
40. McAleer JP, Kolls JK: Mechanisms controlling Th17 cytokine expression and host defense. *J Leukoc Biol* 2011, **90**(2):263–270.

20

Identification of the main allergen sensitizers in an Iran asthmatic population by molecular diagnosis

Fardis Teifoori[1,2,3], Masoomeh Shams-Ghahfarokhi[1*], Idoia Postigo[2,3], Mehdi Razzaghi-Abyaneh[4], Ali Eslamifar[5], Antonio Gutiérrez[2,3], Ester Suñén[2,3] and Jorge Martínez[2,3*]

Abstract

Background: There has been a significant growth in the prevalence of allergy, mainly associated to IgE-mediated disorders such as asthma and rhinitis. The identification of atopy in asthmatic patients through the measurement of specific IgE can help to identify risk factors that cause asthmatic symptoms in patients. The development and use of individualized allergen-based tests by the Component Resolved Diagnosis has been a crucial advance in the accurate diagnosis and control of allergic patients. The objective of this work was to assess the usefulness of molecular diagnosis to identify environmental allergens as possible factors influencing the development and manifestation of asthma in a group of asthmatic patients from Iran.

Methods: Studied population: 202 adult asthmatic patients treated at the Loghman Hakim Hospital and Pasteur Institute of Teheran (Iran) from 2011 to 2012. Specific IgE determined by the ImmunoCAP system were used to both evaluate the patients' atopic condition and the molecules involved in the allergic sensitization. SDS-PAGE IgE-immunoblotting associated with mass spectrometry was carried out to study the cockroach IgE-binding sensitizing proteins.

Results: Forty-five percent of all patients could be considered atopic individuals. Eighty-two percent of atopic patients were sensitized to pollen allergens. The *Salsola kali* (Sal k 1) and the *Phleum pratense* (rPhl p 1 and/or rPhl p 5) major allergens were the most common sensitizers among pollens (71% and 18%, respectively). Thirty-five percent of the atopic population was sensitized to cockroach. Four different allergens, including a previously unknown alpha-amylase, were identified in the cockroach extract. No significant associations could be demonstrated between the severity of asthma and the specific IgE levels in the atopic population. Statistical analysis identified the Sal k 1 as the main protein allergen influencing the development and expression of asthma in the studied population.

Conclusions: Pollen and cockroach were the most relevant allergen sources in the asthmatic population. The *Salsola kali* major allergen was the main cause for sensitization in the atopic patients suffering asthma. Using the Component Resolved Diagnosis, it was possible to identify a new *Blattella germanica* cockroach allergen (*Blattella* alpha amylase 53 kDa) that could sensitize a relevant percentage of this population.

Keywords: Allergy, Atopy, Specific IgE, Component resolved diagnosis, Asthma, Risk factor, Pollen, Mould, Cockroach, Protein, Allergen

* Correspondence: shamsm@modares.ac.ir; jorge.martinez@ehu.es
[1]Department of Mycology, Faculty of Medical Sciences, Tarbiat Modares University, Tehran 14115-331, Iran
[2]Laboratory of Parasitology and Allergy, Center for Research Lascaray Ikergunea, University of the Basque Country, Pº Universidad, 7, 01006 Vitoria, Spain
Full list of author information is available at the end of the article

Background

The World Allergy Organization defines the term atopy as a personal and/or familiar tendency to become sensitized and produce IgE antibodies in response to ordinary exposure to allergens, most frequently proteins. Common allergens associated with atopy are inhaled and food proteins [1]. There has been a significant exponential growth in the prevalence of atopy, including IgE-mediated allergic diseases such as asthma and rhinitis. It is estimated that 30% of the world population is now affected by one or more allergic conditions and is capable of developing specific IgE antibodies to different allergenic proteins from various sources, including pollens, molds, dust mites, insects, epithelia and foods [2].

Asthma is a worldwide problem, with an estimated 300 million affected individuals. The global prevalence of asthma ranges from 1-18% of the population, depending on the country. Indoor and outdoor allergens are important environmental factors that influence the development and expression of asthma. The identification of atopy through specific IgE determination can help to identify the triggers able to develop symptoms of allergic asthma in atopic patients [3]. Geographical variation in the prevalence of sensitization to common aeroallergens is commonly observed across different geographical sources [4] and several studies have reported on the aeroallergen sensitivity of Iranian patients with asthma or rhinitis [5-7] demonstrating significant variation in sensitization sources depending on the report. Despite the different localizations of these studies, all results agree that pollen sensitization is the most prevalent and that Chenopodiaceae, grass and sycamore are the most important allergenic sources. The arthropods most commonly associated with sensitization were house dust mite and cockroach, but their prevalence was very different according to their location.

The development and use of individualized native and/or recombinant allergen-based tests in the routine diagnosis of allergic diseases have been crucial advances in the accurate diagnosis and control of allergic patients [8]. This advance enables the progression from mere taxonomic diagnostic approximations to the molecular classification of allergenic substances [9] and, thus, from individualized allergens to clinical decisions [10]. Component Resolved Diagnosis (CRD) has been shown to be the most accurate methodology for the molecular diagnosis of allergy [3], and the use of this methodology would redefine concepts such as major allergens, cross-reactivity or primary sensitization [11-13]. The proteomics underlying CRD enables a more complete description of the molecular allergen panel, independent of the availability or knowledge of the allergen molecules involved [14].

With this in mind, the objective of this work was to demonstrate which environmental allergenic proteins could be the possible triggers of asthma in a population of atopic individuals suffering asthma symptoms in the north of Iran.

To the best of our knowledge, this is the first report to demonstrate the prevalence of aeroallergens in asthmatic patients from Iran evaluated by CRD.

Methods

Study population

Two hundred and two adult patients (aged 18–83 years, mean = 41 years) treated at the Loghman Hakim Hospital and Pasteur Institute of Teheran (Iran) from 2011 to 2012 were included in this study.

All these patients were diagnosed with asthma following the Global Initiative for Asthma criteria [15]. Respiratory symptoms (cough, dyspnea or chest tightness), spirometry measurements with and without bronchodilator, and methacholine tests (in normal pulmonary function test cases) were performed. Only those patients who were positive for methacholine or pulmonary function tests were selected for inclusion in the study. Oral informed and written consent for participating in this study was obtained from the patients. The study was approval by the Ethics Committee of the Loghman Hakim Hospital. The sex distribution was 40.1% (81) male and 59.9% (121) female.

Atopy study

Atopy for all subjects was analyzed using the Immuno-CAP Phadiatop (ThermoFisher Sci. USA) assay [16], which is a solid-phase immunoassay for serum specific IgE against a balanced mixture of relevant inhaled and food allergens. The recommendations of the manufacturer's protocol were strictly followed. Phadiatop ImmunoCAP results are displayed as qualitative positive or negative responses. Because *Salsola* allergen is not included in the ImmunoCAP Phadiatop, specific IgE to this allergen (Sal k 1) was measured for all subjects separately in an ImmunoCAP-specific IgE assay (ThermoFisher Sci).

Specific IgE quantification

Specific IgE to allergens was quantified by the ImmunoCAP-specific IgE assay (ThermoFisher Sci. USA) following the recommendations of the manufacturer's protocol. ImmunoCAP-specific IgE results are expressed in kU/L. Values ≤ 0.1 kU/L were considered negative results.

Specific IgE to allergen extracts from cockroach *(Blattella germanica)* was used because the difficulty in obtaining commercially available cockroach allergens.

Component resolved diagnosis

Quantitative CRD was performed in the atopic subjects using ImmunoCAP technology (ThermoFisher Sci. USA) following the manufacturer's instructions. The results are expressed in kU/L, and values ≤0.1 kU/L were considered negative results. The following allergens were used: rDer p 1, rDer p 2, rDer p 10, rPen a 1, rPhl p 1, rPhl p 5, rPhl p 7, rPhl p 12, nOle e 1, nSal k 1, nArt v 1, rFel d 1, rAlt a 1, rAsp f 1, r Asp f 6 and *Aspergillus oryzae* alpha amylase.

Identification of *Blattella germanica* allergens
Cockroach extract
Cockroach crude extract was obtained from Bial Laboratories (Bial-Aristegui, Bilbao, Spain).

SDS-PAGE-IgE-Immunoblotting
Sodium dodecyl sulphate-polyacrylamide gel electrophoresis (SDS-PAGE) was performed on a 4% stacking gel and 12.5% resolving gel according to the method of Laemmli [17]. After protein separation, gels were either fixed and stained for crude protein using Coomassie Brilliant Blue R-250 or transferred to a polyvinylidene fluoride (PVDF) membrane [18]. The PVDF membrane was incubated overnight with the patient's sera at 4°C. Bound IgE antibodies were detected using HRP-conjugated goat anti-human IgE and an ECL-Western blotting kit (Amersham ECL Plus Western Blotting Detection System, GE Healthcare UK Ltd, Buckinghamshire, UK) [19].

Mass spectrometry and database searching
The IgE-binding bands revealed by immunoblotting were sent to the Proteomic Unit of Carlos III National Centre for Cardiovascular Disease Research Foundation (Madrid, Spain) for identification by MALDITOF-MS/MS. MALDI-MS and MS/MS data were combined using the BioTools programme (Bruker Daltonics, Billerica, MA, USA) to search protein databases (NCBInr; $\sim 4.8 \times 10^6$ entries; National Centre for Biotechnology Information, Bethesda, MD, USA; SwissProt; $\sim 2.6 \times 10^5$ entries; Swiss Institute for Bioinformatics, Switzerland) using Mascot software (Matrix Science, London, UK). MALDI-MS/MS spectra and database search results were manually inspected in detail using the above programs as well as homemade software and the Structural Database of Allergenic Proteins. The amino acid sequence was assessed by searching the NCBInr database with fragment ion masses from the precursor ion at m/z = 2710.286. Protein scores greater than 81 were considered significant (P < 0.5).

According to the Structural Database of Allergenic Protein (SDAP), possible cross-reactivity between a query protein and a known allergen has to be considered when there is an identification of six contiguous amino acids between the query sequence and any allergen [20]. The alpha-amylase amino acid sequence was assessed by searching the SDAP in this manner, following the database instructions.

Statistical analysis
The data obtained were analyzed with GraphPad Prism 4.0 (La Jolla, CA. USA). Data are expressed as the mean and 95% confidence interval (CI). Means were compared using ANOVA. P values <0.05 were considered statistically significant. Logistic regression (SPSS Statistics 21. IBM) was used to assess the association between the quantification of major allergen-specific IgE and the severity of asthma.

Results
Ninety-two subjects (45%) from the total evaluated sample (202 asthmatic patients) tested positive for Phadiatop and specific IgE to *Salsola kali*. All these individuals were considered atopic. Among the 202 patients studied, 57% presented with severe asthma, 36% with moderate asthma and 7% with mild asthma. The distribution of asthma severity among the atopic patients within the sample was 49% for severe asthma, 38% for moderate asthma and 13% for mild asthma. No statistically significant differences were found between the asthmatic population and the asthmatic population with atopy (p > 0.05).

Table 1 displays the results of the allergy diagnosis based on the CRD concept. Eighty- two percent of atopic patients were sensitized to pollen allergens, with *Salsola kali* major allergen (Sal k 1) as the most frequent allergenic source, which was able to sensitize 71% of the atopic subjects and was associated with higher specific IgE values (26.7 ± 21.0 kU/L). Taking into account the prevalence of sensitization to each allergen in the atopic population, the statistical analysis demonstrated that Sal k 1 was the primary sensitizing allergen in the asthmatic population, showing significant differences when compared with the remaining allergens studied (p ≤ 0.0001).

Thirty-five percent of the atopic subjects had anti-cockroach IgE responses, but the level of specific IgE was lower (2.8 kU/L ± 7). Major allergens from grass pollen (Phl p 1 + 5) showed a sensitization frequency of 18% and a specific IgE mean value of 7.64 ± 10.8 kU/L. Eighty-eight atopic patients (95%) were sensitized to pollens and/or cockroach allergens.

Table 1 Allergy diagnosis based on the allergen components

Allergen	Mean sIgE (kU/L)	SD	Percentage (%)
Sal k 1	26.7	18.1	71
*Phl p*1+ 5	7.64	10.8	18
Fel d 1	6.43	5.8	10.8
Ole e 1	2.9	3.3	7.6
Art v 1	1.4	1.3	7.6

Mean specific IgE values, standard deviation (SD) and percentage (%) of sensitized patients to each allergen in the atopic population (n = 92).

Although significant specific IgE values were discovered for other major allergens, such as Fel d 1 (6.43 kU/L ± 5.8), Ole e 1 (2.9 kU/L ± 3.3) and Art v 1 (1.4 kU/L ± 1.3), the sensitization rates were less than 15%. The remaining sensitizing allergen components (Alt a 1, Asp f 1, Asp f 6, Phl p 7 + 12, Der p 1, Der p 2, and tropomyosin) showed no significant specific IgE values (mean values ≤0.5 kU/L) or important frequencies (values less than 10%). Sensitization by cross-reactive allergens (pollen polcalcins/profilins and tropomyosin) reached 5.4% of atopic individuals (5 patients), with allergen-specific mean values ranging from 0.4 to 0.5 kU/L.

Table 2 depicts the results of a statistical analysis of the association between asthma severity and the levels of specific IgE in the atopic population. No significant associations were observed.

To identify which cockroach allergens were able to sensitize the atopic population, SDS-PAGE immunoblotting associated with MALDI-TOF-MS and MALDI-TOF-MS/MS were performed. Figure 1 shows the allergogram of the 22 from 33 atopic patients sensitized to cockroach crude extracts. Four IgE-binding components of 75.0, 53.0, 42.0 and 36.0 kDa molecular weight (MW), reactive in 63.6%, 86.4%, 72.7% and 54.5% of cockroach-sensitized patients, respectively, were revealed in this way. The prevalence rates of each uncovered cockroach allergen (75, 53, 42 and 36 kDa) in the total atopic population with asthma were 15%, 20%, 17% and 12%, respectively. Mass spectrometry analysis of the four bands allowed for the identification of only the 53 and 42 kDa proteins. Table 3 displays the results of mass spectrometry. These two proteins were identified as alpha-amylase and arginine-kinase, which have theoretical MWs of 57.5 and 40.1 kDa, respectively. No specific IgE to *Aspergillus oryzae* alpha-amylase was found in sera from 8 patients sensitized to *Blattella germanica* alpha-amylase (≤0.1 kU/L). A BLAST alignment of protein sequences of *Blattella germanica* alpha-amylase with *Aspergillus oryzae* alpha amylase showed a query cover and E-value of 50% and 4E-12, respectively. An SDAP search revealed that there was a match of at least of six contiguous amino acids between the alpha-amylase of *Blattella germanica* and the alpha-amylase of *Blomia tropicalis* (Blo t 4.0101), *Dermatophagoides*

pteronyssinus (Der p 4) and *Euroglyphus maynei* (Eur m 4), which are three described mite allergens.

Discussion

Asthma is a common worldwide health problem with a high global prevalence ranging from 1-18% of the population depending on the country. Its association with elevated total serum IgE and with allergic sensitization to local aeroallergens has been well documented [21,22]. Indoor and outdoor allergens are important environmental factors influencing the development and expression of asthma, and the measurement of specific IgE can better define an individual's atopic condition [23].

Several studies have demonstrated that the prevalence of atopy is varied among asthmatic patients. Arbes *et al.* [24] have reported that approximately 50% of the current asthma cases in the US population are attributable to atopy, whereas Sunyer *et al.* [25] have found that the overall attributable fraction of asthma symptoms caused by atopy in Europe is 30%, although varying widely between centres, from 4% to 61%. In our study, the prevalence of atopy in the asthmatic population was of 45%. Despite the prevalence, the variability was wide, and considering the possible role of environmental allergens as a trigger of asthma development, the attributable fraction of asthma symptoms related to atopy in the population studied in this work agreed with the results found by the European studies. Vernon *et al.* [26] have reported that the most cited triggers of asthma are very similar across countries/regions and included allergens (particularly pollens, moulds, dust and pet dander), tobacco, exercise, air pollutants/particulates, weather patterns/changes and respiratory diseases. They concluded that a global checklist should be used in research and clinical practice. Despite this similarity in asthma triggers, the geographical differences in the sensitization to environmental aeroallergens [27] and in the allergen sources (fungi, plants and animals) distributed across each region [28] make the study of allergen distribution necessary in each area.

Component Resolved Diagnosis [11-13] has been shown to be a more accurate methodology for the diagnosis of allergy, allowing for a very fine definition of the causes of allergic sensitization from a molecular perspective. Proteomics appears to provide a crucial added value in the molecular diagnosis of allergy, especially when individualized allergens are not available or when identifying novel allergens [14]. Sensitization to specific allergens and/or to panallergens or cross-reactive allergens offers an accurate evaluation of the diagnosis according to the concepts of cross-reactivity, co-sensitisation and polysensitisation. Taking into account the abovementioned concepts and in accordance with the sample studied and the geographical location of the individuals included in

Table 2 Statistic analysis of the association between the severity of asthma and the level of specific IgE to the individual allergens in the atopic population

Allergen	Odds ratio	P value	% 95 CI
Sal k 1	1.071	0.516	0.870-1.319
Cockroach	0.992	0.969	0.673-1.462
Phl p 1 + 5	1.185	0.517	0.709-1.982
Fel d 1	0.934	0.824	0.511-1.707
Ole e 1	1.002	0.997	0.423-2.372

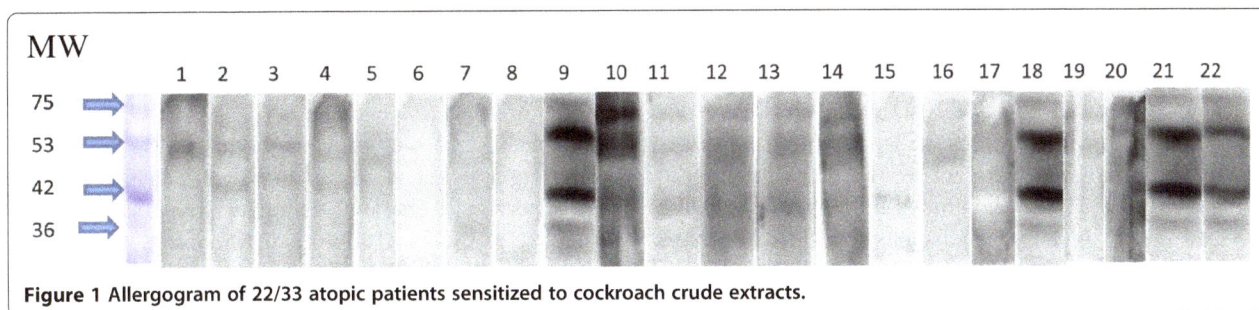

Figure 1 Allergogram of 22/33 atopic patients sensitized to cockroach crude extracts.

this work, we studied a sensitization panel of individual allergen components belonging to allergenic sources distributed throughout the North-Central part of Iran that contribute to the allergen sensitization in these patients. Major allergens implicated in the sensitization of the studied asthmatic population were the *Salsola kali* major allergen Sal k 1 (71% prevalence), the grass major allergen groups 1 and 5 (18% prevalence), the cat major allergen Fel d 1 (10%), the *Artemisia vulgaris* major allergen Art v 1 (7.6% prevalence) and the *Olea europaea* major allergen Ole e 1 (7.6% prevalence). Only five asthmatic patients were sensitized to pollen cross-reactive allergens (profilins or polcalcins) and the panallergen tropomyosin, with very low specific IgE values (≤0.5 kU/L), suggesting that the phenomenon of cross-reactivity is of little relevance in these patients.

The prevalence of sensitization to *Blatella germanica* as an allergenic source was relevant (35%) although the level of specific IgE was lower compared with the other sources described above (Sal k1, Phl p 1 + 5, Fel d 1 and Ole e 1). From the immunoblotting results, 4 different IgE-binding components (75.0, 53.0, 42.0 and 36.0 kDa) from cockroach were identified, with sensitivity prevalence

rates of 15%, 20%, 17% and 12%, in our atopic patient population, respectively.

According to WHO guidelines [29], cross-reactivity between an expressed protein and a known allergen has to be considered in cases in which there are at least six contiguous identical amino acids or when a segment of at least 80 residues shares more than 35% identity at the amino acid level. Using these guidelines, cockroach arginine kinase (42 kDa) and cockroach alpha-amylase (53 kDa) were identified. Allergenic molecules homologous to the identified IgE-binding proteins were used to search the Allergome and IUIS *Allergen* Nomenclature databases (www.allergome.org, www. allergen.org), resulting in the identification of arginine kinase as the Bla t 9 cockroach allergen [30]. No homologue to the alpha-amylase cockroach allergen has been previously described; therefore, a novel major allergen from cockroach sensitizing 86.4% of cockroach-sensitized patients was identified. To test for cross-reactivity with this novel cockroach allergen, sera from reactive individuals were tested for their specific IgE reaction to an available alpha-amylase (*Aspergillus oryzae*) allergen and by searching the SDAP to demonstrate that the fragment identified as a *Blattella germanica* alpha-

Table 3 Protein identification of *Blattella germanica*

	SDS-PAGE protein 1	SDS-PAGE protein 2
Calculated MW	53 kDa	42 kDa
Theorical MW	57.501 kDa	40.109 kDa
Protein description	Alpha amylase	Arginine kinase
Peptide sequence matched	r.saivhlfewkfadiadecerf.l	k.laasdsksllr.k
	k.gfagvqvspvhenviisspfrpwwer.y	k.hppkdwgdvdtlgnldpageyiistrvrcgrsmqgypfnpclteaqyk.e
	v.rncelvglhdlnqgsdyvr.g	k.gqfypltgmtk.e
	k.vnnlntdhgfpsgarpffyqevidlggeaihsteytgfgr.v	r.flqhanacr.f
	k.mavafmlaypygyp.r	k.tflvwcneedhlriismqmgggdlgqvyrrlvtavndiekrvpfshddrlgf.l
	r.qifnmvgfrnavagtavsnwwdngdkqisfcr.g	
	k.gfvafndefnndlk.q	
Sequence covered	36.31%	43.5%
Mascot score	200	292
Mascot expect	3.3E-014	2.1E-023
NCBI accession number	gi|85002763	gi|86160922

Results of Mascot search.

amylase could be included in the allergen group belonging to the alpha-amylase superfamily because of its similarity (six contiguous amino acids) with other alpha-amylase allergens. We found no cross-reactivity with *Aspergillus oryzae* alpha amylase, and BLAST alignments of cockroach alpha-amylase with other reported allergenic alpha-amylases [31] showed limited homology. The SDAP revealed that alpha-amylase allergens from *Blomia tropicalis* (Blo t 4.0101), *Dermatophagoides pteronyssinus* (Der p 4) and *Euroglyphus maynei* (Eur m 4) have the defined requirements for cross-reactivity with the *Blattella germanica* alpha-amylase. However, the lack of IgE reactivity against *Dermatophagoides* allergens found in this report suggests that there is little cross-reactivity between cockroach alpha-amylase and alpha-amylase from mites in this patient population.

The statistical analysis between the prevalence of sensitization by each allergen in the atopic population and the level of sensitization as indicated by specific IgE, suggested that Sal k 1 was the main protein allergen influencing the development and expression of asthma in this population. Several studies have reported on the aeroallergen sensitivity of Iranian patients with asthma or rhinitis [5-7,32], and they found different prevalence rates among atopic subjects and different percentages of allergen sensitization. However, all of these studies agree that pollen sensitization is the most prevalent and that Chenopodiaceae, grass and sycamore are the most important allergenic sources. In the present work, *Salsola kali* and grasses were also found to be the most important allergens, although no sensitizations to major allergens from sycamore were discovered. The prevalence of pollen sensitization found in this work was 37% of the total asthmatic population and 82% of the allergen-sensitized population. The aforementioned authors [5-7,32] reported that indoor allergens were the second most common cause of sensitization after pollens. Mite sensitization ranged from 43% to 18%, and cockroach sensitization ranged from 11% to 29% [33,34]. In our study, however, no sensitization to mites was demonstrated, although the prevalence of cockroach sensitization was 16% among the total asthmatic population and 35% among the allergen-sensitized population. Moghtaderi *et al.* [35] have reported a mold sensitization prevalence of 11%, with *Aspergillus* as the most prevalent source, followed by *Cladosporium, Alternaria, Penicillium* and *Rhizopus*. In this work we did not find significant sensitization to major allergens from the fungi *Aspergillus* or *Alternaria*.

Conclusions

Pollen and cockroach were the more relevant allergen sources in the asthmatic population studied herein, with the *Salsola kali* major allergen serving as the main cause for sensitization in the atopic patients suffering asthma. A new *Blattella germanica* cockroach allergen (*Blattella* alpha amylase 53 kDa) has been identified as a major allergen of *Blattella*.

To the best of our knowledge, this is the first study examining a panel of sensitizing allergens in a population of asthmatic patients living in Iran for molecular diagnostic purposes. Using this methodology, it was possible to identify new allergens from cockroach that could sensitize a relevant percentage of this population.

These results indicate that cross-reactivity between pollens or arthropods do not play any significant role in the sensitization phenomenon of these patients.

Abbreviations
CRD: Component resolved diagnosis; SDS-PAGE: Sodium dodecyl sulphate-polyacrylamide gel electrophoresis; PVDF: Polyvinylidene fluoride; SDAP: Structural database of allergenic proteins; NCBI: National Center for Biotechnology Information; BLAST: Basic local alignment search tool; ANOVA: Analysis of variance; US: United States; WHO: World Health Organization; IUIS: International Union of Immunological Societies.

Competing interests
The authors declare that they have no competing interests.

Authors' contributions
FT: carried out the molecular diagnosis and drafted the manuscript. MS: participated in the study design and coordination and helped to draft the manuscript. IP: participated in the design of the study and coordination, helped to draft the manuscript and performed the statistical analysis. MR: participated in the study design and coordination and helped to draft the manuscript. AE: participated in the study design and coordination and helped to draft the manuscript. AG: participated in the sequence alignment and drafted the manuscript. ES: participated in the study design and coordination and helped to draft the manuscript. JM: conceived of the study, and participated in its design and coordination and helped to draft the manuscript. All authors read and approved the final manuscript.

Acknowledgments
The authors wish to thank Dr. Maryamossadat Tehrani from the Department of Internal Medicine, Loghman Hospital, Tehran-Iran for handling patients, and Niloofar Rashidi and Naser Shahbazi from the Pasteur Institute of Iran for their assistance in preparing patient sera.
This study has been founded by the Government of The Basque Country, Project IT787-13.

Author details
[1]Department of Mycology, Faculty of Medical Sciences, Tarbiat Modares University, Tehran 14115-331, Iran. [2]Laboratory of Parasitology and Allergy, Center for Research Lascaray Ikergunea, University of the Basque Country, Pº Universidad, 7, 01006 Vitoria, Spain. [3]Department of Immunology, Microbiology and Parasitology, Faculty of Pharmacy, University of the Basque Country, Pº Universidad, 7, 01006 Vitoria, Spain. [4]Department of Mycology, Pasteur Institute of Iran, Tehran 13164, Iran. [5]Clinical Research Department, Pasteur Institute of Iran, Tehran 13164, Iran.

References
1. Pawankar R, Canonica GW, Holgate ST, Lockey RF: **WAO White Book on Allergy 2011–2012: Executive Summary.** [http://www.worldallergy.org/publications/wao_white_book.pdf]
2. Pawankar R, Baena-Cagnani CE, Bousquet J, Canonica GW, Cruz AA, Kaliner MA, Lanier BQ: **Allergy and chronic respiratory disease.** *World Allergy Organ J* 2008, 1(Suppl 6):S4–S17.

3. Valenta R, Lidholm J, Niederberger V, Hayek B, Kraft D, Grönlund H: The recombinant allergen-based concept of component-resolved diagnostics and immunotherapy (CRD and CRIT). *Clin Exp Allergy* 1999, **29**:896–904.

4. Newson RB, van Ree R, Forsberg B, Janson C, Lötvall J, Dahlén SE, Toskala EM, Baelum J, Brożek GM, Kasper L, Kowalski ML, Howarth PH, Fokkens WJ, Bachert C, Keil T, Krämer U, Bislimovska J, Gjomarkaj M, Loureiro C, Burney PG, Jarvis D: Geographical variation in the prevalence of sensitization to common aeroallergens in adults: the GA2 LEN survey. *Allergy* 2014, Mar 21. doi:10.1111/all.12397.

5. Assarehzadegan MA, Shakurnia A, Amini A: The most common aeroallergens in a tropical region in Southwestern Iran. *World Allergy Org J* 2013, **4**:6–7.

6. Farhoudi A, Razavi A, Chavoshzadeh Z, Heidarzadeh M, Bemanian MH, Nabavi M: Descriptive study of 226 patients with allergic rhinitis and asthma. *Iran J Allergy Asthma Immunol* 2005, **4**:99–101.

7. Behmanesh F, Shoja M, Khajedaluee M: Prevalence of aeroallergens in childhood asthma in Mashhad. *Maced J Med Sci* 2010, **15**:295–298.

8. Ebo DG, Bridts CH, Verweij MM, De Knop KJ, Hagendorens MM, De Clerck LS, Stevens WJ: Sensitization profiles in birch pollen-allergic patients with and without oral allergy syndrome to apple: lessons from multiplexed component-resolved allergy diagnosis. *Clin Exp Allergy* 2009, **40**:339–347.

9. Mothes N, Horak F, Valenta R: Transition from a botanical to a molecular classification in tree pollen allergy: implications for diagnosis and therapy. *Int Arch Allergy Immunol* 2004, **135**:357–373.

10. Ferreira F, Hawranek T, Gruber P, Wopfner N, Mari A: Allergic cross-reactivity: from gene to the clinic. *Allergy* 2004, **59**:243–267.

11. Valenta R: The future of antigen-specific immunotherapy of allergy. *Nature Rev Immunol* 2002, **2**:446–453.

12. Harwanegg C, Laffer S, Hiller R, Mueller MW, Kraft D, Spitzauer S, Valenta R: Microarrayed recombinant allergens for diagnosis of allergy. *Clin Exp Allergy* 2003, **33**:7–13.

13. Casquete-Román E, Rosado-Gil T, Postigo I, Guisantes JA, Fernández M, Torres HE, Martínez-Quesada J: Profilin cross-reactive panallergen causes latex sensitization in the pediatric population allergic to pollen. *Ann Allergy Asthma Immunol* 2012, **109**:215–219.

14. Postigo I, Guisantes JA, Negro JM, Rodríguez-Pacheco R, David-García D, Martínez J: Identification of two new allergens of *Phoenix dactyliphera* using an immunoproteomics approach. *J Invest Allergol Clin Immunol* 2009, **19**:504–507.

15. Global organization for asthma. http://www.ginasthma.org.

16. Vidal C, Gude F, Boquete O, Fernández-Merino MC, Meijide LM, Rey J, Lojo S, González-Quintela A: Evaluation of the Phadiatop™ test in the diagnosis of allergic sensitization in a general adult population. *J Invest Allergol Clin Immunol* 2005, **15**:124–130.

17. Laemmli UK: Cleavage of structural proteins during the assembly of the head of bacteriophage T4. *Nature* 1970, **227**:680–685.

18. Towbin H, Sthaelin I, Gordon J: Electrophoretic transfer of proteins from polyacrylamide gels to nitrocellulose sheets: procedure and some applications. *Proc Natl Acad Sci* 1979, **76**:4350–4354.

19. Kyhse-Andersen J: Electroblotting of multiple gels: a simple apparatus without buffer tank for rapid transfer of proteins from polyacrylamide to nitrocellulose. *J Biochem Biophys Methods* 1984, **10**:203–209.

20. Postigo I, Gutierrez A, Fernandez J, Guisantes JA, Suñén E, Martínez J: Diagnostic value of Alt a 1, fungal enolase and manganese-dependent superoxide dismutase in the component-resolved diagnosis of allergy to pleosporaceae. *Clin Exp Allergy* 2011, **41**:443–451.

21. Sherrill DL, Stein R, Halonen M, Holberg CJ, Wright A, Martinez FD: Total serum IgE and its association with asthma symptoms and allergic sensitization among children. *J Allergy Clin Immunol* 1999, **104**:28–36.

22. Christie GL, Helms PJ, Godden DJ, Ross SJ, Friend JA, Legge JS, Haites NE, Douglas JG: Asthma, wheezy bronchitis, and atopy across two generations. *Am J Respir Crit Care Med* 1999, **159**:125–129.

23. Jaakkola MS, Ieromnimon A, Jaakkola JJ: Are atopy and specific IgE to mites and molds important for adult asthma? *J Allergy Clin Immunol* 2006, **117**:642–648.

24. Arbes SJ Jr, Gergen PJ, Vaughn B, Zeldin DC: Asthma cases attributable to atopy: results from the Third National Health and Nutrition Examination Survey. *J Allergy Clin Immunol* 2007, **120**:1139–1145.

25. Sunyer J, Jarvis D, Pekkanen J, Chinn S, Janson C, Leynaert B, Luczynska C, Garcia-Esteban R, Burney P, Antó JM: Geographic variations in the effect of atopy on asthma in the European Community Respiratory Health Study. *J Allergy Clin Immunol* 2004, **114**:1033–1039.

26. Vernon MK, Wiklund I, Dale P, Chapman KR: What do we know about asthma triggers? a review if the literature. *J Asthma* 2012, **49**:991–998.

27. Bousquet PJ, Chinn S, Janson C, Kogevinas M, Burney P, Jarvis D: European Community Respiratory Health Survey I. Geographical variation in the prevalence of positive skin tests to environmental aeroallergens in the European Community Respiratory Health Survey I. *Allergy* 2007, **62**:301–309.

28. Ziello C, Sparks TH, Estrella N, Belmonte J, Bergmann KC, Bucher E, Brighetti MA, Damialis A, Detandt M, Galán C, Gehrig R, Grewling L, Gutiérrez Bustillo AM, Hallsdóttir M, Kockhans-Bieda MC, De Linares C, Myszkowska D, Pàldy A, Sánchez A, Smith M, Thibaudon M, Travaglini A, Uruska A, Valencia-Barrera RM, Vokou D, Wachter R, de Weger LA, Menzel A: Changes to airborne pollen counts across Europe. *PLoS One* 2012, **7**:e34076.

29. Food and Agricultural Organization of the United Nations: Evaluation of the Allergenicity of Genetically Modified Foods. Rome: Report of a Joint FAO/WHO Expert Consultation on Allergenicity of Foods Derived from Biotechnology; 2001:22–25.

30. Chuang JG, Su SN, Chiang BL, Lee HJ, Chow LP: Proteome mining for novel IgE-binding proteins from the German cockroach (*Blattella germanica*) and allergen profiling of patients. *Proteomics* 2010, **10**:3854–3857.

31. Vissers M, Doekes G, Heederik D: Exposure to wheat allergen and fungal alpha-amylase in the homes of bakers. *Clin Exp Allergy* 2001, **31**:1577–1582.

32. Bemanian MH, Korkinejad NA, Shirkhoda S, Navabi M, Pourpak Z: Assessment of sensitization to insect aeroallergens among patients with allergic rhinitis in Yazd City, Iran. *Iran J Allergy Asthma Immunol* 2012, **11**:253–258.

33. Ghaffari J, Khademloo M, Saffar M, Rafiei A, Masiha F: Hypersensitivity to house dust mite and cockroach is the most common allergy in north of Iran. *Iran J Immunol* 2010, **7**:234–239.

34. Safari M, Amin R, Kashef S, Aleyasin S, Ayatollahi M: Cockroach sensitivity in iranian asthmatic children under the age of five years. *Tur Toraks Der* 2009, **10**:26–30.

35. Moghtaderi M, Aleyasin S, Amin R, Kashef S: Skin test reactivity to fungal aeroallergens in asthmatic children in Southern Iran- Iran. *J Pediatr* 2010, **20**:242–245.

21

Peripheral blood T cells and neutrophils from asthma patients express class-I MHC-restricted T cell-associated molecule

Carlos Ramirez-Velazquez[1,2], Nonantzin Beristain-Covarrubias[1], Leopoldo Guido-Bayardo[3] and Vianney Ortiz-Navarrete[1*]

Abstract

Background: Class-I MHC-restricted T cell-associated molecule (CRTAM) is a protein expressed by activated natural killer T (NKT) cells, natural killer (NK) cells, CD8 T cells, and certain CD4 T lymphocytes. It is also expressed in Purkinje neurons and epithelial cells. However, no studies have examined the expression of CRTAM in peripheral blood cells during homeostasis or disease. Therefore, we explored whether CRTAM expression is influenced by the presence of allergic asthma.

Methods: We collected whole peripheral blood cells from non-asthmatic control subjects (n = 17) and patients with asthma (n = 17). All patients with asthma tested positive in allergen skin prick tests. We analyzed CRTAM expression in $CD4^+$ and $CD8^+$ T lymphocyte populations. CRTAM expression was also analyzed in $CD177^+$ neutrophils and $IL5R\alpha^+$ eosinophils.

Findings: The percentage of $CD4^+CRTAM^+$ and $CD8^+CRTAM^+$T lymphocytes in peripheral blood was higher in allergic asthma patients compared with healthy controls. Furthermore, the percentage of $CD177^+CRTAM^+$ neutrophils in peripheral blood was also elevated in patients with allergic asthma. However, the percentage of $IL5R\alpha^+CRTAM^+$ eosinophils in peripheral blood was not significantly different in patients with allergic asthma compared with healthy controls.

Conclusions: CRTAM expression on T cells, eosinophils, and neutrophils may be involved in bronchial inflammation in allergic asthma. Determination of CRTAM expression in peripheral blood may be useful for the diagnosis of bronchial inflammation and/or to identify recently activated immune cells.

Keywords: CRTAM, CD355, Asthma, CD4 T cell, CD8 T cells, Neutrophils, Eosinophils

Background

Asthma is a problem worldwide, with an estimated 300 million affected individuals [1]. It is a heterogeneous chronic inflammatory respiratory disease that is characterized by mucus overproduction and airway-wall remodeling that results in bronchial hyperactivity and airway obstruction [2]. Allergens and some pathogens have been implicated in the worsening of asthma. The characteristic patterns of inflammation found in allergic diseases is observed in asthma, including activated mast cells, increased numbers of activated eosinophils, increased numbers of invariant natural killer T cells (NKT), T helper 2 and 17 lymphocytes (Th2 and Th17), and neutrophils. Each of these cell populations releases mediators, contributing to symptoms or enhancing resistance to steroid treatment. Structural cells of the airways also produce inflammatory mediators and contribute to the persistence of inflammation in various ways. Over 100 deterrent mediators are now recognized to be involved in asthma and mediate the complex airway inflammatory response [3-6].

Asthma diagnosis and management is generally based on reported asthma symptoms and is often combined with lung function tests to assess reversible airway obstruction and airway hyperresponsiveness [2]. However, symptoms and lung function measurements may not reflect the underlying airway inflammation. Bronchoscopy

* Correspondence: vortiz@cinvestav.mx
[1]Molecular Biomedicine Department, Centro de Investigación y de Estudios Avanzados (CINVESTAV)-IPN, Av. IPN No. 2508, Colonia San Pedro Zacatenco, México
Full list of author information is available at the end of the article

with biopsies and bronchoalveolar lavage (BAL) are considered the best methods to assess airway inflammation. However, they are too invasive for general application in clinical practice [7]. Although the clinical value of a single FeNO measurement is limited, combining this measure with other markers of airway inflammation may lead to more accurate assessments of disease stage [8]. In addition, asthma appears to encompass a broad collection of heterogeneous disease subtypes with different underlying pathophysiological mechanisms [9]. Thus, there is a need for asthma biomarkers in order to identify relevant clinical asthma phenotypes, optimize diagnosis, and guide treatment.

Class-I MHC-restricted T cell-associated molecule (CRTAM) was initially described as a protein expressed only on activated NKT cells and CD8 T cells [10,11]. This protein, named CD355 during The 9th HLAD workshops [12], has also been identified in a small fraction of phorbol 12-myristate 13-acetate (PMA)/ionomycin-activated CD4 T cells. The interaction of CRTAM with its ligand, Necl-2, promotes cell adhesion, NK cell cytotoxicity, and IFNγ-secretion by CD8 T cells [13,14]. Non-lymphoid cells also express CRTAM, such as Purkinje neurons or epithelial cells, where it is involved in epithelial cell adhesion [11,15]. CRTAM is also essential for the establishment CD4 T cell polarization after TCR engagement and induce the capacity to secrete IFNγ, IL-17 and IL-22 [16]. However, no studies have investigated CRTAM expression in peripheral blood cells in a normal state or during disease (e.g., allergic asthma). Taken in consideration that recently activated immune cells express CRTAM it would be valuable to study its expression in patients with asthma. In this study, we analyzed whether CRTAM is expressed in human neutrophils, eosinophils, CD4 T cells, and CD8 T cells from allergic asthmatic patients.

Methods

Patients and control subjects

We recruited seventeen patients with asthma diagnosis according to Global Strategy for Asthma Management and Prevention: GINA Executive Summary 2008 [17] (Table 1). All patients tested positive to at least one allergen (house dust mites, pollens, or fungal allergens) in allergen skin prick tests (>5 mm; Alerquim, Mexico City, Mexico). Among them we found seven patients with mild asthma, four patients with moderate but persistent asthma and six patients with acute asthma; classified according to GINA. The acute asthma patients were defined as those who show exacerbation in symptoms such as wheezing, breathlessness, and chest tightness 48 hours prior to admission to the emergency department and received only rescue medication. These patients were enrolled within 24 hours of admission to the emergency

Table 1 Characteristics of study subjects

	Asthma patients	Healthy controls
Sex (female/male)	6/11	7/10
Age, y (mean ± SEM)	22.35 ± 3.82	24.12 ± 1.38
Atopy (N°)[1]	17/17	0/17
Total serum IgE levels (IU/mL) (mean ± SEM)	425.2 ± 105.2***	278.89 ± 14.6
FEV1 (% predicted; mean ± SEM)	77.65% ± 4.77***	96.59% ± 1.61

[1]Atopy is defined as at least one positive prick test.
***P < 0.001 compared with non-asthmatic controls.
FEV1: forced expiratory volume in 1 second; Ig, immunoglobulin; SEM, standard error of the mean.

department. Prior to the start of treatment, a blood sample was obtained for this study. Nine asthmatic patients had treatment with allergen- specific immunotherapy for more than 6 months (wt/vol;Alerquim, Mexico City). All subjects were either nonsmokers or ex-smokers, who had quit smoking for at least 12 months prior to the study. Subjects who had used corticosteroids, long-acting β2-agonists, leukotriene antagonists, or antihistamines in the month preceding the study were excluded, along with subjects with history of respiratory tract infection within the 4 weeks preceding the study. Healthy subjects without history of allergy or bronchial symptoms and who tested negative in allergen skin prick tests (Alerquim) comprised the control group. We measured total serum immunoglobulin E and the forced expiratory volume in 1 second (FEV1) in every subject. Three different independent measurements of FEV1 were performed with a dry spirometer (Medgraphics, Minnesota, USA). The optimum value is expressed as a percentage of the predicted value. All asthmatic patients had 12% of reversibility in FEV1 after 200-μg salbutamol [17]. The Ethics Committee of the Fernando Quiroz Hospital approved the study, and each subject gave written informed consent.

Preparation of human mononuclear cells

Whole blood cells were obtained from 17 healthy volunteers and 17 patients with asthma. Peripheral blood mononuclear cells (PBMCs) were isolated using a differential centrifugation gradient (Ficoll-Paque PLUS, GE Healthcare). PBMCs were analyzed for viability using trypan blue, washed, and stained *ex vivo*.

Surface staining

Ex vivo cells from heparinized whole blood (HWB) were stained for 20 min at 4°C with fluorescein isothiocyanate (FITC)-conjugated anti-CD177, phycoerythrin (PE)-conjugated anti-IL-5Rα, and allophycocyanin (APC)-conjugated anti-CRTAM (R&D Systems). Blood erythrocytes were lysed for 15 min at room temperature (RT) in lysis buffer solution [155 mM NH_4Cl, 10 mM $KHCO_3$, and 0.1 mM

EDTA, (pH 7.3)], and analyzed using a CyAn ADP cytometer (Beckman Coulter, Inc. Indianapolis). PBMCs were stained for 20 min at 4°C with FITC-conjugated anti-CD3, allophycocyanin (APC)-Cy7-conjugated anti-CD4, PE-conjugated anti-CD8 (BioLegend), and (APC)-conjugated anti-CRTAM (R&D Systems) and subsequently analyzed using a CyAn ADP cytometer. Isotype control matched monoclonal antibodies were used as negative controls for each fluorochrome.

Flow cytometry analyses

Neutrophils were identified according to size (forward scatter, FSC) and complexity (side scatter, SSC), and the expression of CD177 (BioLegend). The eosinophil IL5Rα marker was used to distinguish eosinophils from neutrophils in HWB to further evaluate CRTAM expression in neutrophils and eosinophils. CRTAM expression was also evaluated in CD3$^+$CD4$^+$ and CD3$^+$CD8$^+$ lymphocytes from PBMCs previously gated according to FSC and SSC. Data analyses were performed using FlowJo 7.6.5 software.

Statistical analyses

Distributions of continuous variables are expressed as the mean ± standard error of the mean (SEM) and median. Nonparametric Mann–Whitney U tests were used to compare continuous variables, Wilcoxon tests were used for comparisons among two groups. Friedman's post hoc tests were used to confirm differences in individual groups. P values less than 0.05 were considered statistically significant.

Findings

CRTAM expression in peripheral blood T lymphocytes

PBMCs were isolated from peripheral blood of allergic asthma patients and healthy controls. Cells were analyzed by flow cytometry according to size (forward scatter, FSC) and complexity (side scatter, SSC), as well as by gating CD3$^+$, CD4$^+$, and CD8$^+$ populations (Figure 1A). Analyses were performed using 4-color flow cytometry based on CRTAM expression in CD4$^+$ and CD8$^+$ T lymphocyte populations (Figure 1B). We observed that the percentage of CD3$^+$CD4$^+$CRTAM$^+$ (21.53% ± 7.4% vs. 2.37% ± 1.08%, P < 0.0001) and CD3$^+$CD8$^+$CRTAM$^+$ (5.98% ± 1.43% vs. 2.06% ± 0.22%, P < 0.0001) T lymphocytes was higher in allergic asthma patients compared with healthy controls subjects (Figure 2). Remarkable we observed a very low percentage CD4+ and CD8+ T cells that expressed the T cell activation marker CD69 for both asthma patients and healthy controls (Figure 1C). CD3 + CD4+ CD69+ (0.6857% ± 0.1060% vs 0.8803% ± 0.1394%,) and CD3 + CD8+ CD69+ (0.07112% ± 0.03457% vs 0.06594% ± 0.01767%,) and it was not difference (P < 0.72)

CRTAM expression in peripheral blood neutrophils and eosinophils

We analyzed neutrophils and eosinophils in HWB from allergic asthma patients and healthy controls by flow cytometry according to size (forward scatter, FSC) and complexity (side scatter, SSC), as well as the expression of CD177 and IL5Rα (Figure 3A). CRTAM expression was evaluated in the CD177$^+$ (Figure 3B) and IL5Rα$^+$ (Figure 3C) population. We observed that the percentage of CRTAM + neutrophils (12.84% ± 4.23% vs. 4.38% ± 2.02%, P < 0.002) was significantly increased in patients with allergic asthma compared with healthy control subjects. However, the percentage of CRTAM + eosinophils (33.45% ± 5.6% vs. 16.78% ± 6.04%, P > 0.051) did not differ in patients with allergic asthma compared with healthy controls (Figure 4).

Discussion

Asthma biomarkers in peripheral blood are easy to obtain, and the procedure, itself, is less invasive than sputum induction and bronchoalveolar lavage (BAL). Because inflamed tissues release chemoattractants and cytokines that recruit activated immune cells from the peripheral blood, the dynamic process of immune cells entering and leaving the bloodstream can be used as an indirect readout of disease state [7].

Many studies have shown that inflammatory cells, such as monocytes and granulocytes, respond to inflammatory signals by upregulating several activation markers [6,18,19]. Many of these markers, including CD11b/CD18 (Mac-1), CD63, CD66, and CD67, are typically found in granules that fuse with the plasma membrane upon activation of the cells with inflammatory mediators [20]. However, previous studies that compared the presence of markers on blood cells and tissue cells obtained from sputum and BAL did not take into account that cells homing to the tissue under homeostatic conditions exhibit the same phenotype [21,22]. Thus, the expression of these markers in peripheral blood has not led to a clear link between granulocyte expression profiles and asthma type.

In this study, we found an increase in peripheral blood neutrophils that express cell surface CRTAM from patients with allergic asthma. Peripheral blood eosinophils expressing CRTAM were also increased in patients with allergic asthma but the difference was not significant (P = 0.051). No differences were noted between the severity of disease (acute, mild or moderate asthma) and CRTAM expression or treatment with specific immunotherapy (data not shown). It is currently not known what induces CRTAM expression in these polymorphonuclear leukocytes or how CRTAM functions; however, because it belongs to a family of proteins involved in cell adhesion, it is likely that CRTAM is

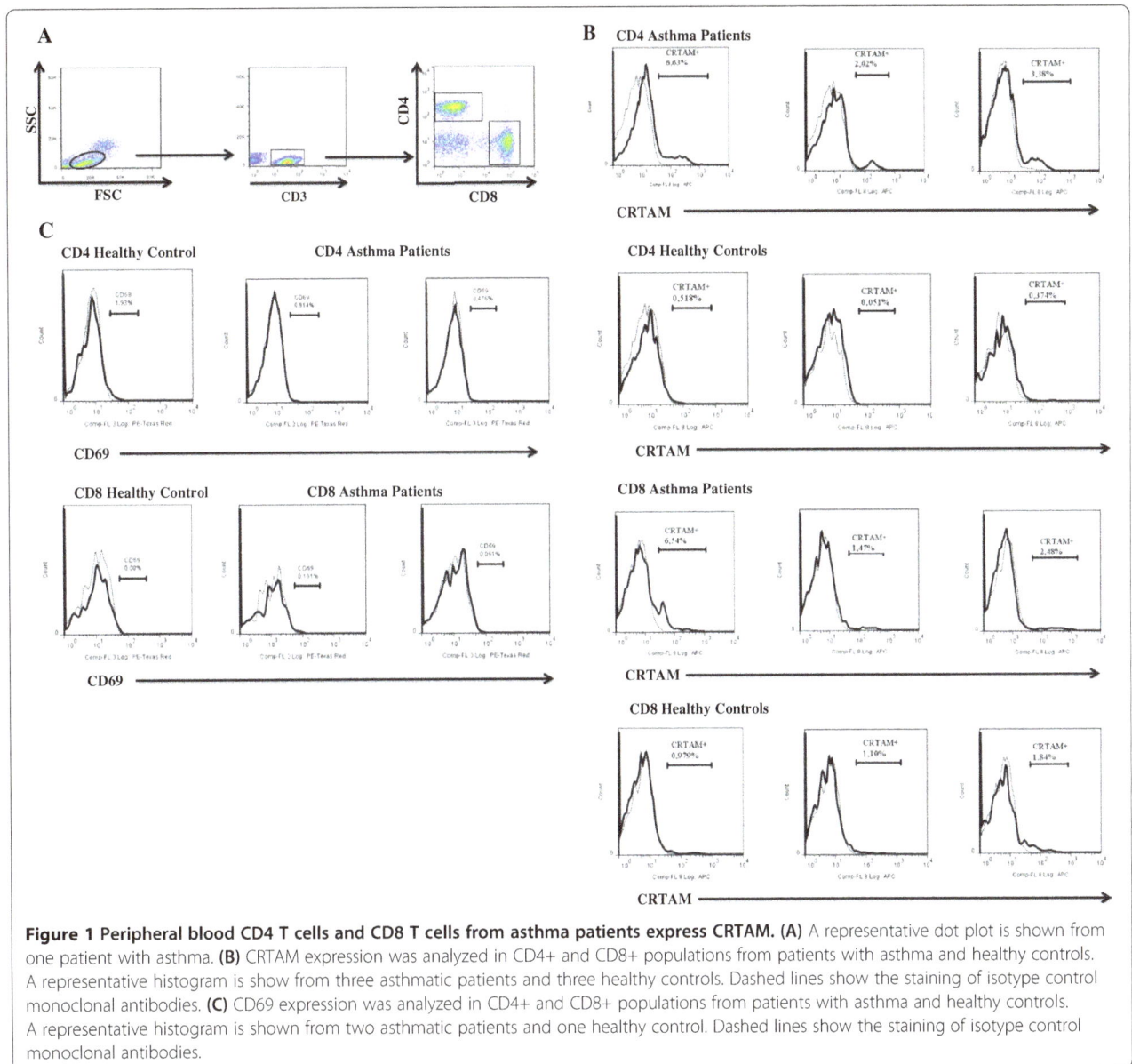

Figure 1 Peripheral blood CD4 T cells and CD8 T cells from asthma patients express CRTAM. (A) A representative dot plot is shown from one patient with asthma. **(B)** CRTAM expression was analyzed in CD4+ and CD8+ populations from patients with asthma and healthy controls. A representative histogram is show from three asthmatic patients and three healthy controls. Dashed lines show the staining of isotype control monoclonal antibodies. **(C)** CD69 expression was analyzed in CD4+ and CD8+ populations from patients with asthma and healthy controls. A representative histogram is shown from two asthmatic patients and one healthy control. Dashed lines show the staining of isotype control monoclonal antibodies.

involved in leukocyte transmigration through venular walls. Further studies will be necessary to define these fundamental features. We also observed an increase in CRTAM expression in CD4 T cells and CD8 T cells in peripheral blood from allergic asthma patients but it was not associated with the clinical features evaluated (severity or a specific immunotherapy). It has been reported that CRTAM expression is driven by TCR/JNK pathway [23]. Therefore, it is likely that allergens presented by MHC molecules stimulate surface expression of CRTAM on T cells from patients with asthma and the interaction of CRTAM with its ligand Nelc-2 might participate in Th1 and/or Th2 polarization, as has been described for mouse T cells [16]. However the frequency

observed of CD3 + CD4+ CRTAM + T cells represent more than 20%. It is very likely that among this CRTAM + subpopulation are included antigen specific and also a bystander activated CD4 T cells. Future studies are need to determine whether expression of CRTAM is induced by another stimulus (e.g. cytokines or chemokines). In this context recently have been published that CRTAM gene associate with an increase of asthma exacerbation and the presence of a low circulating vitamin D levels. Studies on cell lines confirmed the influence of vitamin D and CRTAM gene expression [24]. Suggesting that others signaling pathways play a role for the expression of CRTAM. Further studies are required to elucidate these important aspects on

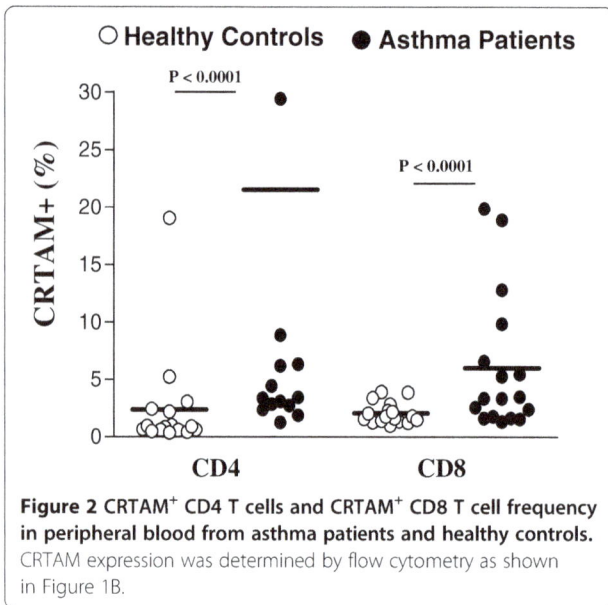

Figure 2 CRTAM⁺ CD4 T cells and CRTAM⁺ CD8 T cell frequency in peripheral blood from asthma patients and healthy controls. CRTAM expression was determined by flow cytometry as shown in Figure 1B.

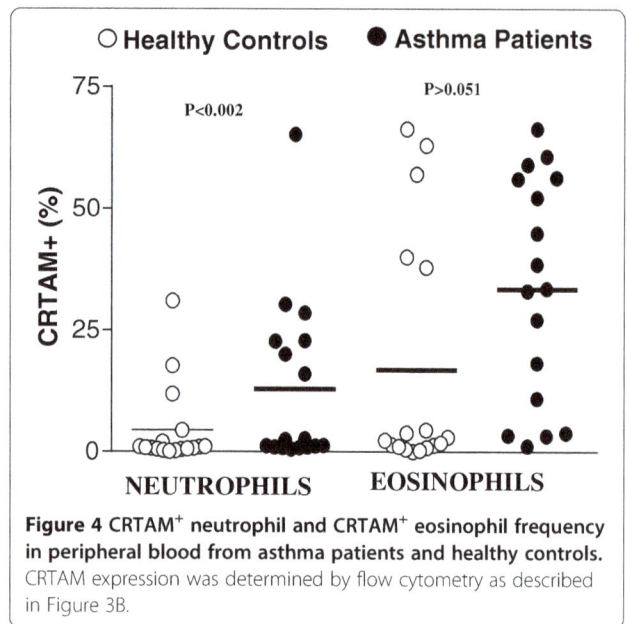

Figure 4 CRTAM⁺ neutrophil and CRTAM⁺ eosinophil frequency in peripheral blood from asthma patients and healthy controls. CRTAM expression was determined by flow cytometry as described in Figure 3B.

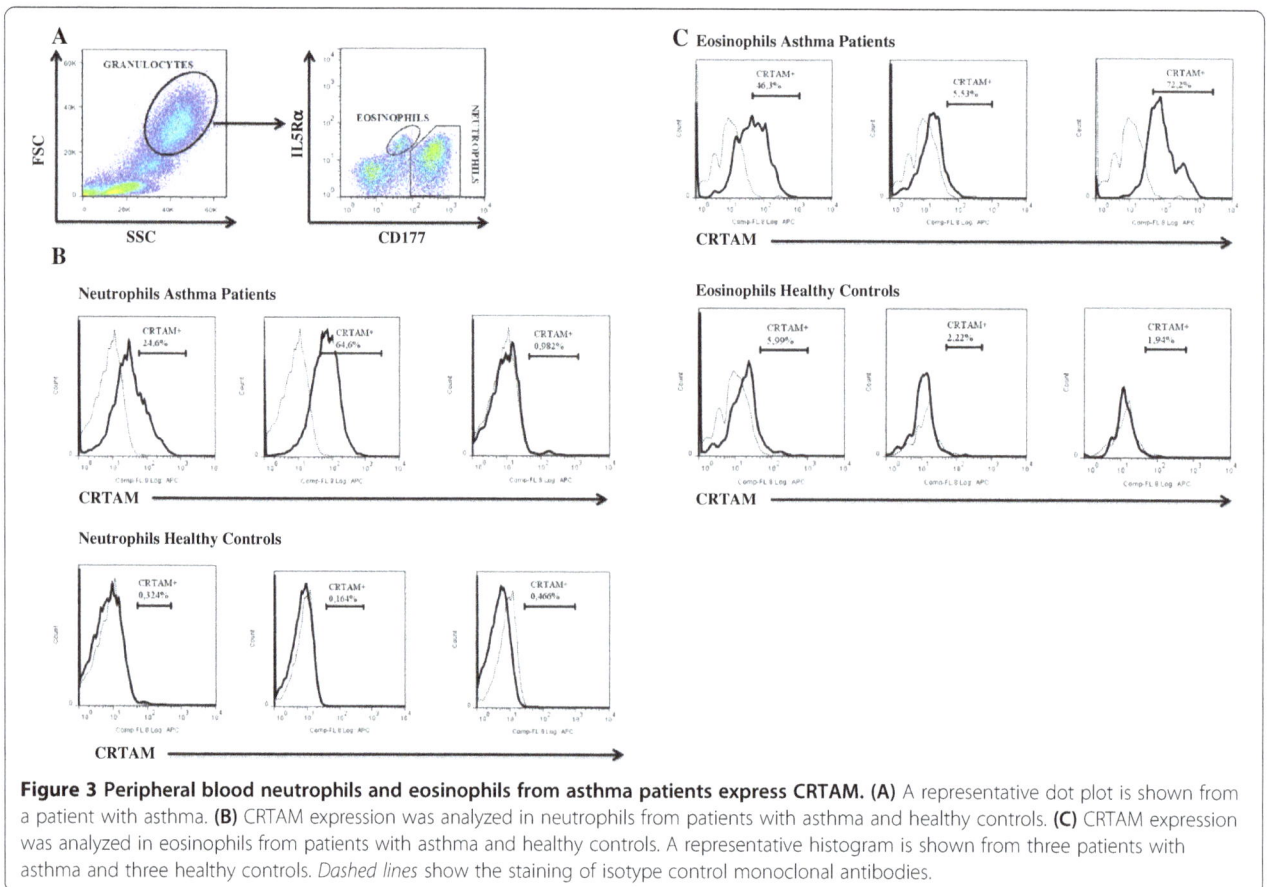

Figure 3 Peripheral blood neutrophils and eosinophils from asthma patients express CRTAM. **(A)** A representative dot plot is shown from a patient with asthma. **(B)** CRTAM expression was analyzed in neutrophils from patients with asthma and healthy controls. **(C)** CRTAM expression was analyzed in eosinophils from patients with asthma and healthy controls. A representative histogram is shown from three patients with asthma and three healthy controls. *Dashed lines* show the staining of isotype control monoclonal antibodies.

CRTAM expression and whether it might contribute during the initial phase of asthma disease and/or during progression.

Conclusions

In conclusion, we propose that CRTAM expression on T cells, eosinophils, and neutrophils may be involved in bronchial inflammation in allergic asthma. Expression of CRTAM in peripheral blood may be useful for the diagnosis of bronchial inflammation or to identify recently activated immune cells.

Abbreviations

PMA: Phorbol myristate acetate; FACS: Flow cytometry (fluorescenceactivated cell sorting); SEM: Standard error of the mean; FSC: Forward scatter; SSC: Side scatter; PBMC: Peripheral blood mononuclear cell; HLDA9: Ninth International Workshop on Human Leukocyte Differentiation Antigens.

Competing interests

The authors declare that they have no competing interests.

Authors' contributions

CRV and VON designed the experiments; LGB selected the patients; CRV and NBC did the experiments; CRV, NBC and VON analyzed the data and wrote the manuscript. All authors read and approved the final manuscript.

Acknowledgments

The authors are grateful for the support of CONACYT (Grant No. 24312 to VON and Scholarship No. 20700 to CRV), We thank Ismael Carrillo-Martín for discussion regarding the manuscript.

Author details

[1]Molecular Biomedicine Department, Centro de Investigación y de Estudios Avanzados (CINVESTAV)-IPN, Av. IPN No. 2508, Colonia San Pedro Zacatenco, México. [2]Allergy Department, Hospital General Dr. Fernando Quiroz Gutiérrez, ISSSTE. Calle Felipe Angeles y Canario. Colonia Bellavista, Mexico, DF CP 01140, Mexico. [3]Allergy Department, Centro Médico Nacional 20 de Noviembre ISSSTE, Felix Cuevas 540, Colonia del Valle, Mexico, DF CP 03229, Mexico.

References

1. Masoli M, Fabian D, Holt S, Beasley R: The global burden of asthma: executive summary of the GINA Dissemination Committee report. *Allergy* 2004, 59:469–478.
2. Mathur SK, Busse WW: Asthma: diagnosis and management. *Med Clin North Am* 2006, 90:39–60.
3. Buc M, Dzurilla M, Vrlik M, Bucova M: Immunopathogenesis of bronchial asthma. *Arch Immunol Ther Exp* 2009, 57:331–344.
4. Hamid Q, Tulic M: Immunobiology of asthma. *Annu Rev Physiol* 2009, 71:489–507.
5. Barrett NA, Austen KF: Innate cells and T helper 2 cell immunity in airway inflammation. *Immunity* 2009, 31(3):425–437.
6. Ramirez-Velazquez C, Castillo EC, Guido-Bayardo L, Ortiz-Navarrete V: IL-17-producing peripheral blood CD177+ neutrophils increase in allergic asthmatic subjects. *Allergy Asthma Clin Immunol* 2013, 9:23.
7. Vijverberg SJ, Hilvering B, Raaijmakers JA, Lammers JW, der Zee AH M-v, Koenderman L: Clinical utility of asthma biomarkers: from bench to bedside. *Biologics* 2013, 7:199–210.
8. Dweik RA, Boggs PB, Erzurum SC, Irvin CG, Leigh MW, Lundberg JO, Olin AC, Plummer AL, Taylor DR: An official ATS clinical practice guideline: interpretation of exhaled nitric oxide levels (FENO) for clinical applications. *Am J Respir Crit Care Med* 2011, 184:602–615.
9. Lin TY, Poon AH, Hamid Q: Asthma phenotypes and endotypes. *Curr Opin Pulm Med* 2013, 19:18–23.
10. Kennedy J, Vicari AP, Saylor V, Zurawski SM, Copeland NG, Gilbert DJ, Jenkins NA, Zlotnik A: A molecular analysis of NKT cells: identification of a class-I restricted T cell-associated molecule (CRTAM). *J Leukoc Biol* 2000, 67:725–734.
11. Patino-Lopez G, Hevezi P, Lee J, Willhite D, Verge GM, Lechner SM, Ortiz-Navarrete V, Zlotnik A: Human class-I restricted T cell associated molecule is highly expressed in the cerebellum and is a marker for activated NKT and CD8+ T lymphocytes. *J Neuroimmunol* 2006, 171:145–155.
12. Matesanz-Isabel J, Sintes J, LlinA L, de Solort J, Lazaro PE: New B cell CD molecules. *Immunol Lett* 2011, 134:104–112.
13. Boles KS, Barchet W, Diacovo T, Cella M, Colonna M: The tumor suppressor TSLC1/NECL-2 triggers NK-cell and CD8+ T-cell responses through the cell-surface receptor CRTAM. *Blood* 2005, 106:779–786.
14. Arase N, Takeuchi A, Unno M, Hirano S, Yokosuka T, Arase H, Saito T: Heterotypic interaction of CRTAM with Necl2 induces cell adhesion on activated NK cells and CD8+ T cells. *Int Immunol* 2005, 17:1227–1237.
15. Garay E, Patino-Lopez G, Islas S, Alarcon L, Canche-Pool E, Valle-Rios R, Medina-Contreras O, Granados G, Chávez-Munguía B, Juaristi E, Ortiz-Navarrete V, González-Mariscal L: CRTAM: A molecule involved in epithelial cell adhesion. *J Cell Biochem* 2010, 111:111–122.
16. Yeh JH, Sidhu SS, Chan AC: Regulation of a late phase of T cell polarity and effector functions by Crtam. *Cell* 2008, 132:846–859.
17. Bateman ED, Hurd SS, Barnes PJ, Bousquet J, Drazen JM, FitzGerald M, Gibson P, Ohta K, O'Byrne P, Pedersen SE, Pizzichini E, Sullivan SD, Wenzel SE, Zar HJ: Global strategy for asthma management and prevention: GINA executive summary. *Eur Respir J* 2008, 31:143–178.
18. Kanters D, ten Hove W, Luijk B, van Aalst C, Schweizer RC, Lammers JW, Leufkens HG, Raaijmakers JA, Bracke M, Koenderman L: Expression of activated Fc gamma RII discriminates between multiple granulocyte-priming phenotypes in peripheral blood of allergic asthmatic subjects. *J Allergy Clin Immunol* 2007, 120:1073–1081.
19. Johansson MW, Kelly EA, Busse WW, Jarjour NN, Mosher DF: Up-regulation and activation of eosinophil integrins in blood and airway after segmental lung antigen challenge. *J Immunol* 2008, 180:7622–7635.
20. Faurschou M, Borregaard N: Neutrophil granules and secretory vesicles in inflammation. *Microbes Infect* 2003, 5:1317–1327.
21. Mengelers HJ, Maikoe T, Brinkman L, Hooibrink B, Lammers JW, Koenderman L: Immunophenotyping of eosinophils recovered from blood and BAL of allergic asthmatics. *Am J Respir Crit Care Med* 1994, 149:345–351.
22. Fortunati E, Kazemier KM, Grutters JC, Koenderman L, Van den Bosch VJ: Human neutrophils switch to an activated phenotype after homing to the lung irrespective of inflammatory disease. *Clin Exp Immunol* 2009, 155:559–566.
23. Valle-Rios R, Patiño-Lopez G, Medina-Contreras O, Canche-Pool E, Recilla-Targa R, Lopez-Bayghen E, Zlotnik A, Ortiz-Navarrete V: Characterization of CRTAM promoter:AP-1 transcription factor control its expression in human T CD8 lymphocytes. *Mol Immunol* 2009, 46:3379–3387.
24. Du R, Litonjua AA, Tantisira KG, Lasky-Su J, Sunyaev SR, Klanderman BJ, Celedón JC, Avila L, Soto-Quiros ME, Weiss ST: Genome-wide association study reveals class I MHC-restricted T cell-associated molecule gene (CRTAM) variants interact with vitamin D levels to affect asthma exacerbations. *J Allergy Clin Immunol* 2012, 129:368–373.

22

Association between low vitamin D levels and the diagnosis of asthma in children

Mhd Hashem Rajabbik[1], Tamara Lotfi[1], Lina Alkhaled[2], Munes Fares[2], Ghada El-Hajj Fuleihan[3], Salman Mroueh[2*] and Elie A Akl[1,3,4,5]

Abstract

Background: There is conflicting evidence about the association between low vitamin D levels in children and development of asthma in later life. The objective of this study was to systematically review the evidence for an epidemiological association between low serum levels of vitamin D and the diagnosis of asthma in children.

Methods: We used the Cochrane methodology for conducting systematic reviews. The search strategy included an electronic search of MEDLINE and EMBASE in February 2013. Two reviewers completed, in duplicate and independently, study selection, data abstraction, and assessment of risk of bias.

Results: Of 1081 identified citations, three cohort studies met eligibility criteria. Two studies found that low serum vitamin D level is associated with an increased risk of developing asthma late in childhood, while the third study found no association with either vitamin D2 or vitamin D3 levels. All three studies suffer from major methodological shortcomings that limit our confidence in their results.

Conclusions: Available epidemiological evidence suggests a potential association between low serum levels of vitamin D and the diagnosis of asthma in children. High quality studies are needed to reliably answer the question of interest.

Keywords: Asthma, Wheezing, Childhood, Pediatric, Vitamin D, Bronchial hyper responsiveness, Lung function tests, Systematic review, Cohort

Background

Asthma is a highly prevalent respiratory condition in childhood [1]. Development of asthma is associated with many immunological markers [2]. Hypovitaminosis is prevalent worldwide, and an increasing body of evidence supports pleotropic effects of vitamin D on various chronic disorders including those associated with immune regulatory function [3-5]. This includes associations with a number of childhood disorders [6], such as type I diabetes mellitus [7-11], celiac disease, and asthma [12,13].

The hypothesis is that vitamin D has immunoregulatory properties [14,15] that protect from asthma [16,17]. Vitamin D has been shown to play a role in both the innate and adaptive immune responses by promoting phagocytosis and modulating the effect of Th1, Th2 and regulatory T cells [18]. Vitamin D has also been shown to inhibit the production of TH17 cytokines, which are associated with the severity of asthma and low steroid responsiveness [19]. A number of studies have suggested that low vitamin D levels are associated with increased risk of developing asthma [20-22] but other studies failed to confirm these findings [23,24]. One cohort study has shown that vitamin D supplementation in childhood might be associated with an increased risk of developing asthma [25].

Given these conflicting results and the high prevalence of both asthma and vitamin D deficiency in many countries [26,27], we aimed to systematically review the evidence for the epidemiological association between low levels of serum vitamin D and asthma diagnosis in children.

* Correspondence: smroueh@aub.edu.lb
[2]Department of Pediatrics and Adolescent Medicine, American University of Beirut, Beirut, Lebanon
Full list of author information is available at the end of the article

Methods

Protocol and registration

Prior to starting the review process, we registered the systematic review protocol with PROSPERO (CRD42013004204) [28].

Selection criteria

We included studies meeting the following eligibility criteria:

- *Types of studies*: cohort studies. We excluded case–control studies and cross sectional studies.
- *Types of participants*: children less than 18 years old and free of asthma at the time of inclusion in the cohort. We did not consider other kinds of allergic conditions.
- *Types of exposure*: serum vitamin D levels in the child. We excluded studies of vitamin D levels in the pregnant mother or in the cord blood at the time of delivery and studies of vitamin D intake or supplementation.
- *Types of outcome measures*: asthma diagnosed based on doctor's diagnosis, questionnaires, or spirometry measures.

We did not exclude studies based on language or date of publication, but excluded meeting abstracts.

Search strategy

The OVID interface was used to electronically search MEDLINE and EMBASE (from date of inception to February 2013). The search strategy was designed with the help of a medical librarian. The search combined terms for asthma, vitamin D, and pediatric age group. It used both free text words and medical subject heading. We did not use any search filter for study design. Additional file 1 provides the full details of the search strategy.

In addition, we searched the grey literature (theses and dissertations) and the abstracts and proceedings from the following scientific meetings: American Thoracic Society (ATS), American College of Chest Physicians (ACCP), Pediatric Academic Societies, European Respiratory Society, and European Society for Pediatric Research. We also reviewed the references lists of included studies and publications available in the authors' libraries. We searched forward for papers citing our included papers (ISI Web of Science). Finally, we contacted the authors of included studies inquiring about potentially eligible studies that we might have missed.

Selection of studies

Two reviewers (LA, MF) screened the titles and abstracts of identified citations for potential eligibility in duplicate and independently. We obtained the full text for citations judged as potentially eligible by at least one of the 2 reviewers. The two reviewers (LA, MF) then screened the full texts for eligibility, in duplicate, and independently.

Data collection

Two reviewers abstracted data from included studies in duplicate and independently. A senior team member (EAA) provided oversight. For each included study, the following information was abstracted: type, funding, population characteristics, exposure, outcomes assessed and the statistical data.

For both study selection and data collection steps, the reviewers used a pilot tested and standardized screening form and detailed instructions and resolved disagreement by discussion. A senior team member (EAA) provided oversight.

Assessment of risk of bias in included studies

The two reviewers assessed the risk of bias in each included study in duplicate and independently. They resolved disagreements by discussion or with the help of a third reviewer (EAA) who provided oversight. Risk of bias was assessed using the following criteria: [29].

- Failure to develop and apply appropriate eligibility criteria (e.g., selection of exposed and unexposed in cohort studies from different populations).
- Flawed measurement of exposure (i.e., serum vitamin D levels).
- Flawed measurement of outcome (i.e., asthma diagnosis).
- Failure to adequately control confounding variables (e.g., failure of accurate measurement of all known prognostic factors, failure to match for prognostic factors and/or adjustment in statistical analysis).
- Incomplete follow-up.

We graded each potential source of bias as high, low or unclear.

Data analysis and synthesis

We used the kappa statistic to calculate the agreement between the two reviewers for the assessment of trial eligibility. We were not able to meta-analyze the results of the included studies, as two analyzed vitamin D as a continuous variable [13,24], while the third study analyzed it categorized into tertiles [12]. We report both unadjusted and adjusted odds ratios (ORs) where available.

Results

Description of study selection

Figure 1 shows the study flow. Out of 39 potentially eligible studies, three met our eligibility criteria [12,13,24].

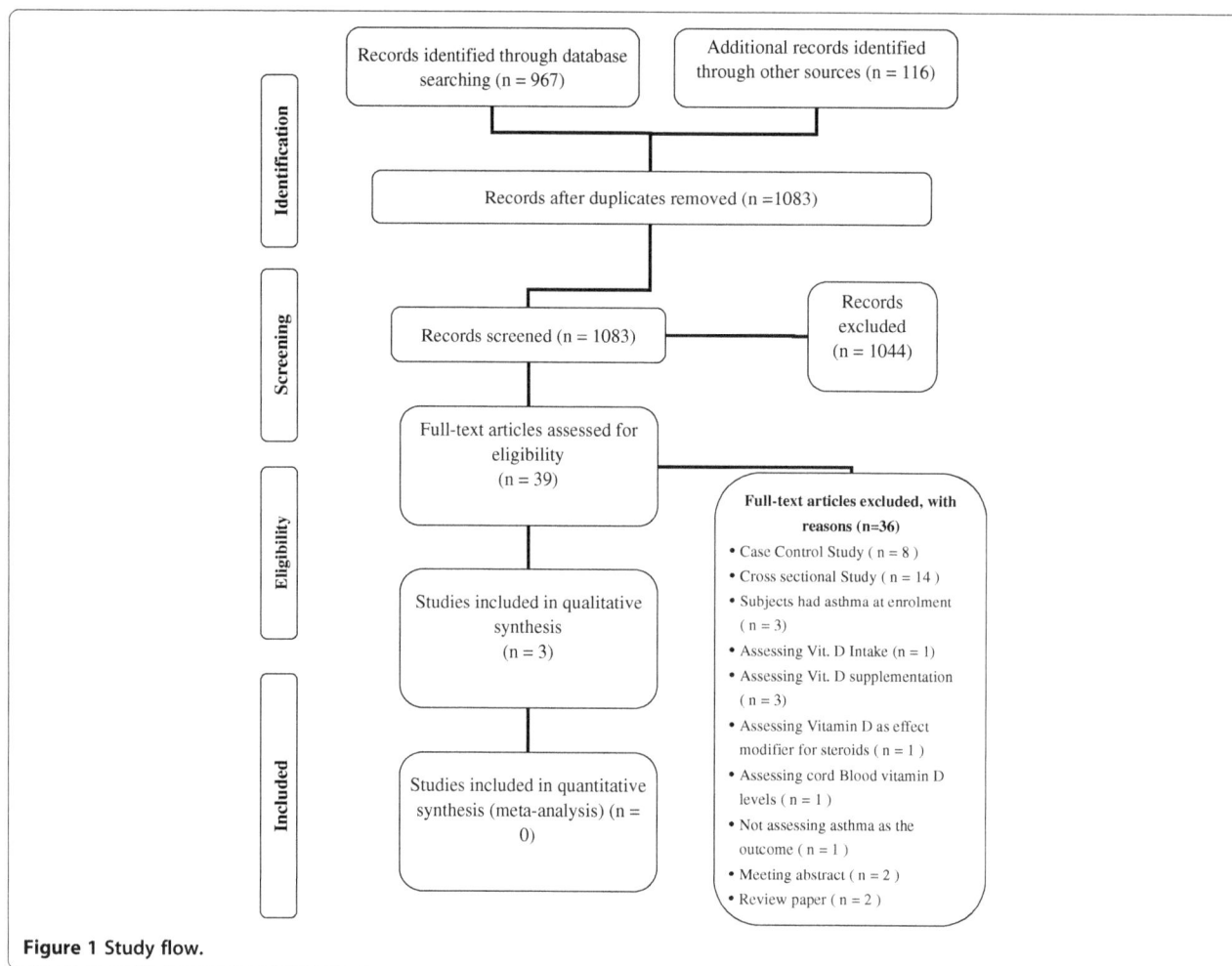

Figure 1 Study flow.

Additional file 2 lists the 36 excluded studies along with the reasons for exclusion.

Study characteristics

Table 1 lists the characteristics of the included studies. All three studies used data collected in the context of larger cohort studies conducted in the late 1980's and 1990's. The first study was conducted in Australia and included a population of 989 six-year-old subjects followed up until 14 years of age. The second one was conducted in the Netherlands and included a population of 372 four-year-old subjects followed up until 8 years of age. The last study was conducted in England and included a population of 3,323 children with a mean age of 9.8 years and followed up until a mean age of 15.5 years.

Risk of bias

Table 2 describes the assessment of the risk of bias in those studies. In our judgment, the risk of bias associated with subject selection in the study by Van Oeffelen et al. was high as only a small percentage of the inception cohort was assessed in this study. The risk of bias

associated with measurement of the exposure (Vitamin D levels) in the Van Oeffelen study was high due to the use of tests for which no validation is described, and due to the low reliability of a single measurement. The risk of bias associated with the outcome measurement (asthma) was low for both the Hollams et al. and Van Oeffelen et al. studies and uncertain for the Tolppanen et al. study in which non-validated questionnaires were used to diagnose asthma. We judged the risk of bias associated with confounding as high in one study due to lack of adjustment (Hollmans et al.). The risk of bias associated with missing data was judged as high in two studies due to high rates of missing data (30% for Hollams et al. and 42% for Tolppanen et al.).

Statistical results
Asthma

Hollams et al. [13] found an unadjusted OR for the association between increasing vitamin D levels and risk of asthma of 0.11 (95% CI 0.02–0.84). Van Oeffelen et al. found an adjusted OR of 0.39 (95% CI 0.27–0.53) when comparing vitamin D tertile 2 to tertile 1 (the lowest

Table 1 Characteristics of included studies

Study name, Funding	Study design	Participants	Exposure	Outcome	Notes
• Hollams [13] Source of funding not reported	• Prospective birth cohort started in 1989 • Follow up: 8 years	• Conducted as part of West Australian Pregnancy Cohort (Raine Study): a longitudinal birth cohort, in which mothers (2900 volunteers) were enrolled for antenatal care at the main local tertiary maternity hospital • Included in this study: 989 children assessed at the age of 6 (no further details provided about selection criteria or process); 693 were included in the analysis. • Perth, Western Australia, Australia	• Serum 25-hydroxyvitamin D levels measured at the age of 6 years • Measured using the enzyme immunoassay kit from Immunodiagnostic Systems Ltd (Scottsdale, AZ, USA)	• Current asthma; defined as wheeze plus use of any asthma medication in the last 12 months, in children with a prior doctor diagnosis of asthma • 8 years period between the point of measuring vitamin D levels and the assessment of asthma • Lung function; assessed by spirometry • Bronchial hyperrsponsiveness (BHR); assessed by methacholine challenge. • Outcomes assessed at the age of 14 years	• Vitamin D levels at age 6 years (Continuous outcome) analyzed as a predictor of subsequent clinical phenotypes at 14 years of age • Reference group: sufficient level of vit D (>75) • Vitamin D values were 'deseasonalized'
Van Oeffelen [12] Funded by the Netherlands Organisation for Health Research and Development, the Netherlands Asthma Foundation, the Netherlands Ministry of Health, Welfare and Sport, and the National Institute of Public Health and the Environment.	• Prospective birth cohort started in 1996 • Follow up: 5 years	• Conducted as part of PIAMA birth cohort of 3963 newborns; pregnant women recruited from the general population when visiting one of 52 prenatal clinics • Included in this study: 372 "selected" 4-year-old children (no further details provided about selection criteria or process); all were included in the analysis Netherlands	• Serum 25-hydroxyvitamin D levels measured at the age of 4 years • Measured using a competitive enzyme immunoassay in microtiter plates (OCTEIA; IDS, Boldon, UK). • Categorized into tertiles (range; median): ○ Tertile 1: 23.1–60.2; 52.0 ○ Tertile 2: 60.7–78.8; 68.3 Tertile 3: 79.0–303.8; 97.0	• Asthma and severe asthma diagnosed using the (ISAAC) [29] questionnaire answered by parents annually until 8 year of age • 4 years period between the point of measuring vitamin D levels and the assessment of asthma • Bronchial hyperrsponsiveness (BHR) measured at 8 years of age; assessed by methacholine challenge	• Vitamin D levels categorized into tertiles (Reference: tertile 1) • Serum extracted and directly stored in a refrigerator at -20C, and defrosted in 2008 to measure of vit. D levels • Storage time of serum samples proved to be no confounder and was therefore not added to the models. • Vitamin D values were 'deseasonalized'

Table 1 Characteristics of included studies *(Continued)*

Tolppanen [22] Funded by the UK Medical Research Council, the Wellcome trust, and the University of Bristol	• Prospective birth cohort started in 1991 • Follow up: 6 years	• Conducted as part of the Avon longitudinal Study of Parents and children (ALSPAC): 14,541 live births from 14,062 enrolled pregnant women who were expected to give birth between 1st of April 1991 and 31st of December 1992 • Lung function measured at a mean age of 15.5 years by spirometry according to the American Thoracic Society/European respiratory Society criteria. The best measurements from three reproducible flow-volume curves were used for analyses • South West England	• Serum 25-hydroxyvitamin D2 and D3 levels measured at a mean age of 9.8 years • Measured using high pressure liquid chromatography tandem mass spectrometer in the multiple reaction mode • Included in this study (mean age of 9.8): 3323 children for the asthma outcome and 2,259 for spirometry (inclusion based on completeness of data on exposures, confounders, and outcome)	• Asthma and wheezing also assessed on a yearly basis (questionnaire to caregiver); not clear whether those data were included in the analysis • The exposures are standardized for age and sex and 25(OH)D3 is adjusted for season and ethnicity • Interassay coefficients of • Variation for 25(OH)D2 and 25(OH)D3 were < 10% across a working range of 1–250 ng/ml • Asthma and wheezing assessed (questionnaire to children) at the age of 15-16 years. • 5-6 years period between the point of measuring vitamin D levels and the assessment of asthma

Table 2 Risk of bias in included studies; each criterion was graded as high, low, or unclear risk

Study name	Developing and applying appropriate eligibility criteria	Measurement of exposure	Measurement of outcome	Controlling for confounding	Completeness of data
• Hollams [13]	• Uncertain risk • Although the risk of bias is low for the original cohort, no further details were provided about selection criteria or process for participants in this current study	• High risk • "Vit D levels was measured in thawed serum cryobanked at age 6 years" (number of years since blood draw not mentioned) • The used enzyme immunoassay kit "method appeared to overestimate the vitamin D levels at age 6 years" • Measuring Vitamin D levels at one point only may not be a reliable measure of integrated 25(OH) D levels over time	• Low risk • Low for lung function and BHR	• High risk • Did not match or adjust for maternal atopy, maternal asthma, maternal age, education or household smoking	• High Risk • Outcome data were missing for 30% of the enrolled cohort
Van Oeffelen [12]	• High risk • Out of the larger cohort, a small "selected" sample included in this study, with no further details about selection provided	• High risk • Serum samples were defrosted to measure concentrations of Vitamin D (number of years since blood draw not mentioned) • Measured using a competitive enzyme immunoassay in microtiter plates • Measuring Vitamin D levels at one point only may not be a reliable measure of integrated 25(OH) D levels over time	• Low risk for asthma (ISAAC score) Low risk for BHR	• Low risk • Confounders were added to all models (gender, maternal atopy, paternal atopy, smoking by anyone in the house, and serum magnesium) • Also considered playing outside and overweight as potential confounders	• Uncertain Risk • Outcome data were missing for 12% of the enrolled cohort
Tolppanen [22]	• Uncertain risk • Except for the loss of follow up, the cohort was from a single community and followed specific eligibility criteria	• High risk • The exposures are standardized for age and sex and 25-hydroxyvitamin D3 is adjusted for season and ethnicity • Measured using high pressure liquid chromatography tandem mass spectrometer in the multiple reaction mode (number of years since blood draw not mentioned) • Measuring Vitamin D levels at one point only may not be a reliable measure of integrated 25(OH) D levels over time	• Uncertain risk for asthma, using spirometry & bronchidilatory responsiveness with non-validated questionnaires to diagnose asthma • High risk for wheezing • Recall bias	• Low risk • Model 1 unadjusted • Models 2 and 3 adjusted for respectively 8 and 9 potential confounders	• High risk • Of 5765 participants in the assessment of the wheezing and asthma outcome 3323 where included (42% missing data) • And of 4488 participants in the spirometric assessment 2259 where included (50% missing data). • Proportion of incident wheezing, and asthma was higher among children excluded owing to missing data

tertile) and an adjusted OR of 0.45 (95% CI 0.32–0.57) when comparing tertile 3 to tertile 1 (see Table 2 for variables used for adjustment) [12]. Tolppanen et al. found no association between vitamin D3 and asthma with an adjusted OR of 1.02 (95% CI 0.93–1.12) and an unadjusted OR of 0.98 (95% CI 0.92–1.05) [24]. Similarly, they found no association between vitamin D2 and asthma with an adjusted OR of 0.89 (95% CI 0.78–1.02) and an unadjusted OR of 0.98 (95% CI 0.89–1.08) (see Table 2 for variables used for adjustment). Hollams et al. also assessed the association between increasing vitamin D levels and severe asthma and found an OR of 0.28 (95% CI 0.06–1.37).

Spirometric outcomes

Both Hollams et al. and van Oeffelen et al. assessed bronchial hyperresponsiveness using the methacholine challenge test. Hollams et al. [13] found an unadjusted OR for the association between increasing vitamin D levels and bronchial hyperresponsiveness of 0.28 (95% CI 0.06–1.37). Van Oeffelen [12] found an adjusted OR of 0.72 (95% CI 0.39–1.35) when comparing vitamin D tertile 2 to tertile 1, and an adjusted OR of 0.66 (95% CI 0.35–1.25) when comparing tertile 3 to tertile 1 (see Table 2 for variables used for adjustment).

Tolppanen et al. assessed lung function through the bronchodilator response to 400 ug dose of salbutamol. They reported the results using "SD change in outcome per doubling of exposure" [24]. This refers to reporting a standardized measure of the lung function outcome (typically equivalent to the mean divided by standard deviation) for every "doubling of exposure". The authors calculated the doubling of exposure after scaling the two forms of 25(OH) D by multiplying the beta coefficients from the regression models by $\log_e$. The highest SD change reached among all analytical models was 0.06, which is typically considered a small effect size.

Discussion
Summary of main results

In summary, our systematic review identified three cohort studies assessing the association between low vitamin D levels in children and the incidence of asthma. Two of the included studies reported results suggesting that lower levels of vitamin D during childhood are associated with later development of asthma [12,13]. The third one found no association with either vitamin D2 or D3 levels [24]. Besides the inconsistent results, all three included studies suffered from major methodological limitations that limit our confidence in their findings. They all suffered to different degrees from selection bias (e.g., unclear selection criteria), inadequate measurement of the outcome (e.g., non-validated questionnaires), confounding (e.g., inadequate adjustment for potential confounders

such as maternal atopy), and incompleteness of outcome data 12%-50% of subjects in the three studies had missing data). The risk of bias associated with exposure measurement was common to the three studies. Indeed, and as detailed in Table 2, vitamin D was measured once, between 5–8 years depending on the study, before the assessment of the outcomes, thus limiting the reliability of the value obtained as a reflection of integrated vitamin D nutritional status over the follow-up time [30]. In addition, the methods of handling the samples (e.g., thawing procedure) may have affected the accuracy of the results. Our confidence in the findings is further decreased by the imprecision of the results as indicated by the wide confidence intervals that include the value of 1 for most odds ratios.

Overall completeness and applicability of evidence

Autier et al. recently published a systematic review of "vitamin D status and ill health" [31]. Although the reviewers included prospective cohort studies, they did not capture any of the studies we included in our review. This makes the possibility that we missed eligible studies unlikely. We have excluded studies of cord blood vitamin D levels because cord blood in part reflects maternal exposure, and evidence of their correlation with actual vitamin D levels during childhood is lacking. Also, we only included cohort studies to minimize the risk of bias in the results of this review. However, we observed that studies we excluded for their study design, and described as "case–control", were actually cross-sectional in nature. Indeed, these studies assessed both the exposure (vitamin D level) and the outcome (asthma) simultaneously at the time of inclusion into the study.

Agreements and disagreements with other reviews

Recently, Theodoratou et al. published an umbrella review that included systematic reviews and meta-analyses of observational studies of vitamin D and multiple health outcomes [32]. They identified no published systematic review or meta-analysis assessing the asthma outcome. We identified two systematic reviews [33,34] and two narrative reviews related to our study [35,36]. Neither of the two systematic reviews identified the studies we included in our review. The systematic review by Nurmatov et al. included studies related to maternal levels of vitamin D as opposed to children's levels'. Most of the studies systematic review by Zhang et al. were either studies of chronic obstructive pulmonary disease or non-cohort studies [34]. The one cohort study of asthma that they included measured cord blood levels [37]. The narrative review by Gupta et al. addressed a range of questions around vitamin D and asthma in children [35]. That review did not include any of the three studies we included. The narrative review by Hollmas [36] identified only one of the three included studies [13].

Implications for practice

The finding of a possible association between lower vitamin D levels and incidence of asthma may imply that vitamin D supplementation may be effective in preventing asthma. However, the considerable uncertainty regarding the validity of this association precludes at this point any translation of the findings into clinical practice. Indeed, we have identified 12 ongoing trials posted on clinicaltrials.gov that are assessing the effects of vitamin D supplementation in children with asthma symptoms.

Implications for research

Future studies should address the methodological limitations of the available evidence. This includes proper assessment of the exposure, by assessing vitamin D status by multiple measurements throughout the study period, and accounting for seasonal variation and other environmental factors. It also requires setting appropriate eligibility criteria, valid measurement of outcomes, controlling for all confounders, and minimizing missing data.

Abbreviations

BHR: Bronchial hyper responsiveness; 25(OH) Vitamin D: 25-Hydroxy Vitamin D.

Competing interests

The authors declare that they have no competing interests.

Authors' contributions

SM, EAA and LA conceived of the study and participated in the design of the study. LA and MF participated in study selection process. MR and TL participated in the data collection process. EA, GEHF and SM participated in data analysis and interpretation of the study. MR and EA helped in drafting the manuscript. All authors reviewed, edited, and approved the final manuscript.

Acknowledgements

We would like to thank Miss Aida Farha for her valuable help in designing the search strategy.

Author details

[1]Clinical Research Institute, American University of Beirut, Beirut, Lebanon. [2]Department of Pediatrics and Adolescent Medicine, American University of Beirut, Beirut, Lebanon. [3]Department of Internal Medicine, Calcium Metabolism and Osteoporosis Program, WHO Collaborating Center for Metabolic Bone Disorders, American University of Beirut, Beirut, Lebanon. [4]Department of Clinical Epidemiology and Biostatistics, McMaster University, Hamilton, Ontario, Canada. [5]Department of Medicine, State University of New York at Buffalo, Buffalo, New York, USA.

References

1. Page TF, Beck-Sague CM, Pinzon-Iregui MC, Cuddihy A, Tyler T, Forno E, Dean AG, Siven J, Pottinger S, Gasana J: Asthma in underserved schoolchildren in Miami, Florida: results of a school- and community-based needs assessment. J Asthma: official j Assoc Care of Asthma 2013, 50:480–487.
2. Chien JW, Lin CY, Yang KD, Lin CH, Kao JK, Tsai YG: Increased IL-17A secreting CD4(+) T cells, serum IL-17 levels and exhaled nitric oxide are correlated with childhood asthma severity. Clin Exp Allergy: J Br Soc Allergy and Clinical Immunol 2013, 43:1018–1026.
3. Holick MF: Vitamin D Deficiency. N Engl J Med 2007, 357:266–281.
4. Holick MF: The vitamin D deficiency pandemic and consequences for nonskeletal health: mechanisms of action. Mol Asp Med 2008, 29:361–368.
5. Makariou S, Liberopoulos EN, Elisaf M, Challa A: Novel roles of vitamin D in disease: what is new in 2011? Eur J Intern Med 2011, 22:355–362.
6. Moreno LA, Valtuena J, Perez-Lopez F, Gonzalez-Gross M: Health effects related to low vitamin D concentrations: beyond bone metabolism. Ann Nutr Metab 2011, 59:22–27.
7. Hypponen E, Laara E, Reunanen A, Jarvelin MR, Virtanen SM: Intake of vitamin D and risk of type 1 diabetes: a birth-cohort study. Lancet 2001, 358:1500–1503.
8. The EURODIAB Substudy 2 Study Group: Vitamin D supplement in early childhood and risk for Type I (insulin-dependent) diabetes mellitus. Diabetologia 1999, 42:51–54.
9. Bener A, Alsaied A, Al-Ali M, Al-Kubaisi A, Basha B, Abraham A, Guiter G, Mian M: High prevalence of vitamin D deficiency in type 1 diabetes mellitus and healthy children. Acta Diabetol 2009, 46:183–189.
10. Bin-Abbas BS, Jabari MA, Issa SD, Al-Fares AH, Al-Muhsen S: Vitamin D levels in Saudi children with type 1 diabetes. Saudi Med J 2011, 32:589–592.
11. Lerner A, Shapira Y, Agmon-Levin N, Pacht A, Ben-Ami Shor D, Lopez HM, Sanchez-Castanon M, Shoenfeld Y: The clinical significance of 25OH-Vitamin D status in celiac disease. Clin Rev Allergy Immunol 2012, 42:322–330.
12. van Oeffelen AA, Bekkers MB, Smit HA, Kerkhof M, Koppelman GH, Haveman-Nies A, Van Der AD, Jansen EH, Wijga AH: Serum micronutrient concentrations and childhood asthma: the PIAMA birth cohort study. Pediatr Allergy Immunol 2011, 22:784–793.
13. Hollams EM, Hart PH, Holt BJ, Serralha M, Parsons F, de Klerk NH, Zhang G, Sly PD, Holt PG: Vitamin D and atopy and asthma phenotypes in children: a longitudinal cohort study. Eur Respir J 2011, 38:1320–1327.
14. Cantorna MT, Mahon BD: D-hormone and the immune system. J Rheumatol Suppl 2005, 76:11–20.
15. Hewison M: Vitamin D and immune function: autocrine, paracrine or endocrine? Scand J Clin Lab Invest Suppl 2012, 243:92–102.
16. Gorman S, Weeden CE, Tan DH, Scott NM, Hart J, Foong RE, Mok D, Stephens N, Zosky G, Hart PH: Reversible control by vitamin D of granulocytes and bacteria in the lungs of mice: an ovalbumin-induced model of allergic airway disease. PLoS One 2013, 8:e67823.
17. Majak P, Jerzynska J, Smejda K, Stelmach I, Timler D, Stelmach W: Correlation of vitamin D with Foxp3 induction and steroid-sparing effect of immunotherapy in asthmatic children. Ann Allergy Asthma Immunol 2012, 109:329–335.
18. Matheu V, Bäck O, Mondoc E, Issazadeh-Navikas S: Dual effects of vitamin D-induced alteration of TH1/TH2 cytokine expression: enhancing IgE production and decreasing airway eosinophilia in murine allergic airway disease. J Allergy Clin Immunol 2003, 112:585–592.
19. Nanzer AM, Chambers ES, Ryanna K, Richards DF, Black C, Timms PM, Martineau AR CJG, Corrigan CJ, Hawrylowicz CM: Enhanced production of IL-17A in patients with severe asthma is inhibited by 1α,25-dihydroxyvitamin D3 in a glucocorticoid-independent fashion. J Allergy Clin Immunol 2013, 132:297–304. e293.
20. Carraro S, Giordano G, Reniero F, Carpi D, Stocchero M, Sterk PJ, Baraldi E: Asthma severity in childhood and metabolomic profiling of breath condensate. Allergy: Eur J Allergy Clinical Immunol 2013, 68:110–117.
21. Robinson CL, Baumann LM, Gilman RH, Romero K, Combe JM, Cabrera L, Hansel NN, Barnes K, Gonzalvez G, Wise RA, Breysse PN, Checkley W: The Peru urban versus rural asthma (PURA) study: Methods and baseline quality control data from a cross-sectional investigation into the prevalence, severity, genetics, immunology and environmental factors affecting asthma in adolescence in Peru. BMJ Open 2012, 2:e000421. doi: 10.1136/bmjopen-2011-000421. Print 2012.
22. Bener A, Ehlayel MS, Tulic MK, Hamid Q: Vitamin D deficiency as a strong predictor of asthma in children. Int Arch Allergy Immunol 2012, 157:168–175.

23. Gergen PJ, Teach SJ, Mitchell HE, Freishtat RF, Calatroni A, Matsui E, Kattan M, Bloomberg GR, Liu AH, Kercsmar C, O'Connor G, Pongracic J, Rivera-Sanchez Y, Morgan WJ, Sorkness CA, Binkley N, Busse W: **Lack of a relation between serum 25-hydroxyvitamin D concentrations and asthma in adolescents.** *Am J Clin Nutr* 2013, **97**:1228–1234.

24. Tolppanen AM, Sayers A, Granell R, Fraser WD, Henderson J, Lawlor DA: **Prospective association of 25-hydroxyvitamin d3 and d2 with childhood lung function, asthma, wheezing, and flexural dermatitis.** *Epidemiology* 2013, **24**:310–319.

25. Hypponen E, Sovio U, Wjst M, Patel S, Pekkanen J, Hartikainen AL, Jarvelin MR: **Infant vitamin D supplementation and allergic conditions in adulthood: Northern Finland birth cohort 1966.** *Ann New York Acad Sci* 2004, **1037**:84–95.

26. El-Hajj Fuleihan G: **Vitamin D Deficiency in the Middle East and its Health Consequences.** *Clin Rev Bone Miner Metab* 2009, **7**:77–93.

27. Braegger C, Campoy C, Colomb V, Decsi T, Domellof M, Fewtrell M, Hojsak I, Mihatsch W, Molgaard C, Shamir R, Turck D, van Goudoever J, ESPGHANCommittee on Nutrition: **Vitamin D in the Healthy Paediatric Population: A Position Paper by the ESPGHAN Committee on Nutrition.** *J Pediatr Gastroenterol Nutr* 2013, **56**(6):692–701.

28. Mroueh S, Alkhaled L, Fares M, Akl E: **Vitamin D for asthma in children.** *PROSPERO* 2013, CRD42013004204 Available from http://www.crd.york.ac.uk/PROSPERO_REBRANDING/display_record.asp?ID=CRD42013004204.

29. Guyatt GH, Oxman AD, Vist G, Kunz R, Brozek J, Alonso-Coello P, Montori V, Akl EA, Djulbegovic B, Falck-Ytter Y, Norris SL, Williams JW Jr, Atkins D, Meerpohl J, Schünemann HJ: **GRADE guidelines: 4. Rating the quality of evidence–study limitations (risk of bias).** *J Clin Epidemiol* 2011, **64**:407–415.

30. Major JM, Graubard BI, Dodd KW, Iwan A, Alexander BH, Linet MS, Freedman DM: **Variability and reproducibility of circulating vitamin D in a nationwide U.S. population.** *J Clin Endocrinol Metab* 2013, **98**:97–104.

31. Autier P, Boniol M, Pizot C, Mullie P: **Vitamin D status and ill health: a systematic review.** *The Lancet Diab Endocrinol* 2014, **2**:76–89.

32. Theodoratou E, Tzoulaki I, Zgaga L, Ioannidis JPA: **Vitamin D and multiple health outcomes: umbrella review of systematic reviews and meta-analyses of observational studies and randomised trials.** *BMJ* 2014, **348**:g2035.

33. Nurmatov U, Devereux G, Sheikh A: **Nutrients and foods for the primary prevention of asthma and allergy: systematic review and meta-analysis.** *J Allergy Clin Immunol* 2011, **127**:724–733. e721-730.

34. Zhang LL, Gong J, Liu CT: **Vitamin D with asthma and COPD: not a false hope? A systematic review and meta-analysis.** *Genet Mol Res: GMR* 2014, **13**:13. (AOP). [Epub ahead of print].

35. Gupta A, Bush A, Hawrylowicz C, Saglani S: **Vitamin D and Asthma in Children.** *Paediatr Respir Rev* 2012, **13**:236–243.

36. Hollams EM: **Vitamin D and atopy and asthma phenotypes in children.** *Curr Opin Allergy Clin Immunol* 2012, **12**:228–234.

37. Rothers J, Wright AL, Stern DA, Halonen M, Camargo CA Jr: **Cord blood 25-hydroxyvitamin D levels are associated with aeroallergen sensitization in children from Tucson, Arizona.** *J Allergy Clin Immunol* 2011, **128**:1093–1099. e1091-1095.

23

The relationship between allergy and asthma control, quality of life, and emotional status in patients with asthma

Hikmet Coban[1] and Yusuf Aydemir[1,2]*

Abstract

Background: Psychiatric comorbidities are prevalent in patients with chronic somatic disorders such as asthma. But, there is no clear evidence regarding the effect of atopic status and the type of sensitized allergen on emotional status. The aim of the present study was to investigate the effects of house dust mites and pollen allergies on emotional status, asthma control and the quality of life in patients with atopic asthma.

Methods: The study included 174 consecutive patients who were diagnosed with asthma accoring to the GINA criteria and who did not receive therapy for their allergy. All patients underwent a skin prick test. The asthma control, quality of life, and emotional status were evaluated using the ACT (asthma control test), AQLQ (asthma-specific quality of life questionnaire), and HAD (hospital anxiety depression questionnaire).

Results: Atopy was detected in 134 (78.7%) patients. Of those patients: 58 (33.3%) had anxiety and 83 (47.7%) had depression. There was no relationship between emotional status, atopic status, and the type of indoor/outdoor allergen. Furthermore, there was no relationship between atopy and asthma severity, asthma control, and the quality of life. The anxiety and depression scores were significantly higher and the quality of life scores lower in the uncontrolled asthma group. The ACT and AQLQ scores were also lower in the anxiety and depression groups.

Conclusions: It was concluded that anxiety and depression are prevalent in patients with uncontrolled asthma, and atopic status did not affect the scores in ACT, AQLQ, and emotional status tests.

Keywords: Atopy, Asthma control, Quality of life, Emotional status, Depression, Anxiety

Introduction

Asthma is a chronic health problem that encompasses the patient's entire lifetime, and causes significant mental and social problems in addition to physical symptoms. It is; therefore, considerably important to evaluate the quality of life of the patients in addition to the symptoms in order to gather full information about the health status of the patients [1].

Psychiatric comorbidities are frequently observed in patients suffering from chronic somatic disorders. These psychiatric comorbidities have a significant negative impact on the quality of life of the patients [1]. Emotional disorders, including anxiety and depression are more prevalent in asthma as compared to the general population [2-4]. Based on review of the literature, the prevalence of anxiety and psychological disorders among bronchial asthma patients can be estimated at 30–52% [5-7]. Similarly, high frequency of anxiety and depression has been demonstrated in atopic patients [8,9]. In that case, the association of asthma and the atopic trait further can contribute to the impairment in emotional status as compared to non-atopic patients with asthma. Also it can be a relationship between the type of allergen and emotional status. These last two topics have not yet sufficiently clear.

The allergens are well-known to cause asthma exacerbations and sustained symptoms [10]; however, there are still very few data regarding the effects of allergens on asthma control, quality of life, and emotional status. To our knowledge, there is no study that evaluated the relationship between the type of internal and external the allergens and emotional status.

* Correspondence: dryaydemir@yahoo.com
[1]Department of Pulmonology, Sakarya University, Sakarya, Turkey
[2]Training and Research Hospital, Sakarya University, 54100 Sakarya, Turkey

The secondary aim of the present study was to assess the emotional status of patients with asthma. Main purpose of our study was to investigate the effects of house dust mites and pollen allergies on emotional status, asthma control and the quality of life in patients with atopic asthma.

Materials and methods

The consecutive 174 patients, who were new diagnosed with asthma according to GINA criteria in Sakarya University Hospital (Turkey) in March-September 2012 period and who have not received at least last one month an antihistamines and immunotherapy for allergy and any inhaled or oral therapy for asthma were included in the present study. The patients who were receiving a therapy for psychiatric disease or those with a chronic disorder (chronic obstructive pulmonary disease, diabetes, coronary artery disease, malignancy) that could affect emotional status were excluded from the study.

A detailed medical history was obtained, and all patients underwent physical examinations. All pulmonary function tests were performed by the same technician on the SpiroAnalyser ST-300 instrument. The severity of asthma was determined based on Global Initiative for Asthma (GINA) criteria [1]. The patients, who provided informed consent, were included in the study, and the questionnaire form evaluating the demographic characteristics, anthropometric measurements, and the features of the asthma were administered to all patients. All patients filled out the ACT (asthma control test), AQLQ (asthma quality of life questionnaire) (Turkish version) and HAD (Hospital Anxiety and Depression) (Turkish version) surveys and the results were recorded on the questionnaire form. An approval was obtained from the university ethics committee.

Assessment of asthma control

The patients were administered a 5-item questionnaire assessing their asthma symptoms, use of rescue medications, and the impact of asthma on daily life [11]. In asthma control test, a score of 25 points indicated full control, 20–24 points indicated controlled disease, 16–19 points indicated partial control, and score below 15 indicated uncontrolled disease. In statistical analysis, patients achieving a score higher than 20 were assessed as a single group (control and full control), and patients achieving a score lower than 19 were assessed as a separate group (partial control and uncontrolled). The validity and reliability of this questionnaire has been previously shown in adult Turkish patients with asthma [12].

Assessment of the quality of life

The AQLQ assessed the scores of the patients regarding their symptoms (12 questions), restriction of activity (11 questions), emotional function (5 questions), and environmental exposure (4 questions). The total score was recorded as the average of the scores in 32 questions [13]. The answers to each question are scored one to seven (1 = maximum impairment and 7 = no impairment). Scoring domains were expressed as the mean score per question. Low scores indicate a poor quality of life. The validity and reliability of this questionnaire has been previously shown in adult Turkish patients with asthma [14].

Assessment of emotional status

The assessment of emotional status was measured by using the HAD questionnaire. The Hospital Anxiety and Depression Scale was developed in 1983 by the Zigmond and Snaith and the validity and reliability were performed [15]. It includes the subscales of anxiety and depression. This scale consisted of a total of 14 questions: 7 of them investigated the symptoms of depression, and 7 of them investigated the symptoms of anxiety. The answers were evaluated in the form of a four-point Likert type scale. The scale was scored between 0 (best) and 3 (worst).

The purpose of the scale is not to diagnose, but to determine the risk group by scanning anxiety and depression in physically ill patients in a short amount of time. The scale can also be used in the follow up of changes in the patient's emotional state. Although the scale uses the word "hospital", it can also be used in the field or in a study performed in outpatient settings. To the aim was to minimize the effects of the existing somatic disease on the scale results in the HAD scale.

For this reason, it does not include any physical signs. In the preparation of scoring, "0 to 1" was recognized as normal, "2" was recognized as borderline symptomatic, and "3" was recognized as having prominent symptoms. It has been proven that the HAD scale is a useful assessment tool, and its score range provides results so as to minimize the false-positive and false-negative data [16]. It has been shown that scores obtained from the scale are not affected by the presence of somatic disease [16]. The HAD scale was used in comparison with other scales and was found to be adequate in terms of the evaluation of anxiety and depression in patients with somatic diseases [17].

Turkish adaptation study of HAD scala has been made by Aydemir et al. According to this study, for the anxiety sub-scale cut-off score has been found 10 and more, and depression subscale cut-off score has been found 7 and more [18]. Measurements displayed that the limit value for anxiety was 10 or higher, while the limit value for depression was 7 or higher. It was evaluated that an anxiety score greater than 10 was HAD-A (+), under 10 was HAD-A (−), and those having depression scores over 7 were HAD-D (+), while those under 7 were HAD-D (−).

Evaluation with allergic skin test

A skin test (ALK-Abello, Madrid, Spain) was performed using 20 different aeroallergens in order to determine atopic status of the patients. The test media contained a mixture of Dermatofagoides farinea, D. pteronyssinus, storage mite, cockroaches, latex, hair, fungi, wheat, oak, olive, trees, mixture of weeds, cat hair, dog hair, grass mixture, and grass-wheat mixture. Histamine was used as a positive control and saline was used as a negative control. The test site was evaluated after 15 minutes, and the result was considered positive if the edema was more than 3 mm in diameter. The house dust mites were considered indoor allergen, and pollens were considered outdoor allergen (trees, mixture of weed, mixture of grass, grass-wheat mixture).

Statistical analysis

The SPSS for Windows 21.0 (IBM) software package was used in the statistical analysis of the study. In the present study, the continuous variables were expressed with mean value, standard deviation, maximum and minimum values. The Shapiro-Wilk test was used for the normality test of continuous variables. Normally distributed continuous variables were compared by means of variables were evaluated with samples t test, nonparametric variables between the two groups were made by Mann–Whitney U test, categorical variables were compared by Chi square test.

Results

Sociodemographic features and general characteristics of asthma

A total of 174 patients were included in the study. The characteristics of the patients are presented in table 1.

Table 1 Asthma and demographic characteristics of patients

	n	(%)
Gender (F/M)	134/40	
Rhinitis	137	(78.7)
Atopy	137	(78.7)
	Mean ± sd	Min/max
Age	43.8 ± 13	18/72
BMI (kg/m^2)	27.49 ± 5.2	17.70/49.30
FVC (%)	84.9 ± 16.5	23/129
FEV$_1$ (%)	84.7 ± 19.3	19/125
FEV$_1$/FVC (%)	84.4 ± 9.6	48/110
PEF (%)	67.4 ± 18.7	12/111
ACT	18.3 ± 5.1	5/25
AQLQ Total	4.3 ± 1.2	1.18/6.84

BMI: Body Mass Index; FVC: Forced Expiratory Volume; FEV$_1$: Forced Expiratory Volume in 1.second; PEF: Peak Expiratory Volume; ACT: Asthma Control Test score; AQLQ; Asthma Quality of Life Questionnaire score.

The prevalance of allergy and psychiatric disorders

The skin prick test was found to be positive for at least one allergen in 137 patients (78.7%), with 45 patients (25.9%) having only a pollen allergy, 32 patients (18.4%) having only a mite allergy, and 60 patients (34.5%) having both pollen and mite allergies. In total, 105 patients (60.3%) had pollen allergies and 92 patients (52.9%) had mite allergies.

The mean anxiety score was 8.07 + 4.42, the mean depression score was 7.00 + 4.54, and the mean HAD score was 15.07 + 7.97. When the cutoff for anxiety and depression was taken as 10 and 7, respectively, 58 patients (33.3%) had anxiety, and 83 patients (47.7%) had depression.

ACT and AQLQ status

The mean ACT score was 18.32 + 5.1. Of the patients, 19 (10.9%) had fully controlled disease, 65 (32.4%) had controlled disease, 78 (44.8%) had partially controlled disease, and 12 (6.9%) had uncontrolled disease. When the cut-off for asthma control was taken as 20, 89 patients (51.1%) had uncontrolled asthma, and 85 patients (48.9%) had controlled asthma.

The mean total AQLQ score was 4.30 + 1.24, the mean symptom score was 4.76 + 1.38, the mean activity score was 4.04 + 1.27, the mean emotional score was 4.50 + 1.57, and the mean environmental exposure score was 3.61 + 1.64.

The relationship between allergic status and ACT, AQLQ, and emotional status

There was no significant difference between patients who had versus who did not have mite and pollen allergy in terms of asthma control, quality of life, anxiety, and depression level (Table 2).

Of the patients, 105 had pollen allergies, 92 had mite allergies, and 60 had both mite and pollen allergies. When analyzed by the type of allergens, there was no significant

Table 2 The relationship between atopy and emotional status, quality of life, and asthma control

Mean (SD)	Non-atopic asthma n = 37	Atopic asthma n = 137	p value
HAD-Anxiety	8.43 (4.35)	7.98 (4.45)	0.607
HAD-Depression	7.57 (4.52)	6.85 (4.43)	0.277
HAD- Total	16.00 (7.51)	14.82 (8.10)	0.302
ACT	17.97 (4.89)	18.42 (5.18)	0.486
AQLQ-Total	4.45 (1.24)	4.29 (1.24)	0.683
AQLQ-Symptom	4.90 (1.34)	4.72 (1.39)	0.550
AQLQ-Activity	4.10 (1.35)	4.02 (1.25)	0.855
AQLQ-Emotional	4.63 (1.49)	4.47 (1.59)	0.771

HAD: Hospital Anxiety Depression Score; ACT: Asthma Control Test score; AQLQ; Asthma Quality of Life Questionnaire score.

difference in terms of asthma control, quality of life, anxiety, and depression level (Table 3).

The relationship between emotional status and ACT and AQLQ

Independent from the type of allergen, the patients with an anxiety score greater than 10 and depression score greater than 7 had significantly worse asthma control and lower quality of life (Table 4).

The relationship between allergic status and general patient characteristics

Atopic patients did not significantly differ in terms of spirometric measurements, BMI, age of asthma, and number of exacerbations; however, prick test positivity was significantly higher among male patients with rhinitis (Table 5).

The relationship between emotional status and general patient characteristics

The general characteristics and spirometric measurements were comparable between the two groups. The number of episodes was the only parameter that differed between patients with and without anxiety (p = 0.039), while the number of episodes (p = 0.002), and asthma severity (p = 0.013), were the two parameters that significantly differed between patients with and without depression.

The relationship between asthma control status and emotional status

The patients with uncontrolled asthma achieved significantly worse scores in emotional status and quality of life domains (Table 6).

Discussion

The present study evaluated the effects of the atopic trait and the type of allergy on the level of anxiety, depression, quality of life, and asthma control. When atopic patients with positive skin prick test were compared to non-atopic patients, no significant difference was found in terms of anxiety and depression scores, asthma control, and quality of life. There was also no

significant difference in terms of the types of pollen and mite allergies.

The exposure to allergens is a well-established cause of asthma episodes and sustained symptoms in atopic patients [19,20]. In this case, atopic patients can be expected to have lower symptom scores and quality of life score, and hence higher anxiety-depression scores. This is due to the fact that anxiety and depression was shown to correlate with disease control [6,21-23]. However, the results provided evidences contrary to this hypothesis. As a matter of fact, whether atopy is associated with increased asthma control is a topic that has not been fully elucidated. In a study that evaluated atopic trait in asthma, no significant difference was found between atopic and non-atopic patients in terms of asthma symptoms, quality of life, hospitalizations, and admission to emergency room [24]. Both groups were found to be similar with regards to asthma severity [25]. In the present study, there was no significant difference between atopic and non-atopic patients in terms of asthma control, frequency of asthma episodes, asthma severity and spirometric measurements.

The major strength of the present study was its cross-sectional design and inclusion of patients with a recent diagnosis that have not received a previous allergic therapy. In studies that are based on the review of patient charts, treatment effect appears as a confounder, in that, therapy may have minimized the effects of allergy. Consequently, the studies that evaluated the effects of therapy have shown improvement in the quality of life score after the therapy in comparison to pre-treatment scores [26]. Another study reported a significant improvement in the quality of life of patients with house mite allergy that underwent immunotherapy [27].

There are a very limited number of studies in the literature regarding allergic sensitization and emotional status. Among these studies, Kohlbeck evaluated 182 atopic and 63 non-atopic children with asthma and reported a 3-fold higher rate of emotional disorders in the asthma group. Similarly to the present study, they did not find any significant differences between atopic asthma group and non-atopic group. In addition, they did not report a

Table 3 The relationship between the type of allergy and emotional status, quality of life, and asthma control

Mean (SD)	Pollen allergy			Mite allergy		
	Absent n = 69	Present n = 105	p value	Absent n = 82	Present n = 92	p value
HAD-A	8.43 (4.42)	7.84 (4.42)	0.327	7.80 (4.27)	8.32 (4.56)	0.444
HAD-D	7.12 (4.31)	6.92 (4.56)	0.561	7.11 (4.28)	6.90 (4.62)	0.486
HAD-T	15.48 (7.83)	14.80 (8.07)	0.418	14.94 (7.59)	15.18 (8.33)	0.947
ACT	17.87 (5.34)	18.62 (4.95)	0.392	18.51 (4,98)	18.15 (5.24)	0.757
AQLQ-T	4.36 (1.32)	4.30 (1.19)	0.675	4.52 (1.20)	4.15 (1.26)	0.099

HAD-A: Hospital Anxiety Depression Scales Anxiety score; HAD-D: Hospital Anxiety Depression Scales Depression score; HAD-T: Hospital Anxiety Depression Scales total score. ACT: Asthma Control Test score; AQLQ; Asthma Quality of Life Questionnaire score.

Table 4 The relationship between emotional status and the quality of life and asthma control

Mean (SD)	Anxiety			Depression		
	Absent n = 116	Present n = 58	*p value*	Absent n = 91	Present n = 83	*p value*
ACT	19.28 (4.82)	16.41(5.17)	*<0.001*	20.18 (4.29)	16.20 (5.19)	*<0.001*
AQLQ-Total	4.68 (1.11)	3.62 (1.20)	*<0.001*	4.80 (1.07)	3.81 (1.21)	*<0.001*
AQLQ-Symptom	5.10 (1.21)	4.07 (1.46)	*<0.001*	5.27 (1.14)	4.20 (1.41)	*<0.001*
AQLQ-Activity	4.31 (1.24)	3.49 (1.15)	*<0.001*	4.44 (1.21)	3.59 (1.18)	*<0.001*
AQLQ-Emotion	5.08 (1.28)	3.36 (1.47)	*<0.001*	5.08 (1.33)	3.88 (1.58)	*<0.001*
AQLQ-Environ.	3.92 (1.63)	3.00 (1.48)	*<0.001*	4.03 (1.59)	3.16 (1.58)	*<0.001*
Asthma severity	1.91 (1.04)	2.21 (1.07)	*0.196*	1.81 (0.98)	2.22 (1.10)	*0.045*

ACT: Asthma Control Test; AQLQ; Asthma Quality of Life Questionnaire score. Environ: environmental.

relationship between emotional disorders and age, gender, BMI, and frequency of rhinitis [28].

In the study by Barone et al. that evaluated 217 patients, the total Anxiety Sensitivity Index score was significantly higher in the atopic group when compared to the non-atopic group; however, no significant differences were found between atopic and non-atopic asthmatics in terms of their scores in Beck Depression Inventory-II. The spirometric measurements and severity of asthma were comparable between the two groups [29].

As a secondary outcome of the present study, ACT and ACLQ scores were found to be significantly lower in patients with anxiety and depression. Our study confirmed that both the prevalence and severity of emotional disorders are related to the degree of asthma control and quality of life. These results are consistent with the works of other authors. Janson observed a correlation between the prevalence of anxiety and depression and the occurrence of asthma symptoms. [30] In another study, anxiety and depression were more frequent among patients with "difficult" asthma [5]. In the study by Trzcińska et al., the prevalence of depression and its severity were significantly correlated with the degree of asthma control [6]. The

results of Di Marco's study show a significant correlation between poor level of asthma control and both anxiety (OR: 3.76) and depression (OR: 2.45), which are frequent disorders in asthmatic subjects [23]. The neurophysiological mechanism of the relationship between depression and asthma has been evidenced in the previous studies [31,32].

Is the asthma control and quality of life worse in those with a psychiatric disorder, or may it be that emotional status is worse in patients with uncontrolled asthma? There is not a straightforward answer to this question as the present study has not been designed as to address this casual relationship. Age, BMI, presence of rhinitis, and as the basic parameters of asthma FEV_1, FVC, and PEF values were similar in patients with anxiety and depression. However, the number of exacerbations were higher in the anxiety group, and the number of exacerbations and asthma severity were higher in the depression group. This discrepancy complicates the interpretation of the results. If these parameters were similar between the groups, this would provide convincing evidence that emotional status has negative effects on asthma control and the quality of life. In our opinion, anxiety and depression are more common in uncontrolled asthma group and the statistical significance of this relationship is stronger.

Table 5 The relationship between atopic trait and various patient characteristics

Mean (SD)	Non-atopic asthma n = 37	Atopic asthma n = 137	*p value*
Age	46.73 (11.82)	43.06 (13.27)	*0.138*
Gender (f/m)	34/3	100/37	*0.016*
BMI (kg/m²)	28.20 (5.47)	27,30 (5.22)	*0.349*
Rhinitis (absent/present)	18/19	19/118	*<0.001*
FVC (%)	85.78 (15.59)	84.65 (16.81)	*0.551*
FEV_1 (%)	85.14 (18.93)	84.79 (19.54)	*0.854*
PEF (%+)	67.46 (17.48)	67.3 (19.05)	*0.760*
Exacerbation/year	0.35 (0,6)	0.66 (1.61)	*0.868*
Asthma severity	2.05 (0,9)	1.99 (1,09)	*0.142*

BMI: Body Mass Index; FVC: Forced Expiratory Volume; FEV_1: Forced Expiratory Volume in 1.second; PEF: Peak Expiratory Volume.

Table 6 The relationship between ACT score and HAD-A and HAD-D

Mean (SD)	Uncontrolled asthma (ACT < 20) n:89	Controlled asthma (ACT ≥ 20) n:85	*P value*
HAD-A	9.18 (4.40)	6.92 (4.16)	*0.001*
HAD-A ≥ 10 n (%)	37 (41,6)	21 (24.7)	-
HAD-D	8.27 (4.18)	5.67 (4.36)	*<0.001*
HAD-D ≥ 7 n (%)	54 (60.7)	29/85 (34.1)	-
HAD-T	17.42 (7.81)	12.61 (7.41)	*<0.001*
AQLQ	5.01 (1.13)	3.67 (0.95)	*<0.001*

HAD-A: Hospital Anxiety Depression Scales Anxiety score; HAD-D: Hospital Anxiety Depression Scales Depression score; HAD-T: Hospital Anxiety Depression Scales total score; AQLQ; Asthma Quality of Life Questionnaire score.

Thus, it is more plausible to suggest that emotional disorders are the result of poor asthma control.

Of the patients in the study group, 78.7% had rhinitis. The prevalenece of house dust mite and pollen allergy was higher in patients with rhinitis. Only 18 patients (13%) had rhinitis combined with a negative prick test. Consistent with the current results, previous studies reported a rate of positive prick test in patients with allergic rhinitis that ranged from 81% to 62.5% [33-35]. No relationship was observed between rhinitis and emotional status.

Another major strength of the study is the use of objective skin prick tests to determine atopic status. And these tests were conducted at the same time with the asthma control, quality of life and psychological status evaluation.

Our study has its limitations; firstly, we used questionnaires to evaluate emotional status, and no actual physician diagnosis was used. Secondly, this study was a single center study, and it is not capable of evaluating various ethnic and sociocultural differences, thus preventing the generalized use of the study results.

The present study is the first, to our knowledge, to systematically investigate the association between emotional status, quality of life, and indoor-outdoor type of atopy in patients with asthma. Finally, it was concluded that house dust mite and pollen allergies did not influence the scores in ACT and AQLQ; therefore, they did not increase the prevalence of anxiety and depression. It was concluded that emotional impairment is prevalent in patients with uncontrolled asthma, and holistic treatment approach should include psychological support and patient education in addition to the provision of medical therapy.

Competing interests

The authors declare that they have no competing interests.

Author's contributions

HC: Conception and design, analysis and interpretation of data, drafting the article. YA: Analysis and interpretation of data, drafting and revising the manuscript. All authors approved the final version of the manuscript.

References

1. Global Initiative for Asthma: *Global Strategy for Asthma Management and Prevention*, NIH Publication No 02-3659; 2005.
2. ten Thoren C, Petermann F: Reviewing asthma and anxiety. *Respir Med* 2000, **94**(5):409–415.
3. Espinosa Leal FD, Parra Román M, Méndez NH, Toledo Nicolás DA, Menez Díaz D, Sosa Eroza E, Torres Salazar AB: Anxiety and depression in asthmatic adults in comparison to healthy individuals. *Rev Alerg Mex* 2006, **53**:201–206.
4. de Miguel DJ, Hernández Barrera V, Puente Maestu L, Carrasco Garrido P, Gómez García T, Jiménez GR: Psychiatric comorbidity in asthma patients. Associated factors. *J Asthma* 2011, **48**(3):253–258.

5. Baumeister H, Korinthenberg K, Bengel J, Härter M: Bronchial asthma and mental disorders; a systematic review of empirical studies. *Psychother Psychosom Med Psychol* 2005, **55**:247–255.
6. Trzcińska H, Przybylski G, Kozłowski B, Derdowski S: Analysis of the relation between level of asthma control and depression and anxiety. *Med Sci Monit* 2012, **18**(3):CR190–CR194.
7. Adams RJ, Wilson DH, Taylor AW, Daly A, Tursan d'Espaignet E, Dal Grande E, Ruffin RE: Psychological factors and asthma quality of life: a population based study. *Thorax* 2004, **59**(11):930–935.
8. Timonen M, Jokelainen J, Hakko H, Silvennoinen-Kassinen S, Meyer-Rochow VB, Herva A, Räsänen P: Atopy and depression: results from the Northern Finland 1966 Birth Cohort Study. *Mol Psychiatry* 2003, **8**(8):738–744.
9. Sanna L, Stuart AL, Pasco JA, Jacka FN, Berk M, Maes M, O'Neil A, Girardi P, Williams LJ: Atopic disorders and depression: findings from a large, population-based study. *J Affect Disord* 2014, **155**:261–265.
10. Simpson A, Tan VY, Winn J, Svensén M, Bishop CM, Heckerman DE, Buchan I, Custovic A, Rietveld S, Everaerd W, Creer TL: Beyond atopy: multiple patterns of sensitization in relation to asthma in a birth cohort study. *Am J Respir Crit Care Med* 2010, **181**(11):1200–1206.
11. Nathan RA, Sorkness CA, Kosinski M, Schatz M: Development of the asthma control test: a survey for assessing asthma control. *J Allergy Clin Immunol* 2004, **113**:59–65.
12. Uysal M, Mungan D, Yorgancıoğlu A, Yıldız F, Akgün M, Gemicioglu B, Turktas H: *The Reliability and Validity of Turkish Version of Asthma Control Test*. Antalya: Turkish Thoracic Society, 15 th Annual Congress; 2012.
13. Juniper EF, Guyatt GH, Epstein RS, Ferry PJ, Jaeschke R, Hiller TK: Evaluation of impairment of health-related quality of life in asthma: development of a questionnaire for use in clinical trials. *Thorax* 1992, **47**:76–83.
14. Sahin B, Tatar M, Karakaya G: *Validity and Reliability of Turkish Version of Asthma Quality of Life Questionnaire*. Antalya: Turkish Thoracic Society 6. th Annual Congress; 2003.
15. Zigmond AS, Snaith PR: The hospital anxiety and depression scale. *Acta Psychiatr Scand* 1983, **67**:361–370.
16. Clark DA, Steer RA: Use of nonsomatic symptoms to differentiate clinically depressed and nondepressed hospitalized patients with chronic medical illnesses. *Psychol Rep* 1994, **75**:1089–1090.
17. Lewis G, Wessely S: Comparison of the general health questionnaire and the hospital anxiety and depression scale. *Br J Psychiatry* 1990, **157**:860–864.
18. Aydemir O, Guvenir T: Validity and reliability of Turkish version of hospital anxiety and depression scale. *Turk J Psychiatry* 1997, **8**:280–287.
19. Carroll WD, Lenney W, Child F, Strange RC, Jones PW, Whyte MK, Primhak RA, Fryer AA: Asthma severity and atopy: how clear is the relationship? *Arch Dis Child* 2006, **91**:405–409.
20. Castro-Rodriguez JA, Ramirez AM, Toche P, Pavon D, Perez MA, Girardi G, Garcia-Marcos L: Clinical, functional and epidemiological differences between atopic and nonatopic asthmatic children from a tertiary care hospital in a developing country. *Ann Allergy Asthma Immunol* 2007, **98**:239–244.
21. Cheng Z, Dai LL, Li F, Liu Y, Kang Y, Chen HJ, Wang X, Zhang H, Ni R: Relationship between anxiety, depression and asthma control. *Zhonghua Yi Xue Za Zhi* 2012, **92**:2128–2130.
22. Di Marco F, Verga M, Santus P, Giovannelli F, Busatto P, Neri M, Girbino G, Bonini S, Centanni S: Close correlation between anxiety, depression, and asthma control. *Respir Med* 2010, **104**(1):22–28.
23. Amelink M, Hashimoto S, Spinhoven P, Pasma HR, Sterk PJ, Bel EH, ten Brinke A: Anxiety, depression and personality traits in severe, prednisone-dependent asthma. *Respir Med* 2014, **108**(3):438–444.
24. Ponte EV, Souza-Machado A, Souza-Machado C, Franco R, Cruz AA: Atopy is not associated with poor control of asthma. *J Asthma* 2012, **49**(10):1021–1026.
25. Inouye T, Tarlo S, Broder I, Corey P, Davies G, Leznoff A, Mintz S, Thomas P: Severity of asthma in skin test-negative and skin test-positive patients. *J Allergy Clin Immunol* 1985, **75**(2):313–319.
26. Storms B, Olden L, Nathan R, Bodman S: Effect of allergy specialist care on the quality of life in patients with asthma. *Ann Allergy Asthma Immunol* 1995, **75**(6 Pt 1):491–494.
27. Yepes-Núñez JJ, Gómez C, Espinoza Y, Cardona R: The impact of subcutaneous immunotherapy with Dermatophagoides farinae and Dermatophagoides pteronyssinus on the quality of life of patients with allergic rhinitis and asthma. *R2Biomedica* 2014, **34**(2):282–290.

28. Kohlboeck G, Koletzko S, Bauer CP, von Berg A, Berdel D, Krämer U, Schaaf B, Lehmann I, Herbarth O, Heinrich J, GINI-plus Study groups; LISA-plus Study groups: **Association of atopic and non-atopic asthma with emotional symptoms in school children.** *Pediatr Allergy Immunol* 2013, **24**(3):230–236.

29. Barone S, Bacon SL, Campbell TS, Labrecque M, Ditto B, Lavoie KL: **The association between anxiety sensitivity and atopy in adult asthmatics.** *J Behav Med* 2008, **31**(4):331–339.

30. Janson C, Björnsson E, Hetta J, Boman G: **Anxiety and depression in relation to respiratory symptoms and asthma.** *Am J Respir Crit Care Med* 1994, **149**:930–934.

31. Van Lieshout RJ, Macqueen G: **Psychological factors in asthma.** *Allergy Asthma Clin Immunol* 2008, **4**(1):12–28.

32. Rietveld S, Everaerd W, Creer TL: **Stress-induced asthma: a review of research and potential mechanisms.** *Clin Exp Allergy* 2000, **30**(8):1058–1066.

33. Zhang L, Han B, Zhang Z, Liu A, Liu G, Du Z, Yao Y, Qi Q: **Skin prick test of inhalative allergens for patients with allergic rhinitis in Yichang.** *Lin Chung Er Bi Yan Hou Tou Jing Wai Ke Za Zhi* 2014, **28**(2):98–101.

34. Lü Y, Xie Z, Zhao S, Zhang H, Liu Y, Chen X, Jiang W: **Prevalence of allergens for Changsha patients with allergic rhinitis.** *Lin Chung Er Bi Yan Hou Tou Jing Wai Ke Za Zhi* 2011, **25**:491–494.

35. Yuen AP, Cheung S, Tang KC, Ho WK, Wong BY, Cheung AC, Ho AC: **The skin prick test results of 977 patients suffering from chronic rhinitis in Hong Kong.** *Hong Kong Med J* 2007, **13**(2):131–136.

Permissions

The contributors of this book come from diverse backgrounds, making this book a truly international effort. This book will bring forth new frontiers with its revolutionizing research information and detailed analysis of the nascent developments around the world.

We would like to thank all the contributing authors for lending their expertise to make the book truly unique. They have played a crucial role in the development of this book. Without their invaluable contributions this book wouldn't have been possible. They have made vital efforts to compile up to date information on the varied aspects of this subject to make this book a valuable addition to the collection of many professionals and students.

This book was conceptualized with the vision of imparting up-to-date information and advanced data in this field. To ensure the same, a matchless editorial board was set up. Every individual on the board went through rigorous rounds of assessment to prove their worth. After which they invested a large part of their time researching and compiling the most relevant data for our readers.

The editorial board has been involved in producing this book since its inception. They have spent rigorous hours researching and exploring the diverse topics which have resulted in the successful publishing of this book. They have passed on their knowledge of decades through this book. To expedite this challenging task, the publisher supported the team at every step. A small team of assistant editors was also appointed to further simplify the editing procedure and attain best results for the readers.

Apart from the editorial board, the designing team has also invested a significant amount of their time in understanding the subject and creating the most relevant covers. They scrutinized every image to scout for the most suitable representation of the subject and create an appropriate cover for the book.

The publishing team has been an ardent support to the editorial, designing and production team. Their endless efforts to recruit the best for this project, has resulted in the accomplishment of this book. They are a veteran in the field of academics and their pool of knowledge is as vast as their experience in printing. Their expertise and guidance has proved useful at every step. Their uncompromising quality standards have made this book an exceptional effort. Their encouragement from time to time has been an inspiration for everyone.

The publisher and the editorial board hope that this book will prove to be a valuable piece of knowledge for researchers, students, practitioners and scholars across the globe.

List of Contributors

William R Henderson Jr
Department of Medicine, Division of Allergy and Infectious Diseases, Center for Allergy and Inflammation, University of Washington, Room 254, 850 Republican Street, Seattle, WA 98109, USA

Ena Ray Banerjee
Department of Zoology, University of Calcutta, 35 Ballygunge Circular Road, Kolkata 700019, West Bengal, India

Ana Carolina Zimiani de Paiva, Fernando Augusto de Lima Marson and Carmen Sílvia Bertuzzo
Department of Medical Genetics, Faculty of Medical Sciences, State University of Campinas (Unicamp), Campinas, São Paulo zip code: 13081-970, Brazil

Fernando Augusto de Lima Marson and José Dirceu Ribeiro
Department of Pediatrics, Faculty of Medical Sciences, State University of Campinas (Unicamp), Tessália Vieira de Camargo, 126, Campinas, SP zip code: 13081-970, Brazil

Felicia C Allen-Ramey and Linda M Nelsen
Merck & Co. Inc., West Point, PA 19486, USA

Joseph B Leader, Dione Mercer and James B Jones
Geisinger Clinic, Center for Health Research, Danville, PA 17822, USA

Henry Lester Kirchner
Geisinger Clinic, Division of Medicine, Danville, PA 17822, USA

Lokesh Guglani
Pediatric Pulmonary Division, Department of Pediatrics, Children's Hospital of Michigan, Wayne State University School of Medicine, 3901 Beaubien St, Detroit, MI 48201, USA

Suzanne L Havstad, Jacquelyn Saltzgaber, Dayna A Johnson, Christine C Johnson and Christine LM Joseph
Department of Public Health Sciences, Henry Ford Health System, Detroit, MI, USA

Dennis R Ownby
Clinical Allergy and Immunology, Georgia Health Sciences University, Augusta, GA, USA

Gert-Jan Braunstahl
Department of Pulmonary Medicine, Sint Franciscus Gasthuis, Kleiweg 500, 3045 PM, Rotterdam, The Netherlands

Jan Chlumský
Department of Pulmonary Disease, Thomayer Hospital, Charles University, Prague, Czech Republic

Guy Peachey
Novartis Pharmaceuticals UK Limited, Horsham, West Sussex, UK

Chien-Wei Chen
Novartis Pharmaceuticals Corporation, East Hanover, NJ, USA

Lennart Bråbäck and Adrian J Lowe
Occupational & Environmental Medicine, Department of Public Health and Clinical Medicine, Umeå University, Umeå, Sweden

Lennart Bråbäck
Department of Research and Development, Västernorrland County Council, Sundsvall, Sweden

Cecilia Ekéus
Department of Women's and Children's Health, Division of Reproductive and Perinatal Health, Karolinska Institutet, Stockholm, Sweden

Adrian J Lowe
Murdoch Childrens Research Institute, Melbourne, Australia
Centre for MEGA Epidemiology , School of Population Health, The University of Melbourne Melbourne, Australia

Anders Hjern
Centre for Health Equity Studies (CHESS), Karolinska Institutet/Stockholm University, Stockholm, Sweden
Clinical Epidemiology, Department of Medicine, Karolinska Institutet, Stockholm, Sweden

Lennart Bråbäck
Department of Research and Development, Sundsvalls sjukhus, Sundsvall SE 85186, Sweden

Xiaoqin Liu, Jørn Olsen and Jiong Li
Section for Epidemiology, Department of Public Health, Aarhus University, Aarhus, Denmark

Xiaoqin Liu and Wei Yuan
Department of Epidemiology and Social Science on Reproductive Health, Shanghai Institute of Planned Parenthood Research, WHO Collaborating Center for Research in Human Reproduction, National Population & Family Planning Key Laboratory of Contraceptive Drugs and Devices, Shanghai, China

Jørn Olsen
Department of Epidemiology, Fielding School of Public Health, University of California, Los Angeles, CA, USA

Esben Agerbo
National Centre for Register-Based Research, Aarhus University, Aarhus, Denmark
CIRRAU-Centre for Integrated Register-based Research, Aarhus University, Aarhus, Denmark

Sven Cnattingius
Clinical Epidemiology Unit, Department of Medicin Solna, Karolinska University Hospital, Karolinska Institute, Stockholm, Sweden

Mika Gissler
Information Department, THL National Institute for Health and Welfare, Helsinki, Finland NHV Nordic School of Public Health, Gothenburg, Sweden

Harri Hemilä
Department of Public Health, POB 41, University of Helsinki, Mannerheimintie 172, FIN-00014 Helsinki, Finland

Cyrille Alode Vodounon, Ylia Valerevna Skibo and Zinaida Ivanovna Abramova
Laboratory Acid Nucleic, Institute of Fundamental Medicine and Biology, Kazan Federal University (KFU-Russian), Kremlyovskaya str. 18, Kazan 480008, Republic of Tatarstan, Russian Fédération

Cyrille Alode Vodounon, Vincent Ezin, Nicolas Aikou and Lamine Baba-Moussa
Laboratoire de Biologie et de Typage Moléculaire en Microbiologie, Département de biochimie et biologie cellulaire, Faculté des sciences et Techniques (FAST), Université d'Abomey-Calavi (UAC-Benin), 05PB1604 Cotonou, Benin

Simeon Oloni Kotchoni
Department of Biology and Center for Computational & Integrative Biology, Rutgers University, Camden, NJ 08102, USA

Cyrille Alode Vodounon, Christophe Boni Chabi and Simon Ayeleroun Akpona
Laboratoire de Biochimie et Biologie Moléculaire, Faculté de Médecine, Université de Parakou, BP: 123 Parakou, Parakou, Benin

Jonathan S Boomer, Amit D Parulekar, Brenda M Patterson, Huiqing Yin-Declue, Christine M Deppong, Seth Crockford, Mario Castro and Jonathan M Green
Department of Internal Medicine, Washington University School of Medicine, St Louis, MO 63110, USA

Amit D Parulekar
Department of Internal Medicine, Baylor College of Medicine, Houston, TX 77030, USA

Nizar N Jarjour
Department of Internal Medicine, University of Wisconsin School of Medicine and Public Health, Madison, WI 53792, USA

Hamdan AL-Jahdali, Abdullah AL-Harbi, Mohd Khan, Salim Baharoon and Salih Bin Salih
Department of Medicine, Pulmonary Division-ICU, King Saud bin Abdulaziz University for Health Sciences, Riyadh, Saudi Arabia

Anwar Ahmed
Department of Epidemiology and Biostatistics, College of Public Health and Health Informatics, King Saud bin Abdulaziz University for Health Sciences, Riyadh, Saudi Arabia

Rabih Halwani and Saleh Al-Muhsen
Asthma Research Chair and Prince Naif Center for Immunology Research, Department of Pediatrics, College of Medicine, King Saud University, Riyadh, Saudi Arabia

Hamdan AL-Jahdali
King Saud University for Health Sciences, Head of Pulmonary Division, Medical Director of Sleep Disorders Center, King Abdulaziz Medical City, Riyadh, Saudi Arabia

Denis Bérubé
CHU Ste-Justine, Université de Montréal, Montréal, Québec, Canada

Michel Djandji
Merck Canada Inc., Kirkland, Québec, Canada
Novartis Canada, Dorval, Québec, Canada

John S Sampalis
McGill University, Montréal, Québec, Canada
JSS Medical Research, Montréal, Québec, Canada

Allan Becker
Section of Allergy and Clinical Immunology, Department of Pediatrics and Child Health, University of Manitoba, Manitoba, Canada

Naomi Tsurikisawa, Chiyako Oshikata and Kazuo Akiyama
Department of Allergy and Respirology, National Hospital Organization Sagamihara National Hospital, 18-1 Sakuradai, Minami-ku, Sagamihara, Kanagawa 252-0392, Japan

Akemi Saito, Takuya Nakazawa, Hiroshi Yasueda and Kazuo Akiyama
Clinical Research Center for Allergy and Rheumatology, National Hospital Organization Sagamihara National Hospital, 18-1 Sakuradai, Minami-ku, Sagamihara, Kanagawa 252-0392,C Japan

Stephen R Hanney and Teresa H Jones
Health Economics Research Group, Brunel University, Uxbridge UB8 3PH, UK

Amanda Watt
RAND Europe, Westbrook Centre, Milton Road, Cambridge CB4 1YG, UK

Leanne Metcalf
Asthma UK, Summit House, 70 Wilson Street, London EC2A 2DB, UK

Mohsen Sadatsafavi and J Mark FitzGerald
Department of Medicine, Institute for Heart and Lung Health, The University of British Columbia, 7th Floor, 828 West 10th Avenue, Research Pavilion, Vancouver V5Z 1 M9, Vancouver, BC, Canada

Brian Rotenberg
Department of Otolaryngology, London, Ontario, Canada

Mohsen Sadatsafavi
Collaboration for Outcomes Research and Evaluation, Faculty of Pharmaceutical Sciences, the University of British Columbia, Vancouver, Canada

Larry D Lynd
Centre for Health Evaluation and Outcome Sciences, the University of British Columbia, Vancouver, Canada

Carlos Ramirez-Velazquez, Elena Cristina Castillo and Vianney Ortiz-Navarrete
Molecular Biomedicine Department, Centro de Investigación y de Estudios Avanzados (CINVESTAV)-IPN, Av. IPN No. 2508, Colonia San Pedro Zacatenco, México, DF CP. 07360, México

Carlos Ramirez-Velazquez
Allergy Department, Hospital General Dr. Fernando Quiroz Gutiérrez, ISSSTE, Calle Felipe Angeles y Canario. Colonia Bellavista, Mexico, DF CP 01140, Mexico

Leopoldo Guido-Bayardo
Allergy Department, Centro Médico Nacional 20 de Noviembre ISSSTE, Felix Cuevas 540, Colonia del Valle, Mexico, DF CP 03229, Mexico

Philippe Bégin and Kari C Nadeau
Allergy, Immunology, and Rheumatology Division, Stanford University, 269 Campus Drive, Stanford, California, USA

Christine Ibrahim, Kulraj Singh, Gina Tsai, David Huang, Jorge Mazza, Brian Rotenberg, Harold Kim and David William Moote
Schulich School of Medicine and Dentistry, London, Ontario, Canada

Gina Tsai, David Huang, Jorge Mazza, Harold Kim and David William Moote
Department of Allergy and Immunology, London, Ontario, Canada

Amrit Singh, Masatsugu Yamamoto, Jian Ruan, Jung Young Choi, Christopher Carlsten and Scott J Tebbutt
James Hogg Research Centre for Heart Lung Innovation, St. Paul's Hospital, University of British Columbia, Vancouver, BC, Canada

Amrit Singh, Masatsugu Yamamoto, Jian Ruan, Jung Young Choi, Christopher Carlsten, J Mark FitzGerald and Scott J Tebbutt
Institute for HEART LUNG Health, Vancouver, BC, Canada

Amrit Singh, Jian Ruan and Scott J Tebbutt
Prevention of Organ Failure (PROOF) Centre of Excellence, Vancouver, BC, Canada

Masatsugu Yamamoto, Christopher Carlsten and J Mark FitzGerald
Vancouver Coastal Health Research Institute, Vancouver General Hospital, Vancouver, BC, Canada

Masatsugu Yamamoto, Christopher Carlsten, J Mark FitzGerald and Scott J Tebbutt
Department of Medicine, Division of Respiratory Medicine, UBC, Vancouver, BC, Canada

Gail M Gauvreau
Department of Medicine, McMaster University, Hamilton, ON, Canada

Sven Olek and Ulrich Hoffmueller
Epiontis GmbH, Berlin, Germany

Louis-Philippe Boulet
Quebec Heart and Lung Institute, Laval University, Québec City, QC, Canada

Fardis Teifoori and Masoomeh Shams-Ghahfarokhi
Department of Mycology, Faculty of Medical Sciences, Tarbiat Modares University, Tehran 14115-331, Iran

Fardis Teifoori, Idoia Postigo, Antonio Gutiérrez, Ester Suñén and Jorge Martínez
Laboratory of Parasitology and Allergy, Center for Research Lascaray Ikergunea, University of the Basque Country, Pº Universidad, 7, 01006 Vitoria, Spain
Department of Immunology, Microbiology and Parasitology, Faculty of Pharmacy, University of the Basque Country, Pº Universidad, 7, 01006 Vitoria, Spain

Mehdi Razzaghi-Abyaneh
Department of Mycology, Pasteur Institute of Iran, Tehran 13164, Iran

Ali Eslamifar
Clinical Research Department, Pasteur Institute of Iran, Tehran 13164, Iran

Carlos Ramirez-Velazquez, Nonantzin Beristain-Covarrubias and Vianney Ortiz-Navarrete
Molecular Biomedicine Department, Centro de Investigación y de Estudios Avanzados (CINVESTAV)-IPN, Av. IPN No. 2508, Colonia San Pedro Zacatenco, México

Carlos Ramirez-Velazquez
Allergy Department, Hospital General Dr. Fernando Quiroz Gutiérrez, ISSSTE. Calle Felipe Angeles y Canario. Colonia Bellavista, Mexico, DF CP 01140, Mexico

Leopoldo Guido-Bayardo
Allergy Department, Centro Médico Nacional 20 de Noviembre ISSSTE, Felix Cuevas 540, Colonia del Valle, Mexico, DF CP 03229, Mexico

Mhd Hashem Rajabbik, Tamara Lotfi and Elie A Akl
Clinical Research Institute, American University of Beirut, Beirut, Lebanon

Lina Alkhaled, Munes Fares and Salman Mroueh
Department of Pediatrics and Adolescent Medicine, American University of Beirut, Beirut, Lebanon

Ghada El-Hajj Fuleihan and Elie A Akl
Department of Internal Medicine, Calcium Metabolism and Osteoporosis Program, WHO Collaborating Center for Metabolic Bone Disorders, American University of Beirut, Beirut, Lebanon

Elie A Akl
Department of Clini cal Epidemiology and Biostatistics, McMaster University, Hamilton, Ontario, Canada
Department of Medicine, State University of New York at Buffalo, Buffalo, New York, USA

Hikmet Coban
Department of Pulmonology, Sakarya University, Sakarya, Turkey

Yusuf Aydemir
Training and Research Hospital, Sakarya University, 54100 Sakarya, Turkey

Index